The MANAGING CARE READER

'*The Managing Care Reader* offers a kaleidoscope of perspectives on care management and the management of care. In a single volume the editors have brought together both the voices of users, carers and front line staff and the analysis of management gurus and those at the cutting edge of management research. Even the most academic material has been presented in easy to read sections, honed to the needs of the busiest student, practitioner or manager. This is a valuable source of reference – but also a good read.'

David N. Jones, formerly Assistant Director Operations, CCETSW and General Secretary, BASW

'Legislation, service standards, structures, delivery systems and user expectations are all changing in the care sector. The familiar boundaries of care no longer seem appropriate. In the midst of such trends and developments the care sector has been slow to acknowledge the crucial role of the manager. Management skills are typically seen as something acquired along the way by the successful practitioner. The management of care has become the management of change in the complex and fast-moving environment of social care. A common theme throughout this unique collection of readings is the complexity of managing social care in all its forms and guises. This book could not be more needed or more timely.'

Des Kelly, Editor of *Social Caring* and Partnership Director, BUPA Care Homes

'Management in social care has never been more important. This excellent Reader looks at management from every perspective – through the eyes of users, practitioners and researchers, as well as those we more conventionally think of as managers. It provides vital information about the Government's modernisation agenda and poses challenging questions about the roles, skills, contexts and contribution of today's managers in complex social work and social care organisations, as well as in interdisciplinary partnerships. I commend it to a wide readership.'

Audrey Mullender, Professor of Social Work, University of Warwick

'This impressive Reader contains a wide range of stimulating papers which succeed in providing considerable food for thought. Existing and aspiring managers will find much here to help them get to grips with the complex demands of management in a social care context. This book helps to fill a significant gap and is therefore a welcome addition to the literature.'

Neil Thompson, Director, Avenue Consulting Ltd and Visiting
Professor, University of Liverpool

Social care is being redefined. The government is placing strong emphasis on training throughout the sector and there is an urgent need for highly skilled people to respond to the challenges of managing within and across traditional service boundaries.

The Managing Care Reader includes material relevant to everyone involved in developing new relationships in the broad area of social care. Alongside readings on social care as traditionally conceived, it offers readings from a wide variety of settings, including health and a range of adult and children's care agencies. It brings together classic management texts and material from current and new care contexts to provide a stimulating range of perspectives on the manager's role. In the management of something as complex as care, this must involve:

- listening to service users
- maintaining professional values
- enabling participation
- facilitating learning.

The Managing Care Reader reflects these imperatives as it focuses in on the experience of being in the front line. In four parts, it looks at how managers experience what they do, their managerial responsibilities in caring work, the key professional issues in changing contexts, and the importance of the organisation as a learning environment. It offers a rich resource for all those undertaking management courses or moving into frontline management roles in the developing world of social care.

Jill Reynolds, Jeanette Henderson, Janet Seden and **Anne Bullman** all work in the School of Health and Social Welfare at The Open University. **Julie Charlesworth** works at The Open University Business School.

The MANAGING CARE READER

Edited by Jill Reynolds, Jeanette Henderson,
Janet Seden, Julie Charlesworth and
Anne Bullman

Routledge
Taylor & Francis Group

LONDON AND NEW YORK

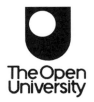

The Open
University

First published 2003
by Routledge
11 New Fetter Lane, London EC4P 4EE

Simultaneously published in the USA and Canada
by Routledge
29 West 35th Street, New York, NY 10001

Routledge is an imprint of the Taylor & Francis Group

Typeset in 10/12 Sabon by Wearset Ltd, Boldon, Tyne and Wear
Printed and bound in Great Britain by TJ International Ltd, Padstow,
Cornwall

British Library Cataloguing in Publication Data
A catalogue record for this book is available from the British Library

Library of Congress Cataloging in Publication Data
A catalog record for this book has been requested

ISBN 0–415–29789–3 (pbk)
ISBN 0–415–29788–5 (hbk)

Open University Course: Managing Care

This Reader forms part of The Open University course *Managing Care*, a 60 points third level undergraduate course. The section of readings is related to other materials available to students and to two further published texts:

- *Managing Care in Context*
- *Managing Care in Practice.*

If you are interested in studying this course or working towards a related degree or diploma please write to the Information Officer, School of Health and Social Welfare, The Open University, Walton Hall, Milton Keynes, MK7 6AA, UK. Details can also be reviewed on our web page http://www.open.ac.uk.

Opinions expressed in the Reader are not necessarily those of the Course Team or of The Open University.

CONTENTS

BIOGRAPHIES

Anne Bullman has worked in several faculties of The Open University as a Course Manager, and is currently working in the School of Health and Social Welfare. Previous co-edited work includes *Changing Practice in Health and Social Care* and *Evaluating Research in Health and Social Care*.

Julie Charlesworth is a Lecturer in Management in The Open University Business School. Her research interests include interagency working, local governance, public management and the role of volunteers in health and social care services. Her publications focus on partnership in health and social care, health improvement, local politics and qualitative research methods.

Jeanette Henderson is a Lecturer in the School of Health and Social Welfare at The Open University. She has experience as a manager in mental health training and development in a social services department. Her research interests are in mental health, especially the meanings and constructions of 'care'. Recent publications include papers on implementing change in mental health, assessing Approved Social Workers' knowledge of mental health legislation, and the impact of 'care' on partnerships.

Jill Reynolds is a Senior Lecturer in the School of Health and Social Welfare at The Open University. She has experience as a manager in the voluntary sector in the UK and Australia. Research interests and publications include education, training and practice issues, feminist practice, and meanings of care and support. Previous co-edited and co-published work includes *Health, Welfare and Practice*, *Mental Health Matters* and *Speaking our Minds*.

Janet Seden is a Lecturer in the School of Health and Social Welfare at The Open University. She has worked as probation officer, children and families field social worker, social worker/manager in a family centre, and lectured at Leicester University. She is the author of *Counselling Skills in Social Work Practice*, and has also published on the assessment of and provision of services for children and their families, social work processes, children and spirituality and practice teaching. Recent work includes publications on Family Assistance Orders and the Children Act, 1989, and on theories underpinning the assessment of children in need and their families.

ACKNOWLEDGEMENTS

The editors and publishers are grateful to the following for permission to include their material in this Reader.

Chapter 5: Dimmock, B. (1996), 'Team and management consultation', in N. Gould and I. Taylor (eds) *Reflective Learning for Social Work: Research, Theory and Practice*, pp. 132–8. Aldershot: Ashgate Publishing Limited. Reproduced by permission of Ashgate Publishing Limited.

Chapter 6: Whitaker, D., Archer, L. and Hicks, L. (1998), 'Working with and being managed by the larger organisation', in Whitaker, D., Archer, L. and Hicks, L. (eds) *Working in Children's Homes: Challenges and Complexities*, pp. 81–100. Chichester: John Wiley & Sons, Ltd. © John Wiley & Sons Ltd. Reproduced by permission of John Wiley & Sons Limited.

Chapter 8: Ells, P. and Dehn, G. (2001) 'Whistleblowing', in Cull, L.-A. and Roche, J. (eds) *The Law and Social Work: Contemporary Issues for Practice*, pp. 106–19. Basingstoke: Palgrave. © The Open University 2001. Reproduced with permission of Palgrave Macmillan.

Chapter 10: Tannen, D. (1995) 'Women and men talking on the job' and ' "She's the boss". Women and authority', in *Talking From 9 to 5*, pp. 21–3, 161–203. London: Virago Press. © Deborah Tannen 1994. Permission granted by Time Warner Books UK for non-exclusive English language rights for distribution throughout the UK and Commonwealth. Permission granted by HarperCollins Publishers Inc. for territories – USA, North America.

Chapter 13: Evans, M. (2001) 'The quest for quality: reflecting on the modernising agenda', *NISW Briefing No. 30*. © Mike Evans. Reproduced by kind permission of Mike Evans.

Chapter 14: Pine, B., Warsh, R. and Maluccio, A.N. (1998) 'Participatory management in a public child welfare agency: a key to effective change', in Patti. R.J. (ed.) Administration in Social Work, Vol. 22(1), pp. 19–31. Binghampton, New York: The Haworth Press, Inc. Reprinted by permission of The Haworth Press, Inc.

Chapter 15: Shaw, C. (1997) *Remember My Messages: The Experiences and Views of 2000 Children in Public Care in the UK*. London: The Who Cares? Trust. © Catherine Shaw and The Who Cares? Trust. Reproduced by permission of The Who Cares? Trust which works to improve the delivery of public care and the day-to-day lives of 60,000 children and young people in residential and foster care in the UK through promoting and acting on their views and experiences. The Trust offers a range of services to young people, carers and professionals including a magazine and telephone helpline. Visit the Trust's website at www.thewhocarestrust.org.uk.

Chapter 16: Piachaud, D. (2001) 'Child poverty, opportunities and quality of life', in Gamble, A. and Wright, T. (eds) *The Political Quarterly*, Vol. 72(4), pp. 446–52. Oxford, London and Massachusetts, USA: Blackwell Publishers. © The Political Quarterly Publishing Co. Ltd 2001. Reproduced by permission of Blackwell Publishing.

Chapter 17: Vernon, A. and Qureshi, H. (2000) 'Community care and independence', in *Critical Social Policy*, 20(2), pp. 255–76. London: Sage Publications. © Critical Social Policy Ltd, 2000. Reprinted by permission of Sage Publications Ltd.

Chapter 18: Pattison, S. (1997) 'Virtues and values', in *The Faith of the Managers*, pp. 100–17. London and Washington: Cassell. © Stephen Pattison 1997. Reproduced by permission of Continuum International Publishing Group.

Chapter 19: Gunaratnam, Y. (2001) 'We mustn't judge people . . . but': staff dilemmas in dealing with racial harassment amongst hospice service users', in Dingwall, R., James, V., Murphy, E. and Pilnick, A. (eds) *Sociology of Health and Illness*, Vol. 23, No. 1, pp. 65–84. Oxford, London and Massachusetts, USA: Blackwell Publishers. © Blackwell Publishers Ltd and the Foundation of Sociology of Health and Illness, 2001. Reproduced by permission of Blackwell Publishing.

Chapter 20: Lewis, J. (2002) 'The contribution of research findings to practice change', in *Managing Community Care*, Vol. 10, Issue 1, February, pp. 9–12. Brighton: Pavilion Publishing. © Pavilion Publishing (Brighton) Ltd. Reproduced by permission of Pavilion Publishing (Brighton) Ltd.

Chapter 21: Marshall, J. (1986) 'Towards ecological understanding of occupational stress', in Erez, M. (ed.) *International Review of Applied Psychology*, Vol. 35, pp. 271–86. London, Beverly Hills and New Delhi: Sage. Reproduced by permission of Blackwell Publishing.

Chapter 22: Adams, J. (2000) 'The last years of the workhouse, 1930–1965', in Bornat, J., Perks, R., Thompson, P. and Walmsley, J. (eds) *Oral History, Health and Welfare*, pp. 98–118. London and New York: Routledge. Reproduced by permission of Taylor & Francis Ltd.

Chapter 23: Clarke, J. (1998) 'Doing the right thing? Managerialism and social welfare', in Abott, P. and Meerabeau, L. (eds) *The Sociology of the Caring Professions, 2nd Edition*, pp. 234–54. London: UCL Press. Reproduced by permission of Taylor & Francis Ltd.

Chapter 24: Foster, P. and Wilding, P. (2000) 'Whither welfare professionalism? (abridged)', in *Social Policy and Administration*, Vol. 34, No. 2, June, pp. 143–59. Oxford, London and Massachusetts, USA: Blackwell Publishers. © Blackwell Publishers Ltd, 2000. Reproduced by permission of Blackwell Publishing.

Chapter 25: Causer, G. and Exworthy, M. (1999) 'Professionals as managers across the public sector', in Exworthy, M. and Halford, S. (eds) *Professionals and the New Managerialism in the Public Sector*, pp. 83–101. Buckingham: Open University Press. © Mark Exworthy, Susan Halford and the Contributors 1999. Reproduced by permission of Open University Press.

Chapter 26: Kitchener, M., Kirkpatrick, I. and Whipp, R. (2000) 'Supervising professional work under new public management: evidence from an "invisible trade"', in Hodgkinson, G.P. (ed.) *British Journal of Management*, Vol. 11(3), pp. 213–26. Oxford, London: Blackwell Publishing. © British Academy of Management. Reproduced by permission of Blackwell Publishing.

Chapter 27: Hudson, B., Hardy, B., Henwood, M. and Wistow, G. (1999) 'In pursuit of inter-agency collaboration in the public sector: what is the contribution of theory and research?', in *Public Management: An International Journal of Research and Theory*, Vol. 1(2), June, pp. 235–60. London: Routledge. http://www.tandf.co.uk. © Routledge 1999. Reproduced by permission of Taylor & Francis Ltd.

Chapter 28: Hornby, S. and Atkins, J. (2000) 'The environment of collaborative care', in *Collaborative Care: Interprofessional, Interagency and Interpersonal, 2nd Edition*, pp. 192–203. Oxford, London and Massachusetts, USA: Blackwell Publishing. Reproduced by permission of Blackwell Publishing.

Chapter 30: Horwath, J. and Morrison, T. (2000) 'Identifying and implementing pathways for organizational change – using the *Framework for the Assessment of Children in Need and Their Families* as a case example', in *Child and Family Social Work 2000*, Vol. 5, pp. 245–54. Oxford, London and Massachusetts, USA: Blackwell Publishing. © Blackwell Science Ltd. Reproduced by permission of Blackwell Publishing.

Chapter 31: Bilson, A. and Ross, S. (1999) 'Social work management – a systems case study', in *Social Work, Management and Practice: Systems Principles, 2nd Edition*, pp. 137–53. London: Jessica Kingsley Publishers Ltd. ©1999 Andy Bilson and Sue Ross. Reproduced by permission of Jessica Kingsley Publishers Ltd.

Chapter 32: Clarke, M. and Stewart, J. (1997) 'Handling the wicked issues: a challenge for government', School Discussion Paper, School of Public Policy, The University of Birmingham. © Michael Clarke and John Stewart.

Chapter 33: Obholzer, A. (1994) 'Managing social anxieties in public sector organizations', in Obholzer, A. and Roberts, V.Z. (eds) *The*

Unconscious at Work: Individual and Organizational Stress in the Human Services, pp. 169–78. London: Routledge. Reproduced by permission of Taylor & Francis Ltd.

Chapter 34: Mintzberg, Henry (1975). Reprinted by permission of Harvard Busines Review from *The Manager's Job: Folklore and Fact*, by Henry Mintzberg, pp. 49–61, July-August 1975. Copyright © by the Harvard Business School Publishing Corporation; all rights reserved.

Chapter 35: Hartley, J. and Allison, M. (2000) 'The role of leadership in the modernization and improvement of public services', in *Public Money and Management*, Vol. 20, April–June, pp. 35–40. Oxford, London and Massachusetts, USA: Blackwell Publishing. Reproduced by permission of Blackwell Publishing.

Chapter 36: Sawdon, C. and D. (1995) 'The supervision partnership: a whole greater than the sum of the parts', in Pritchard, J. (ed.) *Good Practice in Supervision: Statutory and Voluntary Organisations*, pp. 3–18. London: Jessica Kingsley Publishers. Reproduced by permission of Jessica Kingsley (Publishers) Ltd.

Chapter 37: Ayre, P. (2001) 'Child protection and the media: lessons from the last three decades', in *British Journal of Social Work*, Vol. 31(6), December, pp. 887–91. © The British Association of Social Workers. By permission of Oxford University Press.

Chapter 38: Bates, J. (1995) 'An evaluation of the use of information technology in child care services and its implications for the education and training of social workers', in Preston-Shoot, M. (ed.) *Social Work Education*, Vol. 14(1), pp. 60–76. London: Carfax. © Social Work Education, 1995. http://www.tandf.co.uk. Reproduced by permission of Taylor & Francis Ltd.

Chapter 39: Gould, N. (2000) 'Becoming a learning organisation: a social work example', in *Social Work Education*, Vol. 19(6), pp. 585–96. http://www.tandf.co.uk. London: Carfax. © Social Work Education, 1995. Reproduced by permission of Taylor & Francis Ltd.

While the authors and publishers have made every effort to contact copyright holders of the material used in this volume, they would be happy to hear from anyone they were unable to contact.

GENERAL INTRODUCTION

This book is a resource for managers in the changing contexts of modern social care. There is an urgent need for highly skilled people to respond to the challenges of managing across traditional service boundaries of social services, health, education, housing and voluntary and independent sectors. As service arrangements become more complex, an increasing number of people are identifying elements of managing in their work, or expecting an early move into a managerial role after initial qualification. There is a serious shortage of educational material that can help both the experienced and the novice manager grapple with changing demands for improvements in care.

If you are already a manager in the broadly defined care sector; if you are expecting to take on supervisory responsibilities; or if you are simply interested in how the complex mix of changing contexts of public, private and voluntary services is organised, you will find much here to explore. Managers' experiences and dilemmas are presented directly and through the medium of research. Different readings help managers to identify the professional and practice issues in their responsibilities for others' work and encourage managers to play a part within an overall need for organisations where workers can learn and develop. With the exception of two readings from the US, all the work in this book is from a UK context.

We have searched for and commissioned material that resonates with the concerns of managers. Above all we wanted to raise the profile of practice – both the centrality of practice to managers' work – how care is offered and undertaken – and the practice of managers. This rich collection of articles will help you to tease out questions of how good managers develop and what makes for good management in this complex work.

The collection is unusual in its inclusion of readings that relate to a wide range of care settings: there is writing relating to education and early years settings; residential care for children and for adults; health and nursing care; voluntary sector projects through to fieldwork social services settings. If services are to work holistically to help people with needs that span organisational compartments, then today's managers require a working knowledge of issues faced in different contexts. There are lessons to be learnt by stepping outside familiar territory to find out how things are done elsewhere. The volume is also exceptional in offering a range of perspectives from service users and carers on what they want to see from managers and care organisations. How do things look from the viewpoint of the person who wants a kind of help that may not yet have been invented – or perhaps a kind of help that may need to be rediscovered since service objectives were redefined?

We have avoided allocating material to separate areas of theory and practice, so theoretical and research perspectives jostle with the views of managers and of service users. The book is in four parts and each has an introduction giving an overview of the chapters it contains. You will find that you get as much from dipping into the book according to your needs and interests as from reading it from end to end in the order laid down. The mixture of readings coming from research, management theory and practice, social policy and personal experience is likely to mean different readings have distinctive appeal either in general or for specific purposes. You may want to vary your reading between those offering a depth of academic content and those providing a more immediate and in some instances lighter personal flavour. Or you may want to pursue particular themes or kinds of managerial task. You will find the contents listing and the introductions to each part helpful in guiding such choices.

Managers in the frontline provides perspectives from managers who stand at the intersection of the organisation and the provision of care and services, sometimes themselves engaging in direct work as well as managing the practice of others. Articles offer insights into how managers balance the demands of clients, the organisation and government policy.

Managing to care focuses on the primary function of offering caring and inclusive services. Managers who care also need to value workers and recognise potential stresses in the nature of the work.

Managing in changing contexts takes the reader on a route that looks back at some earlier models of managing care, and offers contrasting conceptualisations of how the manager's role has changed under recent policy initiatives.

Managing for a learning and developing organisation identifies new challenges for managers and supervisors and looks at the manager's responsibility for helping others to learn and develop within organisations that are often contradictory and complex. It also, as the title implies, examines the potential for organisations to learn from frontline practice.

Some of the chapters in this Reader were specially commissioned to fill a gap in the existing literature. Most are reprinted, and in order to be able to include the wealth and diversity of perspectives that are represented here, readings are either extracts from the original work or abridged from a longer piece. The original sources of reprinted work are noted at the front of each reading. The symbols used to signify an abridgement has been made are [. . .] where an extensive cut has been made, and . . . where only a few words have been missed out in order to make sense in this version. If you want to follow an author's detailed argument, we recommend that you read the work from which it originated. We hope that this Reader will introduce you to many new authors whose ideas excite or intrigue you, and that these 'tastes' will whet your appetite to become better acquainted with their work.

PART I

MANAGERS IN THE FRONTLINE

Jeanette Henderson

This opening section brings together a collection of work that has the challenges, joys and dilemmas of day-to-day frontline management as its theme. The roles and tasks undertaken by managers in care services are many and complex. One way to make sense of this complexity is to group these roles around three broad areas of work – operational, strategic and professional. The operational aspects of management are the day-to-day tasks that underpin the delivery of care services. In a single day a manager can be dealing with staff care, service user consultations, supervision and appraisal and the myriad routine tasks required to develop and maintain a team of care workers.

Managers are increasingly involved in strategic developments linked to the implementation of legislation and policy. Strategic demands on managers are to be found in the organisational aims and targets in developing services alongside partners in a wide range of agencies.

The professional aspect of work stems from the particular challenges posed in managing people who deliver care services. A manager in children's services could be dealing with complex child protection issues requiring a keen knowledge of legislation, supporting and supervising their staff to take difficult decisions which will have profound effects on the lives of service users. The professional experience managers have gained working as practitioners in care services will be invaluable. So, experience of direct work with people using care services underpins management in this area.

Frontline managers are faced with a challenging, at times frustrating, sometimes conflicting and often exciting set of roles. Part I seeks to illustrate this complexity and we begin with extracts from diaries kept by frontline managers. Jacqui takes us through two days in which she responds to potential petty cash shortages, staffing problems and concerns over a child's welfare. Anita shares her feelings and expectations on the day before she begins her first job as a frontline manager and her experiences on her first day. Finally, Bronwyn's diary illustrates her role over a longer period of time. The sheer energy and skill with which the three managers tackle their role shines through in these first-hand accounts which illustrate the operational, strategic and professional elements of managers' daily lives.

Links between service users and managers are considered in the following three chapters. Jim Read discusses the experiences of people who have used services when they become managers in the same or a similar setting. On the one hand, service users have essential knowledge about what makes services responsive to their needs, yet on the other the very fact of using services makes it difficult for some employers to accept them as managers. Service users are also citizens and Peter Beresford and Suzy Croft argue for a model of participation that recognises service users' citizenship. Ensuring honest and meaningful participation is a key role of the frontline manager, and Lou Townson and Rohhss Chapman stress that consultation must be more than just a management exercise.

Managers and workers in care settings may experience tensions related to the content of their work as well as the personal and organisational interactions that affect them. Acting as a consultant to managers and teams who are not working together as effectively as they could enables Brian Dimmock to make some reflections on team and management consultancy and emphasises the importance of team 'stories' in enabling change. Some of the experiences that might form such team stories are considered in the next chapter by Dorothy Whitaker and her colleagues. They use material from research with workers in residential care homes, about being managed as part of a larger social care organisation.

Voluntary sector organisations may be large or small and present particular challenges to frontline managers. Julie Charlesworth explores the tensions in managing unpaid workers and managers' relationships with executive committees. For example, a manager could be managing an unpaid worker who is also a member of an executive committee, and in turn the executive committee manages the manager!

Whistleblowing is an emotive subject for managers, workers and the general public. People who blow the whistle are often applauded, yet may experience various forms of discrimination as a result of their actions. As well as relating the experiences of whistleblowers, Phillip Ells and Guy Dehn provide policy background and case study material to illustrate the practical implications of the Public Interest Disclosure Act 1998 and the protection it provides.

Another area that managers find challenging is that of 'managing' death. Jeanne Katz looks at the management challenges presented by deaths of residents in residential care. Losses, she argues, are felt by residents and staff alike, and managers need to talk about, work with and be aware of them.

Deborah Tannen focuses on communication in the workplace and argues that communication styles and patterns are often influenced by gender. Women, she suggests, may soften critical feedback to such an extent that the message is lost. This approach denies colleagues the opportunity to learn from mistakes as well as forming the basis for potential conflicts at a later stage.

The conflicts or tensions illustrated by Jeanette Henderson and Janet Seden's study suggest that managers are expected to perform many different roles which do not always work in harmony and one of the dilemmas that brings this disharmony into sharp focus is that of charging for services. It seems that for the managers interviewed by Greta Bradley and her colleagues, dealing with financial assessment symbolises the pressures they face in modernising care services.

These chapters illustrate the complexity, sense of achievement and challenges of managing in care services and give a taste of the diversity and richness of the role.

ONE

DAYS IN THE LIFE ...
MANAGERS' DIARIES

JACQUI, MANAGER OF A FAMILY CENTRE

Monday

At 8.30 a.m. we began the morning meeting where we established what staff we had in and how many children and families were due. If we're short staffed we must request cover from another unit who may be able to spare a staff member, which is not very often. Anyway, this morning we were OK, just one on annual leave. I also use this time to go through the diary for the next couple of days so everyone is aware of what is going on.

The meeting finished at 8.45 a.m. and I intended spending the first hour or so sorting out and sending in a claim for more petty cash. We used to order provisions from large suppliers but since most of the children only attend for sessions there is no need to order large supplies of food. From January we started to use local supermarkets. However, this means that we must always have cash ready for the cook to go shopping. The claim needs to be sent and then we have to wait for a cheque to arrive and allow it time to clear. If the claim wasn't sent today the money would run out, hence no food and one angry cook! This has happened on two occasions and it makes us as managers look very incompetent in her eyes.

I was just about to start this laborious task, when the cook came in wanting to talk to me urgently. She launched into a whole host of complaints about one of the other staff, whose job it is to clean the kitchen. She believes that his cleaning is not up to standard and wants me to talk to him about it. I assured her that we would follow this up and she went off a little happier.

I attempted to get back to my earlier task and was just in the middle of adding up about thirty receipts when the phone rang. We haven't had any clerical staff since last November, due to budget savings. We did get a clerk for a few weeks but she didn't stay long as the pay affected her benefits so she was no better off.

The phone continued to ring several times after that and I was just about to give up trying to sort out the money, when my deputy arrived. This allowed me to get on, although it took far longer than it normally does, because it wouldn't balance. Eventually it did get finished and I had to ask one of the staff to hand deliver it to the Finance Department to ensure they would receive it on time.

We have had several new families starting at the centre recently and I feel at times that because I am out of the unit so often I begin to lose touch with what is happening. There were a few minutes before lunch so I spent them in one of the group rooms with the staff, talking about how the families had settled and introducing myself to them. I hate it when the children and their parents don't know who I am. I know that some of the parents who use the centre think I am the secretary and I have been called 'Office' by more than one child!

After lunch, I had a meeting with the other two managers, my deputy and senior nursery officer. We needed to catch up with one another to feed back information (including the incident with the cook this morning). I'm going to be out of the unit for the next two days, on a course about the Assessment Framework we must implement soon. Certain things are outstanding and we spent quite a long time going through the 'attention tray' and deciding what was priority. I then spent the rest of the day following up queries and preparing for the course tomorrow.

Thursday

It never fails to amaze me that I can be out of the unit for a short time and it always seems so long when I get back! I walked in and was greeted by my new senior nursery officer having a major panic attack because she didn't have a key to the key safe and was unable to open the filing cabinets! I really must talk to her in supervision, if she gets so worked up by something so trivial, she will never cope in a real crisis.

In the morning meeting everyone wanted to know about the course and whether it would affect their work but it wasn't the time to feed back. I wanted to discuss it with the other managers first.

It's been a busy day today. There were a lot of things to fit in. Two staff were on leave and one had rung in sick. We requested another nursery officer but there was no one available. Supervision with two members of staff had to be cancelled – we were unable to spare them from the group rooms and one staff member had to run a parent group on her own when normally there are two facilitators. There has been a development with our advert for a new clerk. It has been stopped by the redeployment panel and they say that they have someone who will meet our requirements. I just hope they do and can start ASAP! I spent sometime looking through the post that had arrived over the last few days and then priced up some fax machines.

A social worker visited this afternoon regarding a family we are concerned about. After a lengthy meeting we agreed that we would monitor the situation for another week and if they did not attend or there were further concerns then a case conference would be called. The mother did not come which in itself is cause for concern.

One member of staff asked for annual leave tomorrow. We have a policy that only two are allowed on leave at any one time and the staff member who was off sick today may still be off tomorrow. How could I agree to more leave? She wasn't pleased about being refused but as a manager you can't please everyone all the time and this can make you decidedly unpopular!

ANITA, MANAGER OF A COMMUNITY MENTAL HEALTH TEAM

Sunday

It's the night before I start my new job as a manager. On Thursday night I had my leaving night from my old job, and an awful lot of people turned out to say goodbye to me. It made me realise just how strong the network was that I was leaving behind, how many people I could call upon to help me out. I'm now sitting here thinking goodness me, I'm going into a new job, I've got no networks of people to call on within the area that I'm now working. Although I suppose the people who I previously worked with will still be there to help out if necessary. It's also made me extremely anxious. I realise that I was probably quite good at what I did, and I've absolutely no guarantees whatsoever that I'm going to be any good as a manager.

Looking at it objectively I know I have the skills necessary for being a manager. I'm anxious that I'm not going to be given a chance to prove that I'm able to do the job. However on a more positive note I'm really looking forward to it, even though I haven't a clue what's on the agenda. The team manager of the team geographically next to me is responsible for my induction. I'm really quite lucky because I met her approximately seven years ago when I was doing further training in social work. I gave her some advice then on divorce solicitors and she's obviously never forgotten that. I'm really pleased for that one thing I did all those years ago because it means that somebody is actually paving the way for me.

Monday

I started my first day as a manager today. I arrived thirty-five minutes early. I'd set off from home extra early because I wasn't entirely sure how long the journey would take in traffic. There was nobody from my team around, so I let myself into the building with the district nurses. The office, which had been pointed out to me as being mine, was still functioning as a waiting room. There were chairs and a coffee table and a pile of old magazines in there. My office furniture, I later understood, had been delivered elsewhere. The staff arrived at nine o'clockish – the administrator who has been extremely helpful, and two of the nurses.

I discovered that the social workers who had previously been based in a different building hadn't arrived as predicted. This is because the computers haven't arrived and social workers need the computers to input their work. When I asked what the problem was with getting computers it seems that everybody had requested one, and the budget couldn't allow for this. However the good news is it looks like the building's networked, so one of my tasks is to set off looking for computers. I'm sure nobody will mind sharing as long as we have some on the site.

We borrowed a desk from another office for me, found a chair which had been ordered for me, and discovered that my furniture had been delivered to another site twenty-seven miles away, but hopefully will eventually be delivered to my office. I didn't have a telephone so I borrowed one of those from somebody else's office. The administrator had ordered me all the things that go on desks, like filing systems, pens, paper and so on. By half-past-nine I had somewhere to sit and some papers to shuffle around.

I went in to talk to the staff to discover that one of the nursing staff is going off on a long-term sickness absence on Friday, probably for about six months. Part of me is actually pleased because this lady is very experienced but has been turned down for a management job. I had anticipated not having an easy ride, however it does leave the problem of being one nurse down. I also discovered that the audit which I had originally been told was planned for September takes place on Friday of this week. I definitely have no concerns about the audit now because no manager – however good – is going to change anything in four days. The positive side of that is that by the time the next audit comes round we can only have improved.

I asked about team meetings which take place on Fridays. In my previous job I took a lot of responsibility for the team meetings. I suppose it was my hobby horse and had been for quite a number of years. I always insisted on them having an agenda, being chaired, and having a definite function. The team meeting in this team seems to be very woolly with an unclear function. I asked about the time the meeting starts and nobody was even clear about that. I think given my fanaticism about meetings, maybe that's something I really would like to have a look at, however not in the first instance. I think I'll sit through a few and try and get a feel of what people expect.

I have two budget sheets which I sat and looked at today. I've never had to study a budget sheet in my life. I think I picked up the gist of what they were saying, as in I still have some money, accumulated money from the past couple of months, however I'm not entirely sure what I'm allowed to do with it. The job advert said we could have training in budget management, I hope they meant it.

I spent quite a lot of time today actually just sitting, jotting down ideas, things I needed to know, people I'd like to meet. However it's very difficult when you don't even know the names of the people or the structure of the organisation. Tomorrow I'm meeting with another team manager for my induction. She's responsible for this because both the social services manager and the health service manager are on holiday.

BRONWYN, MANAGER OF A VOLUNTARY SECTOR PROJECT

Tuesday

Senior staff meeting – it's the only time I catch up with 'what's going on'. Lots of changes to one of the departments, lots of new forms to fill in and so on. A colleague caught me at lunch time to say that a member of her staff who is currently doing some sessional work for me is to be 'pulled out'.

Met with another manager at tea break to discuss a very difficult staffing issue we share. It felt good to air this and realise we had similar feelings. Agreed that we need jointly to take it forward.

A local university wants to do research on volunteer projects on outcomes/effectiveness of services. I put my project's name forward as I think it would be helpful to have some academic evaluation of our work.

Wednesday

Team meeting day. Feeling really pissed off. As I was at managers' meeting all previous day, I have so much admin to do I can't join the meeting. I normally guard time for team meetings, but it's the end of financial year. As usual whatever 'good housekeeping' I try to employ I'm overspent – luckily it's not by vast amounts. No-one taught me accountancy on my CQSW!

Member of staff distressed. A mother had left the building very upset and the staff member didn't know what to do. Agreed that we'd give the woman time to get home and ring. It's such awful shit we deal with day to day. Member of staff feeling slightly better, but I could see she was concerned.

Friday

Our only means of fire escape from the top of the building is by a door to the building next door. The administrator was concerned that this hadn't been checked recently. We tried to release catch between doors – wouldn't budge. Tried one on next floor down and managed to activate what I thought was fire alarm. Ran down four flights of stairs to de-activate it, but I couldn't get it to stop.

Rang head office as phone number for company that services alarm was unobtainable. Realised it wasn't fire but burglar alarm that was ringing – rushed back down stairs and turned it off. Got back up the four flights to see two police officers coming up front path – forgot alarm is wired to local station. Red faced (not only from exertion), I explained what had happened.

Went back to office to find man there – how did he get in? He was from the local security firm and has office keys. He'd come in the back way, he told me proudly – my heart beating like a hammer with shock. We're really careful with access to the building because of the work we do and here was this guy pleased as punch that he'd got in without us knowing! He set to work securing the two doors, cut his hand and fell through the door into next door offices. They were very upset at all the noise and disturbance.

Wednesday

Chaired a review meeting. Lots of workers involved and the meeting took two hours. It was exhausting with so many feelings ricocheting around. I felt I was walking on egg shells.

Meeting with one of my consultants. Looked at the future of our work together and came up with a plan for, hopefully, attracting quite a lot of money to the project. Need to write up discussion and a proposal for a service level agreement.

Monday

What a stressful day! Couldn't see the wood for the trees. I had driven in quite cheerfully. I felt 'got at' the minute I walked in. I had taken the previous Thursday afternoon and Friday off so a pile of work awaited. A major referral had somehow got lost, so I had to deal with a very grumpy referrer.

Had supervision with a member of staff who is not the easiest person to relate to.

Had supervision with a member of staff newly transferred to this team. This was a more positive experience but still felt difficult. I don't have the answers to many of the practical details that still need to be sorted.

Thursday

Met two management colleagues for a meeting that should have been with our joint manager. She was still on sick leave but we decided to proceed as so much seems to be happening in the organisation we felt it would be useful to share what we did/didn't know. One colleague has just come back after secondment to another part of the country and was astonished by the changes. It helped me realise just how much change we've tried to accommodate over the past year. It also helped reduce the guilt feelings that I'm often not on top of the work and am still pretty clueless about some aspects of the reorganisation. I realised how much I did know. I think we're all operating from a principle of 'let's get the work of our teams done, and we'll deal with the organisational bits when we can'. Not always a comfortable position.

A new building surveyor came and needed to be in all the nooks and crannies – with me accompanying to give a running commentary on the last time things had been inspected, repaired, decorated and so on. It's at times like this that I really feel the responsibility of looking after the 'whole' project. It's not only the clients and the team, but the actual environment that needs close attention.

TWO

MENTAL HEALTH SERVICE USERS AS MANAGERS

Jim Read

Prior to the 1980s, it was unusual for people who had been diagnosed as mentally ill to play an obvious role in public life. People who were able to continue with their normal lives, or who recovered after a period of time out, did everything they could to hide their experience from all but their most trusted friends and family. Feelings of shame and well-justified fear of other people's reactions were incentive enough to cover up and keep quiet.

Since then there have been some changes. With the increased emphasis on community care, there are more people receiving treatment and using services who are also looking for something useful to do with their time. Encouraged by legislation and sympathetic staff, they have stepped out of the patient role to take part in consultation exercises, act as advocates and share their personal experiences in training sessions for staff. Some have taken a more radical position. More likely to call themselves mental health system survivors than service users, they have challenged the medical model of 'mental illness' and developed self-help alternatives.

All this activity has created employment opportunities where having been diagnosed and treated as mentally ill is actually a requirement, or at least a desirable attribute. Current or former service users are employed as advocates, co-ordinators of user forums and in other jobs. Within the mental health voluntary sector, it has become commonplace for staff to be open about their own experiences of distress and service use, and this includes people in senior positions. This reading is based upon interviews with three such people who have become managers in voluntary sector organisations.

Lisa is the director of City and Hackney Mind. It employs about 30 full-time staff and another 20 sessional staff or part-timers, and has an annual budget of around £1,250,000. Projects include supported housing, computer training, employment, support for people coming off medication and a drop-in used mainly by young Black men.

Robert had recently left his post of director of a voluntary sector project. The project employs about 36 staff with an annual budget of just under £1 million. Activities include a drop-in, employment project, independent living scheme, registered care home, counselling and advocacy.

Alison is project development manager for CHANGE, a charity set up to provide user-led crisis services in Birmingham. She is responsible for two crisis houses and a scheme of crisis sponsor homes (where people in crisis can move in with a family or residents of an ordinary home). There are 10 staff and an annual budget of £250,000.

Routes to employment

None of the people I interviewed had taken a conventional route into management.

Lisa had previously been a teacher and stopped when her daughter was born. There followed several years doing casual work such as cleaning and decorating while she coped with her distress and periods in hospital. As life got a little easier, Lisa became a founder member of one of the first user-led groups in the country, Hackney Mental Health Action Group. Lisa then became a volunteer at City and Hackney Mind and, soon after, she applied successfully for the post of advice worker. As her confidence grew, Lisa became the first chair of MindLink, national Mind's service user network, and joined Mind's Council of Management, later becoming vice chair. Meanwhile, her responsibilities at City and Hackney Mind grew as she became manager of a couple of projects. I asked Lisa how she became the director:

> I was a bit bored in my previous job. I didn't have enough to do and being under-used contributed to me having another breakdown. The director left and it was suggested that I acted up into the post until a new director was appointed. No-one was appointed the first time around and I ended up doing it for several months. By then I realised that I could do the job. I was 50 years old, I felt I hadn't done a lot with my life and decided to apply for it.

Robert had been director of a Black resource centre in Manchester:

In those days I put a lot of energy into work and it took over my life and that was one of many factors that led to me having a breakdown. I had various spells in and out of hospital and various stages of thinking, 'I've got to get back on my feet'. But I also felt I didn't have the energy to do it. I felt the system – the hospital, the medication, the electric shock treatment – robbed me of energy, of confidence, of memory. I was having to reinvent things I could previously do with my eyes closed. I felt the need to move back into work. I needed to earn money. I was in a huge financial mess. I wanted to get back into management because I didn't want to slip down the career ladder.

I got a part-time job managing a community centre. It was relatively easy and that gave me confidence. Later I got a job as director of a small team of people working with user/survivor groups across London. Then my last job came up.

Alison had started work in the insurance industry. She became so bored and demoralised that she found it difficult to motivate herself to go into work and was eventually sacked. She found herself working as a temporary receptionist for a mental health team:

I absolutely loved it there and they loved me. So when the permanent job came up, I applied for it and the reason they didn't give me that particular job was because they thought I wasn't actually interested in it. I was interested in everything else except answering the telephone!

But they obviously recognised that I had some potential and one of the guys on the interview panel said, 'We've got another job coming up as administrator for the homeless team', which was a lot more involved, a lot more responsibility. It was actually setting up this new homeless team and I thought, 'This sounds fantastic', so I applied for that job, which I got. I then became a psychiatrist's secretary and the administrator for this new team, and demanded that I spent one day a week working with homeless people. I did that and it was always the people I was interested in.

After a couple of years, I got promoted to become PA to Professor Max Birchwood (well known for his work on early intervention in psychosis) and got involved in more user conferences. Up until then, I hadn't told many people about my mental health problems. But when I went to work for him, I did tell him. And so he helped me and I spoke at a big conference he organised.

During this time, Alison also wrote a book about her experiences (Reeves,

1998). How did she get her current job, which began as manager of one crisis house with two other staff?

> I was asked to go on the interview panel. And I looked at the job and decided I wanted to apply for it!

Worries and reality

I asked what they had been most apprehensive about when they started their jobs and whether their concerns had been justified. Lisa began:

> I was worried about the finances and about cracking up. I thought the personnel stuff would be easy – I thought, 'I'm emotionally literate because of all my therapy and talking to friends'. In fact, although the finances are hard and time consuming, it doesn't freak me because it's practical and impersonal. It turned out to be the personnel stuff that I do find difficult and it affects my mental health. For example, there was a manager who had been promoted beyond her abilities. I had to make a judgement that she wasn't up to the job and then I had to deal with the fall-out from that situation. She hated me and that was hard.
>
> I haven't cracked up and overall the job has been good for me in just the way I anticipated, including a period when I have been dealing with difficult personal problems. Being an operational manager is good for me. In some way I'm saved by the demands it makes. If I did more of a policy job, for example, I would have too much time to think. If I can get myself to work, people make demands on me all the time and it gets me out of it.

Robert remembered:

> I went in with rose coloured spectacles. I didn't realise there were so many skeletons in the cupboard. I didn't realise there was a history of managers under-performing and covering up. From day one, I became aware that funding for various projects was running out, and there had been no reports to funders for several years.
>
> It was frustrating trying to change the organisation so that the services were what I would want to have. I was really dissatisfied with the standard of services on offer. I put pressure on myself. I've always said that I would never go to the drop-in but I would like one that I would feel comfortable going to, comfortable bringing my family to. I

really wanted to make dramatic changes. It was so frustrating. You would think as director that you would have the power to sweep through these changes. But the reality is so different. People get into a set pattern of working; members get into a set pattern of how things need to be, and it is so difficult to push back those barriers. I found that frustrating and as a survivor, I found it even more difficult.

Alison said she was terrified:

On the one hand, I always knew I could do it, but on the other, I'd never run a crisis house before or worked with people as a 'professional'. Supposing there was someone we couldn't help, who would feel let down by the service? That was the most terrifying part and still is. But I'm a lot less fearful now than I was then.

Ultimately, it comes down to believing in humanity – the human potential to overcome anything. The more you let go of the outcome of what you are doing, the better the result will be; if you just try to be with someone and try to relate to them and believe that one human being to another we can have a positive impact with our presence. Once you start wanting a particular outcome then you can get disappointed, and even feel angry with the person because they didn't do what you wanted them to do. You have to untangle all the crap in your own head and put it in the background.

Getting the right balance

What role does work play in their life?
Lisa:

It plays a big part in my life because it helps me to maintain my self-respect when I feel awful. It keeps me occupied, but not like a crossword puzzle. It is more creative than I thought it would be and I'm always having to make decisions.

But that doesn't mean she works all the time:

It is better for me to be over-occupied rather than under-occupied but I'm not a workaholic. I can't remember when I last went in at a weekend.

Robert said:

> I was conscious of the need to learn lessons from my first job and not
> let it take over my life. I was able to step back and leave my work at
> work, even though there were many pressures not to.
>
> There were many situations that reminded me of my own experi-
> ence in the mental health system. I reacted in horror to seeing certain
> medications still being used or incidents where someone would be
> stripped, in an isolation room and staff not wanting to go near them.
> I think it was good that I understood that reality. It took me back but
> not totally back. I could see that I had moved on and was in control.
> None of the situations floored me or knocked me back.

Finally, Alison:

> When I met my current partner, I felt my identity was too entwined
> with Anam Cara. It was almost as if I didn't have another identity. He
> isn't involved in mental health. We have a genuine interest in each
> other's jobs but I make a concerted effort not to take work home. I am
> disciplining myself to see that my work is only part of my identity. I
> feel privileged to have been given a very special chance, and I took it. I
> am the one leading it but it would be nothing without the other
> people.

Support

I asked about sources of support, formal and informal. First, Lisa:

> I've found myself a good external supervisor. He helps to significantly
> reduce the tension I feel about personnel stuff. I see him about once a
> month, which isn't often enough. All staff have a budget of £600 a
> year for external supervision. The two chairs of the management com-
> mittee have both been managers themselves, which is good, but they
> haven't had time to give me systematic supervision. Some of the staff
> are very supportive. Some of my friends are good at enabling me to be
> reflective about what I do and that is very helpful, but friends tend to
> take your side, which isn't necessarily what I want.

Robert felt

> Very much alone – totally unsupported by the management commit-
> tee. I should have pushed for a budget for external supervision for
> myself. I needed to have somebody who could be supportive, some-
> body who could help me look at things from different angles. The
> informal support came through my family, and friends who have used
> mental health services.

Alison said:

> It's been difficult. I've had a few mentors but none have really lasted. I
> have needed to find someone who understands the mental health
> system and also has the right values, and then need to feel I can ask
> them for time. We did pay someone for a while but I felt I shouldn't
> be taking money from a charity. A couple of the Trustees give me
> practical and emotional support which I really value. They are all busy
> people but I think they can see that I need to have more support as we
> grow and change.

Reflections

Alison, Lisa and Robert have all demonstrated what can be achieved
despite having experienced severe distress and being diagnosed as mentally
ill. They are living proof that you don't have to live quietly and carefully in
order to avoid risking another breakdown. Lisa's idea that she needed to
take on a more demanding role, for her mental health, is a particular challenge to traditional attitudes.

Rachel Perkins, clinical director of adult mental health services for an
NHS Trust and herself a service user, has written:

> The accounts of service users/survivors are replete with the bleak prog-
> nostications of professionals, the 'you'll nevers'. 'You'll never get
> better, be able to work, have a place of your own, raise children, cope
> with stress, stop taking medications, manage without help.'
>
> (Perkins, 2001)

People making use of services that are managed by people who are open
about their own struggles and labels get a very different message, about –
in Alison's words – 'the human potential to overcome anything'.

Although Robert had a tough time in his job, he doesn't think that there was prejudice against him as a mental health system survivor. But when I asked him what it was like for him as a Black man of African heritage, he replied:

> Being a Black man within a predominantly white organisation throws up a heap of issues; subtle forms of racism where you have people come in at different levels in the organisation and questioning your ability.

This is a sharp reminder of the multi-faceted nature of discrimination.

Robert, and to a lesser extent, Lisa and Alison, had found it difficult to find the right kind of support. I think this reflects a general ambivalence about how much people in charge of organisations should be expected to 'just get on with it' and how much they should feel entitled to support. It is certainly hard to think about it for oneself. This suggests that management committees need to take the initiative. In the voluntary sector, there is perhaps a more obvious case for paid, external supervision, given that supervision from the management committee is rarely as frequent and skilled as it should be.

There is also a question about whether service users or mental health system survivors should have extra support. Some people may qualify for it under the terms of the Disability Discrimination Act. Others would view it as quite unnecessary to be treated differently from anyone else. Everyone can benefit from a healthy working environment. One third of the staff of the Manic Depression Fellowship (MDF) have a diagnosis of manic depression. MDF has introduced several procedures for supporting the staff to look after themselves including actively discouraging people from working long hours and provision for relieving people of front-line work when they are feeling fragile. Levels of sick leave are not higher than in other organisations (Jackson, 2001).

So will the practice of positively choosing to employ people who have been diagnosed as mentally ill within mental health services become more widespread? Unfortunately, there is plenty of evidence that employers' attitudes will first have to change a great deal.

Mind surveyed nearly 800 people who had used mental health services, asking them about their experiences of unfair treatment (Read and Baker, 1996). It was notable how many of the people reporting discrimination at work were from the 'caring professions' such as social work and nursing. One person said:

> I am a qualified nurse with lots of experience. Unfortunately I had two years out of work due to anorexia and bulimia caused by rape. I found

it very difficult to obtain a nursing post when I was initially quite open and honest about my illness. Eventually I had to lie about why I had been out of nursing to obtain employment. I have now returned to nursing, at a lower grade prior to being off sick, and work full time, although my employer does not know I have a psychiatric history.

(Read and Baker, 1996)

Tom Sandford, Mental Health Adviser to the Royal College of Nursing, has written of the effects of the Allitt Inquiry Report on nurse recruitment. (The inquiry followed the deaths and injuries to children caused by the nurse, Beverley Allitt.) He argues:

This ambiguity [of the recommendations] has led to the exclusion from nurse training, or the prevention of a return to nursing, of people with a range of mental health problems which may pose absolutely no cause for concern.

(Sandford, 1997)

In stark contrast to the generally negative attitude to be found in statutory services, the South London and St George's Mental Health NHS Trust has embarked on a programme spearheaded by Rachel Perkins, to ensure that 10 per cent of its workforce has experienced a mental health problem.

Perhaps there are two challenges for people making decisions about whether to employ people who have been diagnosed as mentally ill (and may still be using services) in positions of responsibility in mental health services. The first is to see that they may be perfectly competent to do this work. The second challenge is to recognise that they may bring something extra. Mental health services have been strongly criticised for failing to meet the needs of people who use them. Who better to put them right than people who know what it is like to experience mental distress, to seek help from (or be compelled to use) services and know, only too well, the difference between good ones and bad ones?

REFERENCES

Jackson, C. (2001) 'Size Doesn't Matter', *Mental Health Care* 4 (9), 290.
Perkins, R. (2001) 'The "You'll Nevers" . . .' *Openmind* 107, Mind.
Read, J. and Baker, S. (1996) *Not Just Sticks and Stones*, Mind.
Reeves, A. (1998) *Recovery: A Holistic Approach*, Cheshire, Handsell.
Sandford, T. (1997) 'Nursing Wounds', *Openmind* 87, Mind.

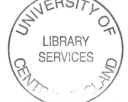

THREE

INVOLVING SERVICE USERS IN MANAGEMENT: CITIZENSHIP, ACCESS AND SUPPORT

Peter Beresford and Suzy Croft

Involving service users in service management means much more than seeing 'user involvement' as an add-on to the conventional management mix. It has implications for the whole ethos and philosophy of management, and all areas of management responsibility. The search for practical skills and understanding to support user involvement in service management is important, but it must always be linked with these broader issues. It is essential that managers are equipped to move from seeing user involvement as a bolt-on (optional) extra, to something integral to *everything* they do.

In this chapter we explore and connect key practical, philosophical and theoretical issues for increasing user involvement in service management. To do this we draw on the knowledge and experience developed by pioneering service user organisations and supportive workers (Beresford and Croft, 1993; Croft and Beresford, 1993; Oliver and Barnes, 1998).

There is now a substantial body of evidence to show that service users particularly value provision in which they have an effective say and control. This is true of both individual self-run personal assistance schemes supported by direct payments (Turner, 1998) and of collectively-run, user-controlled services (Barnes *et al.*, 2001). We know from earlier work that service users believe that a real shift to 'user-led' services demands a different, much more participatory approach to management (Begum and Gillespie-Sells, 1994). We are also beginning to find out how to counter longstanding exclusions and ensure that black and minority service users can better be involved in shaping services (Evans and Banton, 2001).

While we should not confuse user involvement in service management with user-controlled services, there is much that the former can learn from the established examples provided by the latter. Although the two approaches occupy different positions on the continuum from non-involvement to user control, there is a real potential to make conventional services more participatory and to build the learning from service users' pioneering initiatives into mainstream management and service provision.

A first, key step is clarity about what is meant by 'user involvement'. As with related concepts like 'empowerment' and 'partnership', there is a tendency to fight shy of clear definition, as if the good intentions and positives implied by such terms are sufficient in themselves. The chequered history of user involvement in public policy is a strong reminder that this is not the case. We must be clear what is meant by the term; how we are using it and what may be on offer to service users.

Two approaches to participation or user involvement have emerged in recent years. These can probably be best described as the 'consumerist/managerialist' and 'democratic' approaches. They have different origins, concerns, aims and philosophies.

The consumerist/managerialist approach is concerned with people as 'consumers'. It has been developed largely by state and service system organisations. The main aim has been to improve the efficiency, economy and effectiveness of organisations and services by drawing on the ideas and experience of service users to improve management and decision making (Leggett *et al.*, 1999). This approach to participation originated with the political New Right and was associated with a shift from state welfare and an increasing emphasis on the market and individual responsibility. It is closely linked with the philosophy and rhetoric of consumerism, including the purchase of service and ideas of 'consumer/customer choice', 'voices', 'involvement' and 'exit' (Beresford and Croft, 1986; Winkler, 1987). There are ambiguities in consumerist approaches, with their emphasis on individual consumer rights and choice co-existing with the imperatives of profitability and the market economy.

The democratic approach to participation is concerned with people as citizens and emphasises the rights, entitlements and say of citizenship. It has been developed by the movements of health and social care service users, including those of disabled people, people with learning difficulties, older people, people living with HIV/AIDS and mental health service users/survivors. This model is concerned with bringing about direct change in people's lives, through *collective* as well as individual action, by enabling people to have more say over what happens to them (Priestly, 1999). Service users' interest in participation has been part of broader political and social philosophies which prioritise people's inclusion, autonomy, agency, independence and the achievement of their human and civil rights. The disabled people's movement, for example, bases its approach to participation on the social model of disability, using both parliamentary and direct action to achieve its aims (Campbell and Oliver, 1996).

A number of differences can be identified between these two approaches to participation. The first approach generally starts with policy and the *service system*; the second is rooted in people's *lives*, and their aspirations to improve the nature and conditions of their lives. Both approaches may be concerned with bringing about change and influencing what happens. However, in the consumerist/managerialist approach, the search is for external input which the initiating agencies (state, service providers or policymakers) *themselves* decide how to use. The democratic approach is concerned with ensuring that participants have the direct capacity and opportunity to make changes. This latter approach highlights issues of power and the (re)distribution of power. These are not explicit concerns of the consumerist managerialist model of involvement.

These two approaches to participation are not readily reconciled. The first is managerialist and instrumental in purpose, without any commitment to the redistribution of power or control; the other liberatory, with a commitment to personal and political empowerment. The latter's concern is with bringing about direct change in people's lives. This is highlighted by the disabled people's movement's campaigning for anti-discrimination and human rights legislation, and establishment of the 'independent living' movement to ensure that service users are able to maintain control over their personal support through direct payments and self-run personal assistance schemes. While the logic of the democratic approach is for 'user-led' and 'user-controlled' services, a consumerist managerialist approach is compatible with the retention of a provider-led approach to policy and services. The democratic approach is explicitly political, while the consumerist/managerialist approach tends to be presented as politically neutral.

It has been the consumerist/managerialist approach to user involvement which has predominated in recent years. Its significance has increased under New Labour administrations, with increased requirements for formal partnerships and participation in health and welfare policy and practice. But this has also coincided with growing suspicion and caution about getting involved on the part of service users and their organisations. There are increasing concerns about the regressive potential of participatory initiatives associated particularly with consumerist/managerialist approaches to user involvement, where data collection rather than empowerment is the primary aim (Campbell, 1996, 2001; Oliver and Barnes, 1998).

This highlights the importance of being clear about the differences between these two approaches to user involvement, the implications this is likely to have for involving service users in service management, and the most effective ways of advancing this. So far a consumerist/managerialist approach to user involvement seems to hold very limited promise. But the indications for a democratic approach seem much more encouraging.

A range of priority activities can be identified which are consistent with developing a democratic approach to involving service users in service management. These should not be seen as providing some kind of 'ideal model' of user involvement. User involvement is a complex, heavily politicised and value-based activity which is not generally amenable to simplistic ideas of 'best practice'. At the same time, the considerable body of experience developed by service users, their organisations and supportive service providers, does provide a framework of principles for good practice. While these may be no guarantee of success, in our experience initiatives that ignore them are seldom helpful.

Moving forward

Taking these basic steps does seem to help to avoid some of the usual problems encountered in seeking to develop user involvement. Routes to improved practice in involving service users in management and service development include the following.

■ User involvement in professional practice

The first and fundamental issue is that there is user involvement in professional and occupational practice. This means that practice comes to be seen as a joint project. The service user can feed into and influence practice – through the whole process, as long as they are able and wish to. Concerns which they signal at one stage continue to influence practice throughout its course. Practice should always be based on seeking the thoughts, views and ideas of service users. It is a systematic process of discussion and negotiation – which is what best practice has always been. People's personal, direct contact with service provision as service users should be recognised as the starting point for all expressions of participation. The improvement of practice is a key measure of all participation.

■ User involvement in training

The constant message from service user organisations is that there is no more effective way of changing practice and service culture than through involving service users in training. This should extend systematically through all aspects of training; from providing direct input in professional and in-service training to being involved in developing course curricula, providing course materials and evaluating and assessing courses. This is now beginning to happen in social care training and education. The challenge is to ensure it happens coherently and systematically across professions and occupations.

■ Involvement in policy development

User involvement must mean being able to influence services and practice as you experience it, individually, as a service user. But it also must mean that personal knowledge and experience is collected, collated and integrated in a strategic way into the planning and development of policy and services more widely.

■ Support for people to get together

This leads to another of the prerequisites that service user organisations highlight as making real user involvement possible – sustaining opportunities for people in similar situations to get together. In this way people are able to gain information, gain confidence, develop and share ideas. There must be more support for self-help, support and independent user groups and organisations. Self-help and support groups can also provide opportunities for feedback, ideas and proposals for improving policy and provision. Being able to get together – for those who want to – provides essential opportunities to develop collective user involvement to complement the views of service users gained as individuals.

■ Encourage the recruitment of people with experience as service users and involve them in staff selection

If the 'them and us' of service user involvement is to be fully and effectively challenged, then it is crucial that service provider, commissioning and research organisations develop equal opportunities employment policies which value and support the employment of people with experience as welfare service users, for example, as disabled people and mental health service users. In some health and social care services, such experience is seen as an added skill rather than a deficit. As yet, inadequate disability access and support services and disablist attitudes continue to restrict recruitment and promotion of service users. The implementation of the Disability Discrimination Act, the Human Rights Act and the establishment of the Disability Rights Commission may begin to provide a framework and opportunities for change.

■ Recognise the resource implications of user involvement

User involvement costs money and takes time. These costs must be recognised and funded. In time, they will, we hope, be recognised as requirements for all organisations. In the meantime, additional support needs to be costed into budgets where there is a real commitment for participation to ensure that service users' costs and requirements are met. For example, where they contribute their time and skills, service users are recompensed like other members of the workforce or management team.

■ User involvement in developing quality standards and outcome measures

In recent years there has been considerable emphasis on improving quality and developing quality standards, 'performance indicators' and 'outcome measures'. Ideas have come mainly from policymakers, practitioners and managers. We know that patients' and service users' concerns and priorities are not always the same as those of service system professionals. Quality can mean different things to the two groups. User involvement should be extended to involving service users on equal terms in both the development of quality standards and outcome measures and in evaluating and interpreting them. This is beginning to happen in social care.

■ User involvement in monitoring and evaluation

Now that government has placed renewed emphasis on 'evidence-based' policy and practice, the evaluation and monitoring of practice and provision are being given much greater priority. Users' experience is identified as one of four key evidence sources in the government's Quality Strategy for Social Care. The government is now making it clear that service users should be centrally involved in research and evaluation. 'Consumers In NHS Research' has been established to support this goal and has extended its remit to include user involvement in health, public health and social care research. User involvement in research and user controlled research methodologies are increasingly coming to be seen as part of the spectrum of mainstream research and evaluation. This is another key area of management demanding service user involvement. How else will we know what questions to ask and what the focus of research and evaluation should be?

■ The ethics of user involvement

It is essential not to forget the ethical issues raised by user involvement, especially where people face real problems and difficulties in their lives. There must be proper conditions for involvement and there must be *choice* about getting involved. But there are also ethical issues around *not* involving people. Here issues of support and of using sensitive and imaginative approaches to involvement are crucial. We know that, generally, most people want to have a say over what happens to them. So far the signs are that this is no less true of people facing great difficulties in their lives including, for example, people with multiple impairments or life-threatening illnesses and conditions. Choice is crucial here.

■ Equal opportunities in user involvement

Finally, it is essential that initiatives for user involvement challenge rather than mirror prevailing exclusions and discriminations. User involvement must address difference and ensure that people are involved on equal terms regardless of gender, sexuality, age, disability, distress, class, culture or 'race'. This raises additional issues that must be addressed with specific initiatives taken to ensure equal opportunities. First, that black people, members of minority ethnic groups, refugees and asylum seekers are afforded specific support to be involved on equal terms. Second, that people who communicate differently – whether because they have visual impairments, are deaf or have learning difficulties and do not primarily communicate in writing or verbally can contribute from their perspectives on equal terms.

Access and support

As this checklist suggests, for it to work effectively, involving service users in service management needs to be approached in a holistic and strategic way. This must be recognised if broad-based and systematic involvement is to be achieved. Two components seem to be essential if people are to be able to get involved effectively and if all groups are to have equal opportunities for involvement. These prerequisites are *access* and *support*. Both are necessary. Experience suggests that, without support, only the most confident and experienced people and groups are likely to get involved. Without access, efforts to get involved are likely to be difficult and unrewarding however assertive or experienced we are. Access means that there are structured, ongoing methods of being involved; of engaging with services and agencies and of being included in their decision-making structures and processes.

Support means that people can expect to have whatever help, encouragement, skills and assistance they may need to contribute what they want to. This involves some of the issues we have already highlighted, and includes:

■ support for personal development – to increase people's confidence, expectations, self esteem and assertiveness;
■ support to develop skills – needed to participate effectively;
■ practical support to be involved including information, childcare, respite support, transport, meeting places, advocacy, expenses, payment for participation and so on;
■ support for equal opportunities – so that all groups can participate on equal terms;
■ support for people to get together and work in groups, including

organisational, development and training costs to support collective action.

These offer a practical basis for building in user involvement and developing a new truly participative ethos of management.

REFERENCES

Barnes, C., Morgan, H. and Mercer, G. (2001) *Creating Independent Futures: An Evaluation of Services Led by Disabled People. Stage Three Report,* Leeds, Disability Press.

Begum, N. and Gillespie-Sells, K. (1994) *Towards Managing User-led Services,* London, REU (Race Equality Unit).

Beresford, P. and Croft, S. (1986) *Whose Welfare? Private Care or Public Services,* Brighton, Lewis Cohen Urban Studies Centre, Brighton University.

Beresford, P. and Croft, S. (1993) *Citizen Involvement: A Practical Guide for Change,* Basingstoke, Macmillan.

Campbell, J. and Oliver, M. (1996) *Disability Politics: Understanding Our Past, Changing Our Future,* Basingstoke, Macmillan.

Campbell, P. (1996) 'The History of the User Movement in the United Kingdom', in Heller, T., Reynolds, J., Gomm, R., Muston, R. and Pattison, S. (eds), *Mental Health Matters,* Basingstoke, Macmillan.

Campbell, P. (2001) *The Richard Sutton Memorial Lecture,* Bromley Psychosocial Rehabilitation Forum, 23 November.

Croft, S. and Beresford, P. (1993) *Getting Involved: A Practical Manual,* London, Open Services Project/Joseph Rowntree Foundation.

Evans, R. and Banton, M. (2001) *Learning From Experience: Involving Black Disabled People in Shaping Services,* Leamington Spa, Council of Disabled People, Warwickshire.

Leggett, G., Pountney, K., Panizza, S. and Siddiqui, S. (1999) *How Are We Doing?: Service Users and Carers' Views,* Chelmsford, Essex Social Services Department.

Oliver, M. and Barnes, C. (1998) *Disabled People and Social Policy: From Exclusion to Inclusion,* London, Longman.

Priestly, M. (1999) *Disability Politics and Community Care,* London, Jessica Kingsley.

Turner, M. (1998) *Final Report of the User Defined Outcomes Project,* London, Open Services Project.

Winkler, F. (1987) 'Consumerism in Health Care: Beyond the Supermarket Model', *Policy & Politics,* 15, l–8.

FOUR

CONSULTATION: PLAN OF ACTION OR MANAGEMENT EXERCISE?

Louise Townson and Rohhss Chapman

(This is a revised version of an article that appeared in *Community Living* magazine in April 1999)

At first glance, it can be easy to confuse the concept of self-advocacy with 'service user' consultation as if they were inseparable, because consultation involves people expressing a view. However, from an independent advocacy perspective, user consultation is very different to self-advocacy. The former is a management-led process and the latter is person led. There is a fundamental difference in origin, process and aim.

Words can be confusing when there are a variety of available definitions for a single idea. A common assumption about consultation is that it is about services gathering information to improve their work, to provide something better and more responsive for people. Policymakers, service staff, managers at all levels and people receiving services can be confused because of shifting or changing definitions. People, depending on the values they hold, may view consultation differently. For example, some people consider that consultation implies some sort of action. Others may regard consultation as a more passive act.

The Disabled Persons Act set out that representatives of disabled people's organisations should take part in the planning and delivery of services, and that further consultative processes should be established. The NHS and Community Care Act also promote the idea of people having a voice in the services they receive. The government-led initiative on Best Value requires County Councils to provide 'best value' in their services for people following the broad concept of 'the 4 C's': compare, *consult,* compete and challenge. The White Paper, *Valuing People* (Department of Health, 2001) states:

> It is no longer acceptable for organisations to view people with learning disabilities as passive recipients of services; they must instead be seen as active partners.
>
> (p. 51, 4.27)

The White Paper does not make a lot of use of the word 'consultation' but speaks more about action and inclusion in decision making. This brings to the fore the active element of consultation mentioned earlier.

According to one of the authors, Louise Townson of Carlisle People First, an organisation run by and for people with learning difficulties, assumptions that people make around consultation leading to improvement can be misleading. The forums she refers to here are small, representative groups of people with learning difficulties within local day services. The groups are independently facilitated by People First and meet with service management on a regular basis. These meetings are locally known as 'workers' forums'. Louise is also speaking here about information gathered by 'consultation' in Cumbria for a Best Value pilot project:

> The support [of consultative forums] has to be independent of services so there isn't a conflict. Then people can make their own decisions and not be worried about what they say. People should have control of their own information but it's the services who actually have that. It should be us because it affects us.
>
> Services probably make reports on what people have said but what happens to that information people don't know because they don't get to see it. It probably just gets filed away somewhere. Sometimes changes are made and sometimes they are not. Because you don't know what everyone has said it means you never really know if anything has been done or not. It makes people feel their input doesn't make any difference. It makes people think twice about wanting to be involved because they think their views won't be considered. This makes people feel worthless.
>
> Reports and feedback should happen that people can understand. There are lots of ways of doing this. It should show what changes have been made with the information given and if there are no changes it should be explained rather than fobbing people off.

Significantly, in the field of learning difficulties, the move toward 'service-user' consultation has involved statutory services coming into contact with established People First and self-advocacy groups in working together for perhaps the first time. Partnership is a key theme of the 'Valuing People' White Paper and successful implementation is hoped to be secured through new appointments specifically to address such issues.

However, in practice, as we noted above, coming to a common understanding of 'consultation' and its benefits may be difficult when both parties view meaningful and worthwhile 'consultation' in different ways. This became apparent at a meeting in the north west of England attended by the authors. When the meaning of consultation was discussed it became clear that the People First view was that consultation should imply action toward change, a two-way process. This view was challenged by statutory services who viewed 'consultation' as the passing of information. It is therefore imperative that all parties come to an agreed understanding as to what consultation – in their own particular way of working – will be.

In a number of areas people with learning difficulties are invited onto pre-existing working groups rather than being involved from the outset and developing a new model together. Managers need to be clear about the amount of change (or lack of it) consultation may be able to achieve. In turn, this requires them to be open about the limitations they are thus imposing on representatives with learning difficulties. Alternatively services may need to think outside the status quo and change their approach altogether, coming up with new models that work for everyone involved. As Louise argues:

> Services should be honest about what [consultation] means and know what other people think it means. Services need to make a commitment to people to change things to the way people want their services to be. Like it says in the White Paper there should be 'nothing about us without us'. If they don't want to change we might decide not to bother wasting our time with them. The services are for us, we should be the ones having the say.

Some people who receive services feel that consultative forums are a 'tagging on' exercise – this is because the service already exists. The ideas coming out of discussion forums are only seen to be implemented for minor changes or to validate current practice. This does not deal with the initial design and commissioning of services, who is employed, what and how things should happen on a daily basis. In the comments below the 'forums' discussed are made up of staff and managers representing various services and also include some representation of carers and people with learning difficulties. Since the introduction of Valuing People these are known as Partnership Boards. Louise goes on to state that:

People [with learning difficulties] should be on committees right through to the top level deciding about what should happen ... They should be represented all the way through. Consultation should be there from start to finish. People with learning difficulties should be doing the evaluations because they are the only ones who really know what it feels like to get the service. They are the experts.

If things are not going to change then what is the point? It is just wasting everyone's time. People should be involved from the outset, in saying how things should happen, from start to finish.

Getting Direct Payments should help with people getting what they want but really it shouldn't make any difference because the service should be providing what people want anyway, regardless of whether they have a Direct Payment or not.

For Louise and People First and other self-advocacy groups, *process* is as important as outcome. Carlisle People First had representation on the Joint Commissioning group in North Cumbria as it worked its way through the Best Value pilot project for people with learning difficulties. People with learning difficulties are now represented on the Partnership Board and various Task Groups set up under the directives of Valuing People. Despite this being a recent national initiative through the White Paper, People First has been articulating the need for this type of participation for years.

How such participation is achieved is another question. Any measures clearly need to be informed by the practice already established within self-advocacy groups, especially if people with learning difficulties are to be fully involved. Self-advocacy groups argue that they are the experts of knowing what their services should be like and that, out of all people involved, their place is of primary importance. Carlisle People First would like to see a co-worker with learning difficulties in the post of the Integrated Commissioning Manager. In contrast, stories from advocacy networks around the country tell us that consultative groups are often made up of staff and managers who decide the working principles and procedures and who should be invited onto groups to represent people with learning difficulties.

In Carlisle, People First have conducted their own research in the past around dispersal of day-centres and have also been running independently facilitated Workers' Forums within day services for 10 years. They, like other groups around the country, describe themselves as the local voice of people with learning difficulties and expect to choose their own members as representatives.

Despite the problems outlined, this particular group is optimistic about a new way forward in providing services. Louise feels there has been a significant change in the past few years. Genuine partnership should pave the way for active consultation leading to change, as people with learning difficulties will be influencing decisions around definitions, process and practice.

However, there are wider issues for managers and services to take into consideration. At the moment it is becoming clear within the advocacy movement that if services around the country want this particular expertise they will have to pay for it. It is time-consuming work and the main concerns of People First and self-advocacy groups are the ideas and priorities of their members. These ideas may or may not have much to do with the services they currently receive. The fact of the matter is that managers and services need consultation for their own purposes as well as for the people they serve.

Will people with learning difficulties be valued and respected in the same ways as other representatives who are paid for their time and expertise? Will self-advocacy that is locally funded tie groups into providing representation for services rather than self-advocacy for members? This is a difficult question for self-advocacy groups because they are constantly in need of finance but may find their work is compromised. Through group advocacy, as opposed to service consultation, members can push their viewpoint for as far as and as long as they are able to achieve their aim.

Consultation as viewed by services, on the other hand, may be about the floating of ideas and compromises (and self-advocacy groups have the opinion that compromises tend to favour those with power). Consultation may turn out to be about simply relaying information. At worst, it may be a tick-box exercise on a form.

Organised self-advocacy works for its members because groups can control what happens to the information they receive. The group can decide where the information will go – into a complaint, to a councillor, an MP, the newspaper, whatever it takes until change is made. In a service consultation process, information is passed over and entrusted to other people in the hope that something will happen. If self-advocacy groups participate in this process they may run the risk of losing their power to make change happen in wider ways.

The concern, from an independent advocacy perspective, is that forums can be set up and manipulated by services as a management tool. People's concerns and frustrations can be defused in the false belief that their group meeting will be able to activate the changes they ask for. When a response is not forthcoming, there is little comeback, especially if the forum is service conceived and led. People First and self-advocacy groups need to think long and hard about the manner in which they get involved in 'service-user' consultation and who it is there to benefit. In order for this to work for managers and self-advocacy groups, Louise provides some ideas:

> People with learning difficulties who get the services need to be on the management boards. People need to know what is going on and why,

rather than be told 'it's not your concern'. People should be paid for the work they do and given the same respect as other people.

In Carlisle the model developed around the workers' forums separates that work from the main self-advocacy organisation. The advocacy worker is managed by the directors of the organisation (people with learning difficulties). This allows partnership to develop that uses a People First process but does not influence the workings of the main organisation.

Some people say that the demands of the self-advocacy movement are out of touch with 'the real world'. But the real world is whatever we make it and like the word 'consultation', there are many ways of viewing it. There are excellent examples around the UK of organisations that are run by, and cater for, people with learning difficulties in key roles and in control. Managers have a lot to learn from these groups. Louise is clear about what needs to happen:

It's time people stopped hiding behind excuses, we have the White Paper to back us up now.

REFERENCES

Department of Health (2001) *Cm 5086: Valuing People: A New Strategy for Learning Disability in the 21st Century*, The Stationery Office, London.
Disabled Persons (Services Consultation and Representation) Act 1986.
National Health Service and Community Care Act 1990.

FIVE

REFLECTIONS ON TEAM AND MANAGEMENT CONSULTATION

Brian Dimmock

Source: *Reflective Learning for Social Work: Research, Theory and Practice*, Gould, N. and Taylor, I. (eds), Aldershot, Ashgate, 1996.

[...] The consultation style we have developed from using the reflecting team approach involves focusing on the 'stories' which emerge from whichever group is convened.

Typically, we ask those taking part in the team development or consultation exercise to discuss issues which have been identified by them as germane to their problems or needs. We then discuss our ideas about their conversation, with each other and with them. Sometimes we will structure this quite formally; we discuss it, they comment on our discussion, we react to their comments. At other times, we will engage directly in conversation with them and then try and get agreement on the themes and issues which emerge. Our 'expertise' is in facilitating this process, theirs is in their circumstances and their work. The following summary of two different contexts in which the approach is used is drawn from our practice as team/management consultants.

As team and management consultants we could rely on the status of being 'experts' and then attempt to use the power this gives us to impose demands on who takes part, and to diagnose the problem and propose a cure. However, we prefer to accept that ultimately we are relatively powerless in the face of a complex organization with its own unique and complex history. Our approach is to offer to listen to whoever wishes to take part in an initial meeting to discuss how we might be of help. Our role is to listen and to give some immediate feedback to those taking part in the form of a dialogue with them and between ourselves, with the participants observing and commenting. From this initial process we then attempt to establish the focus for the work and how it will proceed. As far as possible we try to ensure that all negotiations about this process are conducted through the proper organizational structures.

The two contexts outlined below are to some extent 'ideal types', but in practice they overlap and we may combine work from each. They represent our 'story' of the experience we have had in this work and they are bound to differ from accounts that others who have taken part would give. The first is 'The troubled team in a time of change'; the second is 'Team development – it's not that we're not a good team it's just that we think we could be so much better'. Whichever of the two contexts are considered, the issues outlined above will apply.

The troubled team in a time of change

In the case of team consultation in personal social services work, managers often call in consultants when a team is seen as being in turmoil, conflict and disarray. In a sense, managers are saying that there is an element to the team's needs which can best be provided by outsiders, or that their own ability to help the team members through the problems they are facing is affected by their own role, perhaps because there are disciplinary proceedings going on, or because the problems have been such that a 'them and us' culture has developed around the boundary of managers and practitioners.

Bringing in consultants can be seen as a way for managers to avoid taking responsibility for problems, or trying to recruit allies. It may also be viewed as an attempt to 'pathologize' team members ('this team needs help, they've been through a lot'). There is also the possibility that it is a way for managers to avoid conflicts between themselves about what to do, or for some managers to recruit allies in their own struggle to define the problems in a particular way. Such negative connotations tend to rely on assumptions about the motivation of others, which is an inexact science at the best of times.

An example

In one case we were asked to help a child protection team (which included social workers, family care workers and administrators) who had been systematically bullied, harassed and intimidated by a team manager. After three years, some of the team members managed to get together and report his abuse to senior managers. Team members were in a varied state of anger and shock, with high rates of sickness and other signs of serious stress. They were at pains to point out that despite all this they had always been determined to maintain their high standards of work. At the time of the consultation, the team manager was suspended pending disciplinary action and investigation of the complaints. In the meantime, radical changes to the team's functions and jobs were being planned.

Having finally managed to act to deal with their manager, the team members who were instrumental in 'blowing the whistle' found that those not involved did not share their views entirely, or agree with their chosen way forward. They began to feel that managers felt that they were 'trouble-makers' and that their heroic efforts to keep the work going were not recognized. In addition, in order to do what they had done they had to develop the kind of solidarity which left little scope for recognizing their own differences and conflicts. A powerful analogy developed with the role of the abused child who reports the abuser and is then 'blamed' by others.

Our approach to this was to suggest that some time be spent together 'telling the story' of the events which led up to the 'whistle blowing'. As the story emerged it was apparent that there were several stories and versions of events – a collective version emerged, but each individual's story was also told and placed in relation to others. Similarities and differences emerged. Women were intimidated differently from men; social workers were threatened in different ways from administrators and family care workers; each individual's fear, and ultimately how they found inspiration to act courageously, were compared and contrasted. A subtle web of overlapping and conflicting motives emerged as the basis for the collective will to act. Instead of seeing themselves as a beleaguered band of survivors, the full story of the extent of the obstacles they faced and the effort needed to act created the opportunity to change the story. The differences between them were no longer seen as a threat to solidarity, but as a useful diversity. As their differences emerged, their 'threat' to others diminished, as they could be seen as individuals rather than a hostile collectivity.

In our view, attempting to present an 'expert' diagnosis of the problems encountered in these circumstances would have created powerful resonances with the style of the team manager, whose approach to his task was to ensure the survival of 'his' team in the face of encroaching change. He did this by seeking allies within the team and beyond, making and breaking temporary alliances and coalitions without fully sharing his own vision with others. There was a powerful identification between himself and the work of the team, and differences with his approach were seen as personal attacks on him. To prevent this he developed a controlling style which restricted the truth to his own version of events. An 'expert' approach to such a management problem might easily involve trying to sell a solution through seeking allies in much the same way as the team manager had gone about his task. Although it might be presented with a different personal style to the previous 'authoritarian' one, it would inevitably be identified with the consultant, rather than as the collective efforts of consultant and consultees.

It's not that we're not a good team, it's just that we think we could be so much better

The engagement of consultants to help with team development may be an attempt to recapture lost feelings from an earlier stage in the team's life, in some ways analogous with marital enrichment for couples who miss the enthusiasm and inventiveness of their earlier love-making. It can also be seen as a solution to a sense of bewilderment and confusion, or an attempt to take stock before, during or after change. Where are we? who are we? what are we? how do others see us? are the kinds of questions being asked. In our experience there are usually one or two enthusiasts within the team for this approach, and the others go along with it either through inertia, curiosity or a lack of desire to question the sense of the suggestion. Approaches to it vary from intensive group activities in wild countryside, to group dynamic exercises involving cushions, lengthy silences and emotional outbursts. Managers may see it as a reward for hard work, a way of easing in difficult changes, or the kind of indulgence which those who have had social work training appear to think is essential from time to time.

Our attitude to team development is that any sane organization which expects its staff to undertake difficult and stressful work will want its staff to take time out to think and reflect on what they are doing and how they can retain their enthusiasm and creativity. At its best and simplest it is time/space for each individual to tell their own story of the team, and for the 'team's' story to be updated and agreed. It is not akin to the kind of commercial or quasi-religious activity which is designed to increase the identification of the individual with the organization. If organizations become only a series of changing enthusiasms, then staff will always have the fear that their own current identification with the organization will easily be replaced with new enthusiasms which belong to others. This engenders obedience, not creativity.

The role of the reflective management consultant is again a facilitative one. It will allow time for the 'accepted' story of the team to be told, and for the differences and new versions to find space. Somehow, participants must be given the opportunity to say, 'I used to think that, but now I think this', or 'I'm more interested in this now, and although I know you all see me as an expert on that, I'm finding it hard to stay enthusiastic'. The consultant's job is to judge the pace at which participants wish to go, and to make them feel safe to try out new or controversial aspects of their own story of the team. It is helping the team to harness differences and conflict by giving them space to explore diversity.

An example

An opportunity arose for us to work with four different teams from within one organization. The organization was undergoing considerable change which was making an impact on teams in quite different ways. Changes in the focus of the work and in the management structure were all putting teams under pressure. Managers recognized that teams could benefit from time to build their new identities to face the challenging times ahead.

We offered to work with all the teams together, with scope to work with individual teams both during this joint work and in subsequent sessions if this was felt desirable. Our thoughts were that bringing the teams together might help to decrease isolation in that common issues would reduce the sense that 'there must be something wrong with us, I bet other teams don't have these problems'. It would also increase the range and diversity of experience, especially if we could help to find ways of making this available across teams. The problem was the numbers involved and our sense that we would find it difficult to help such a large group develop the degree of trust in each other and us to be able to make use of the opportunities.

Tempting as it was, we managed to avoid indulging in a series of exercises which would have been interesting, but no more than the sum of the parts of the different groups' experience. While sharing this dilemma with those attending, a solution emerged. We would demonstrate some of the simple techniques of reflective conversations, and then teams would act as reflective consultants for each other, with us observing and offering a further 'layer' of reflection to the pairs of teams and the group overall.

By trusting in the ability of the consultation process we were able to avoid 'applying' exercises and models of 'team development' and instead found a way of creating opportunities for participants to get some feedback and learn how to use the reflecting team model at the same time. Subsequent work with all four teams individually showed that this exercise had significantly increased energy, enthusiasm and self-belief, and enabled sufficient trust and 'optimism' to emerge to enable more complex and entrenched barriers to development to be tackled.

Further reflections

Although each team and the organization of which it is a part is unique, some common themes have emerged through our work as 'reflective consultants' in the personal social services. These are summarized below.

The fit between the demands of the work and the organizational culture: Donald Schön (1983) has argued that some human service personnel cannot act as reflective practitioners in his sense, as they lack the necessary 'professional autonomy'. In our experience there is a growing tension between attempts to define practice in terms of laws and procedures (see for example DOH 1988, 1991), and the requirements of working with human beings who as well as being makers of rules are also capricious, unpredictable and creative. In itself there is nothing problematic about this tension, but it becomes a problem when its existence is denied. The boundary between practice/service delivery and management is often the point at which such tensions are played out, and the role of the front-line manager is often the key to handling this tension successfully.

Front-line managers – fish or fowl?: The changing culture of personal social services organizations towards market economics is gradually shifting the identity of 'team managers', away from issues of practice and towards the management of resources (Walker 1992). However, whatever the culture of the organization, the team manager has to identify with both her 'team' and her fellow managers. Our experience is that this tension is a vital indicator of the ability of the organization to communicate effectively, especially at a time of rapid change. In most of our work with service delivery teams there has been a tendency to try and avoid exploring this tension, and the team manager often finds herself confused about what feel like conflicting loyalties. This is particularly the case in national organizations where teams are geographically isolated from their regional or national parent organization. The role of the reflective consultant is to help teams to see the potential of exploring these issues.

Gender, generation, culture and hierarchy: Our work with child protection teams illustrates well the importance of exploring the fit between the work of the organization and the style of its management. Put simply, the demands of the work require extreme sensitivity to issues of generation, gender and race. At one level, these may be reflected in the organization's aims and objectives. On the other hand, the demands of the 'marketplace', legislation, and organizational procedure and precedent may require rapid adaptation and change, with maximum flexibility to re-allocate resources, or demand new skills and responses from staff. For these two aspects of organizational culture to exist in a creative tension requires great attention to the pace of change and the ability to engender trust and good communication. No amount of 'macho' style management or the commissioning of 'expert' reports from management consultants can substitute for painstaking and time-consuming consultation. In our experience time and money can be saved by approaching this with a more 'reflective' model of managing organizational change.

Managers are human too: The problem for middle managers appears to us to be that they are often ill-supported, and that their own needs for opportunities to reflect on the human dilemmas they face are subordinated to a task-centred, results-driven culture. Often, there are no formal or even informal opportunities for peer group support and sharing of feelings, with time devoted much more to the problems faced by other staff than to the pressures they experience themselves. This can make it difficult for them to appreciate the demands of service delivery staff who demand resources for their own support and consultation needs, when in some organizations middle managers are not expected to have such needs themselves. A culture can quickly develop in which status among middle managers is gained through ability not to crack under sustained pressure rather than the skills of sensitive communication and an ability to empathize with others.

Last word

'Expert' approaches to consultation seem to us to emphasize the independence, autonomy and control of the consultant, values which could be seen as representing a masculine world view. This is in contrast to valuing relationships and connections which might be associated with the feminine. In our experience, it is the relationships between these value systems and how this is played out which so often forms the focus for a reflective style of consultation.

REFERENCES

Department of Health (1988) *Protecting Children: A Guide for Undertaking a Comprehensive Assessment*. London, HMSO.

Department of Health and the University of Bristol School of Applied Social Studies (1991) *Looking After Children: Guidelines for Users of the Assessment and Action Records*. London, HMSO.

Haley, J. (1987) *Problem Solving Therapy*, 2nd edn. San Francisco, Jossey Bass.

Schön, D. (1983) *The Reflective Practitioner*. New York, Basic Books.

Walker, A. (1992) 'Community care policy: from consensus to conflict', in J. Bornat, C. Pereira, D. Pilgrim and F. Williams (eds) *Community Care: A Reader*. Basingstoke, Macmillan.

WORKING WITH AND BEING MANAGED BY THE LARGER ORGANISATION

Dorothy Whitaker, Lesley Archer and Leslie Hicks

Source: *Working in Children's Homes: Challenges and Complexities*, Chichester, John Wiley & Sons, 1998.

[. . .] The Children's Homes which participated in [our] research were located in the public sector, in Social Services Departments. The Homes were supported and managed by their Departments. These Departments were typically organised hierarchically. There was a unit manager for every Home, and several layers of management above the unit manager. There was an external line-manager, and, above him or her, middle and top managers, and the director. Councillors (people elected to be members of the county or metropolitan council) were sometimes influential. Though not officially in the management hierarchy, field social workers, responsible for the young people living in the Home, exercised certain management functions. Training officers also figure in the work life of staff groups, but less importantly as far as day-to-day operations with young people are concerned.

What is said here does not take into account the full range of tasks and responsibilities of line-managers, field social workers, or higher managers, which we are not in a position to comment upon. We emphasise here the experience of residential staffs as they come into contact with key people in the larger organisation, and are 'managed' by some of them.

Relationships with line-managers and higher managers

The external line-manager is the link person between a residential staff group and higher management in the Department. He or she is expected to be aware of activities in the Home; to communicate Departmental policy to staff and see to it that policy is carried out; to communicate changes in policy to staff; to communicate staff needs, and staff reactions to policy, upwards; and to provide supervision and consultation – sometimes only to the unit manager and sometimes to the staff group as a whole. Staff members thus know their line-manager well and are usually in regular contact.

Staff groups usually have a much more remote relationship with higher management. They usually know who their significant higher managers are, by name and by role or title. Direct interaction does not often occur. In some cases 'higher management' seems to remain a somewhat ill-defined category of people, rather than differentiated individuals with different and nameable responsibilities.

Communication problems

Staff sometimes feel that it is difficult to convey their viewpoints to line-managers and through them, to higher management. They may also feel that managers do not provide information soon enough:

> This week, not from our senior management, we read in the local paper that the unit that's supposed to be replacing this will probably be scrapped, because of lack of money. We've all read that in the paper. Wonderful to hear it from the paper, at the same time as Joe Public.

> One of the kids read in the local paper that we are going to be closed. He said 'did you know . . . ?' and we didn't. It was the first we had heard of it. [Note: This proved to be incorrect – the kernel of truth in the press report was that management was considering changing the function of the Home – a possibility that was not communicated to the staff until much later, and which eventually did take place.]

When information is conveyed down the hierarchy at the early stages of an idea being formed, a line-manager is sometimes seen by staff to communicate uncertainties, as distinct from keeping staff informed of the progress of an idea or plan:

> He's [the line-manager] just created a lot of anxiety in my mind. He'd

have been better off saying nothing until he'd got something concrete to say.

The researchers came to appreciate that when a change is in prospect, the line-manager has a delicate decision to make as to when to inform the staff – avoiding being either 'too soon' or 'too late' with the news – a matter of perspective and judgement. The line-manager may also be under instructions from higher management not to pass information on to staff.

Communicating with external line-managers when the intention is to reach higher management is often viewed by staff as problematic. Staff sometimes expressed the view that they feel that they have to overstate their case in order to have it heard. This can become a tactic for 'dealing' with management:

> Previously . . . we've actually had [four extra] young people in. . . . We had to make sure it was reduced to more reasonable numbers, or the roof would have been off. [We] had to be blunt with management, use scare tactics, so that they would agree. But it meant there was no forward planning. They had to be scared into doing it, which is quite appalling really.

[. . .] Overstating a situation, or considering allowing it to develop to crisis point may be regarded as an 'effective' tactic, but it also makes staff vulnerable to being blamed for inadequate practice or for not acting soon enough.

From staff members' point of view, the question often is: Is the external line-manager 'one of us' or 'one of them'? At times, most usually when information is passed down the hierarchy, staff groups identify line-managers closely with their higher management system. At other times, staff want line-managers to identify with them and be *their* representatives when passing information upwards, or sideways to team managers or the Child Protection Team. This is reflected in the ways that staff describe their managers: sometimes line-managers are referred to as 'management' – in other words, in terms which do not distinguish between different levels of management. Such a conflation in perception of roles frequently raises difficulties for staff when communicating with the line-manager at an *individual* level – they find it hard to view their line-manager as being unequivocally free to represent their interests.

A sense of being supported, or not

Some unit managers and staff have close supportive and positive relationships with their line-managers:

It hasn't always been plain sailing between my line-manager and me, but I think we understand each other pretty well now, and I do ask his advice, because I know that he will – he won't say 'Well, you've got to do this, you've got to do that', he makes me look at things and he makes me see things for myself, which I find very useful.

Other staff have mixed feelings about their line-managers:

A unit manager had written to a senior manager with reference to her need for another member of staff. After supervision with her line-manager she reported the line-manager had said 'There will be an answer'. The unit manager speculated, 'that means there will be no extra staff, or her [the line-manager's] response would have been different'.

(Researcher's notes)

Feeling supported by their line-managers is important for reducing stress and a sense of isolation in staff groups. If staff members feel supported, they feel they are more visible to others in the wider organisation.

Staff members need support and appreciation from higher managers, and sometimes get it, but often do not. It appears to be a rare event, much appreciated when it happens:

It *is* nice to know that you will get support from upper management when you need it. It sometimes feels like their attitude is, right, that's your unit, you get on with it, if you need support, look to the staff. Sometimes you want support from management, reassurance, and not always leave it to the officer-in-charge and the team leaders to support their team. Not just verbal reassurance, to be *for* the staff, not just for the young people. Acknowledgement, and also to offer the staff support in other ways. To be able to say if something goes wrong, not just how is the young person, but how are the staff as well. Sometimes it seems the attitude is forget the staff, you get paid to do that. They don't see what you're doing above and beyond the call of duty, because you're in this job because you care.

Support from managers is particularly appreciated when an allegation is made against a member of staff:

The service manager came down yesterday to go through an incident, a complaint against a member of staff. There was nothing found, it was all clean and no problem at all, but a complaint hanging over you causes anxiety: will I get the sack, will I get the mortgage paid, what's happening? It was nice of him to come down and spend an hour and a half just to go through the scenario and reassure everyone. It was an unusual thing for the service manager to do: the first time [I've known it]. [. . .]

A sense of being understood, or not

Members of a residential staff group could feel that both their line-manager and higher managers underemphasised the importance placed by staff on the composition of their teams. A stable team, which brings with it opportunities for good internal communication and support from colleagues for day-to-day work, is important to residential workers. Sometimes, this was made more difficult by a line-manager requesting that a member of staff cover for another team, or by managers somewhere higher up in the hierarchy operating a central pool of relief staff, resulting in different relief staff turning up at a Home at different times, often unknown to the staff or to the young people. One staff member said:

> It's come to the point where you really have to be selfish and basically say [I'm] not interested in other units, our priority is our staff team. It's not very nice when you see other units and other colleagues floundering with problems, because you like to offer skills, knowledge, expertise or whatever that you've got, but a part of you says not, that's down to management to sort it out, and of course you know it won't get sorted out . . . the stress factor here's enough for me to keep the lid on this, and if we start overlapping from other dimensions, it's going to cause loads of problems. [. . .]

The impact of decisions made by middle managers

Staff members report that they pay a price when decisions are made or new policies are introduced without taking the likely full consequences for care staff into account. For example:

> Somebody [in management] can say you can have X people [working a shift], and that involves you working two weekends out of three . . . the only way the rotas will run successfully with the numbers you require on duty means that two weekends out of three you don't see your wife and kids, so it doesn't matter what happens, it all eventually filters down and by the time it gets to us, we're suffering. [. . .]

'Being managed' and carrying out departmental policies and procedures

There is consensus among those concerned with the residential care of children that Homes and staff groups need to be managed externally in order for good standards of care to be set and maintained. The way this works out in practice is summarised in the following key points.

In practice, it is the line-manager who occupies and embodies the external management role, and is the usual point of contact between a staff group and a Department's management system. The line-manager conveys news, especially about new policy decisions, to unit managers and staff. He or she occupies a lynch-pin position between a residential care staff and others in the organisational hierarchy.

The line-manager usually also takes on supervisory functions, either with the whole staff group or with the unit manager. He or she thus combines the functions of manager and supervisor. The following quotation, from the Central Council for Education and Training in Social Work, sums up the prevailing view about the importance of the line-manager in assuring standards:

> The importance of the role of professional support and line-management of group care units cannot be over-emphasized. . . . Research has confirmed the strong connection between the appropriate external management of group care practice and the ability of the staff to fulfil the complex tasks required of them.
>
> (Baldwin, 1990, quoted in CCETSW, 1992: 22)

However, staff members can be reluctant to seek supervision from line-managers if this means exposing what might be regarded as weaknesses to someone who has power over promotion or contracts.

External line-managers sometimes fulfil their management and supervisory roles appropriately, and sometimes do not. For example, the researchers considered that a line-manager behaved appropriately when he clearly and explicitly informed a member of staff of the Department's investigatory procedures after an allegation had been made, and extended support without glossing over the seriousness of the situation. A line-manager who told a boy that he would be moved if his behaviour did not improve was clearly behaving inappropriately.

The external line-manager is located clearly within the Department's hierarchical structure, and the role itself is usually well-defined. However, in a very real sense, field social workers and those responsible for placements are also exercising a managerial role, especially with regard to the placement and subsequent movement of young people. In addition, field social workers 'manage' in the sense of holding onto certain decisions with respect to a young person while he or she is in residential care.

Decisions about staffing and staff selection, redeployment, and promotion are located within middle management. It is here also that procedures are established for lodging complaints and for the investigation of allegations made against members of staff.

Staff selection procedures can be a sore point for staff groups, especially where equal opportunities procedures are inflexibly applied, or unsuitable staff are placed in a Children's Home because managers are responsible for their redeployment.

Being the object of investigations when an allegation is made is a source of great stress for the accused person and the staff as a whole. A supportive attitude on the part of managers is much appreciated.

How rotas are worked out can present difficulties for staff. In theory, members of the residential staff work to rotas which they themselves devise and agree upon. In practice, rotas are influenced by management decisions, either directly or through knock-on effects. Staff members may end up working two weekends out of three, and/or very long hours.

To facilitate 'being managed', staff are required to follow Departmental and administrative procedures, e.g. keeping logs, devising care plans and updating them, recording all visitors to the Home, and reporting incidents to the Child Protection team. In general, staff see the need for such procedures, but sometimes experience problems related to the escalation of paperwork, which often has to be done late at night during sleep-in duty, because of the pressure of other tasks.

While staff groups accept the need for Departmental inspections, they can be time-consuming and can induce stress if not handled sensitively. [. . .]

The problems and tensions referred to . . . can have a cumulative effect on staff, eroding morale over a period of time and leading to a pervasive sense of helplessness. Staff come to expect little of their management and may give up trying to have a say over their own work-life, or communicating their views, or objecting to decisions which they feel sure will have negative consequences, or defending courses of action which they are convinced are the right ones. [. . .]

REFERENCE

CCETSW (1992) *Setting Quality Standards for Residential Child Care: A Practical Way Forward*, London, Central Council for Education and Training in Social Work.

SEVEN

MANAGING UNPAID WORKERS

Julie Charlesworth

Introduction

> [...] a volunteer is a person who gives his skill, his energy and his time. It is, in fact, the gift of himself, the gift of an understanding human being, who believing it is right that this gift should be made, decides that he is going to be the giver and devotes himself to the giving. It is for him to say how much he will do, how much he will give, how much he will participate and then to abide absolutely and entirely by that undertaking.
>
> (Reading, n.d.: 11)

The world of volunteering has moved on somewhat from this understanding (from the 1970s) of the role of volunteers. Some aspects may still ring true in terms of people's motivations for, and expectations of, volunteering but people's reasons for volunteering vary considerably. Perhaps the desire to obtain useful skills for future paid employment or to fill spare time after retirement are as important as more altruistic concerns. The biggest change is that volunteers are now increasingly integrated into a wider and complex structure of professionalisation and formalisation of the voluntary sector. In addition to performing their duties as volunteers, they are likely to be formally recruited, managed, trained and monitored, and brought into legal frameworks of contracts and partnership.

Although many voluntary organisations, particularly larger ones, have arguably moved closer in structure and management to public sector and even for-profit organisations, the role of the volunteer continues to symbolise one of the sector's main differences and, consequently, raises major management questions. As the basis for the 'exchange relationship' with their organisation remains fundamentally different to that of paid workers, in that it is not based on financial reward, do unpaid workers need to be managed in different ways to paid ones? Moreover, in the constantly changing and integrated care environment and the part played by voluntary organisations in providing state-funded services, is there still a role for volunteer workers and what should that be? This reading explores the complexities and ambiguities associated with the place of unpaid workers in the provision of care and outlines the differences and similarities between managing paid and unpaid workers. This is particularly important given the increasing emphasis on partnership between different organisations and sectors, greater accountability and involvement of service users, and attention to monitoring and evaluation of services. Furthermore, in response to concerns that the supply of volunteers is decreasing, and in line with its vision of active citizenship and caring communities, the government launched a major initiative in 2001 to encourage more volunteering in public services and the community (Toynbee, 2001).

Who volunteers and why?

The role of volunteers and voluntary organisations in providing care has a long and varied history. The great interest in doing such work during the nineteenth century helped set the foundations for much of state provision today (Whelan, 1999). In order to understand differences between paid and unpaid workers, it is useful to consider who the volunteers are, where they might be located and why they have chosen to volunteer. Voluntary organisations vary enormously, including service providers, advocacy groups, self-help groups and intermediary/umbrella organisations (Handy, 1988). Volunteers may be trustees, fund-raisers, core professionals, providing direct services, administrators, and be service users as well as volunteers. Furthermore, depending on the size, purpose and income of the organisation, they may fulfil several of these roles at the same time. To add to the confusion, volunteers could be affiliated to a national voluntary organisation but work in a statutory organisation and be managed by a paid manager from outside their organisation. Volunteers' time commitment also varies from a substantial input to just a few hours a month. Volunteers could be relatives, friends or partners of service users, or service users themselves. Or they may have no connection whatsoever to the organisation and have been recruited through a volunteer bureau because the work sounded interesting.

Volunteers have always been a diverse group, with differences in participation based on age, gender, class, ethnicity, education, income and geography. Surveys of volunteering in the UK suggest that around 22 million people volunteer every year, and it is most common with people in their late thirties to forties, and from higher socio-economic groups (Institute for Volunteering Research, 2001). There are frequent concerns about the overall supply of volunteers and this is affected by changes in social, economic and demographic factors, which also have an impact on the types of people who volunteer. In recent decades, for example, the traditional image of the middle-aged woman as a volunteer has been affected by more women entering the paid labour market and therefore not considering voluntary work. Although older age groups have been less well represented, stricter health and safety regulations have also affected the numbers of volunteers in their seventies and eighties in recent years. However, trends such as earlier retirement and more part-time work may encourage more participation (Heath and Davis Smith, 1992).

People's motivations for volunteering are often complex and do not just relate to a sense of duty or citizenship. They may be looking for ways of utilising spare time or seeking training in a new area of work as a stepping stone to paid employment. Surveys suggest that skills development is becoming more important, particularly among young people, but the most common reason for volunteering was because 'they had been asked' (Institute for Volunteering Research, 2001). The reasons why people volunteer are important to organisations as they ultimately affect retention of unpaid workers. Wardell et al. (2000) suggest that people volunteering for altruistic reasons could be more likely to leave if they have to engage with contracts and other formal structures which they feel get in the way of the cause. However, it could also be the case that if volunteers' commitment to an organisation is strong, they would be more prepared to carry on despite organisational and wider change. Volunteers are unpaid, so their personal motivation and level of commitment are key factors in recruitment, retention and management of volunteers.

Volunteers may interpret their commitment in different ways, perhaps to a cause, an organisation and service users but for some volunteers, it is also 'work' in the same way as having a paid job. Thus, in common with paid workers, volunteers would not consider failing to turn up for work unless they were ill or on holiday. People often derive status and identity through paid work and this is equally valid for volunteer work. Like paid work, volunteering can also offer a focus to the week and a way into new social networks. In these ways, it is clear that perceived differences between paid and unpaid work become blurred.

The supply and motivation of volunteers is also affected by government agendas, and whether they operate in favour of, or against, encouraging people to participate in voluntary activity and what that contribution might be. Experiences under Conservative governments, with their emphasis on competitive mixed economies of care, varied. One thing is clear – increased use of contracts fundamentally changed the basis of the relationship between local statutory and voluntary organisations. Under New Labour, the emphasis on partnership and 'compacts' with the voluntary sector has aimed to improve this often strained relationship. The government is now trying to encourage more people to volunteer, particularly from younger age groups, and is pushing the benefits of volunteering in terms of learning new skills, gaining experience relevant to paid work and 'citizen duty'.

This should lead to an enhanced and improved role for voluntary organisations and thus for volunteers but there is a paradox. In some areas, the continuing drive for cost-cutting and streamlining services has led to a loss of contracts for voluntary organisations. Even where contracts continue, they continue to be subject to funding cuts or delays in payment. Furthermore, the drive to partnership has increased the amount of work voluntary organisations are being asked to do and usually with no extra funding provided; some of this burden may fall on trustees and other volunteers. More skills are required of both paid and unpaid workers, such as costing services, tendering, performance management and managing interorganisational relationships (Hudson, 1995). Increasing opportunities for volunteers can also make paid workers and their unions concerned about the knock-on effects for their jobs and responsibilities and unsettle the relationship between paid and unpaid workers, with implications for managing both groups of workers.

Management issues

It is clear that there are both similarities and differences between paid and unpaid workers, which potentially lead to difficulties and tensions for managers. These have become heightened with the increasing professionalisation of the voluntary sector and its involvement in wider interorganisational structures. This section examines the complexities of governance and management structures within voluntary organisations and the attempts to formalise managing unpaid workers, whilst at the same time remaining sensitive to their different exchange relationship and motivations.

The Charities Act (1992 and 1993) attempted to provide a clearer and stricter regulatory framework for charities through giving the Charities Commission a more supervisory role, improving standards and reminding trustees of their roles and responsibilities (Cornforth, 2001). Larger voluntary organisations tend to structure their governance and management through boards of trustees (also called management committees) and various subcommittees, and attempt to separate the two functions. Boards are expected to provide accountability, devise strategy, resolve tensions and advise the managers, whilst the management function is supposed to inform and make recommendations to the board (Hudson, 1995). However, in smaller organisations these supposedly distinct roles often become blurred, which can lead to confusion over responsibilities and lead to conflict between workers. Even where there are attempts to separate the functions, it is often difficult to explain to very committed volunteers and paid staff not on the board that their role in governance issues needs to be limited, otherwise processes may become too unwieldy to reach decisions.

As voluntary organisations have become more formally structured, there is a danger of becoming too remote from service users' views. Many organisations have increasingly involved service users as trustees to overcome this problem, and some organisations, particularly self-help groups, are largely comprised of service users. As discussed by Locke *et al.* (2002), representation by service users on boards was often considered legally problematic in the past. Charity law used to stipulate a clear distinction between trustees and service users, in that a beneficiary of the service could not also be a trustee, but recent guidance has clarified that a third of representatives on boards can now be service users. However, they also suggest that there are other opportunities for service users to participate and that representation on the board is not always the most appropriate involvement. For example, larger organisations also have subcommittees and other forums where service users can make their views heard, and this can also result in wider representation. Although the board is often perceived as the site of power and thus the place where people feel they can have the most influence, Locke *et al.* highlight the power of other networks, particularly informal ones, and the role of senior, usually paid, staff.

All of this highlights complex management issues. For example, where service users and other volunteers, who were previously 'frontline' workers, are elected to serve on boards, this may cause tension amongst their former colleagues. This could be problematic in smaller organisations where boards fulfil both management and governance functions and where board members may also continue with their old roles. Furthermore, volunteers with the requisite skills and experience are often able to apply for paid positions, perhaps as co-ordinators or managers in their organisation and if appointed, this could also lead to tension. Other difficult situations could arise where a volunteer has been fulfilling a key role informally on an unpaid basis and the organisation decides the work requires a paid member of staff and advertises it, but the unpaid worker fails to secure the post. This may result in resentment or that volunteer may then leave the organisation. These complex situations inevitably require sensitive management in order to ensure that volunteers continue to feel appreciated and that working relationships and services are not disrupted.

On a day-to-day basis, volunteers involved with service delivery are managed or co-ordinated by (paid or unpaid) managers, usually within their organisation. There is often a specific volunteer co-ordinator responsible for a large number of volunteers, which makes managing difficult, but in other situations volunteers work closely with professionals and managers. Some volunteers enjoy a large amount of autonomy in their work but as care work becomes subject to tighter regulation, volunteers are more likely to be directly and formally managed. As mentioned earlier, there are instances of volunteers being managed by a paid manager from outside their organisation. For example, a WRVS volunteer working in a hospital may feel a strong commitment to helping service users and allegiance to their national organisation but resent intrusion from hospital managers 'telling them what to do'. On occasion, tension could arise between paid and unpaid workers working together. For example, volunteers may feel threatened or insecure if a paid and trained professional is brought into work with them and where different patterns of working or cultures may clash (Hornby and Atkins, 2000). Such examples highlight the complexity of managing volunteers and developing solutions (where appropriate) to understanding, and dealing with, differences between paid and unpaid workers. Therefore, managing volunteers should be the responsibility of management at all levels of the organisation and not just left to paid or unpaid co-ordinators without any support when dealing with difficult issues (Willis, 1992).

Many voluntary organisations have acknowledged the similarities with paid workers but understand that differences also exist and have given consideration to the nature of the employment contract with volunteers. Depending on the size and function of the organisation and the specific responsibilities of the job, volunteers may have either a formal or informal contract. A formal contract tends to entail procedures such as written job descriptions, selection interviews, induction and training, monitoring and evaluation. However, a tension remains with job descriptions in that sometimes it is more appropriate to write the description to fit the particular skills and experience of a volunteer who approaches an organisation with an offer of help. With recruitment of volunteers still largely dependent on word of mouth, this is likely to continue.

Having more formal procedures may help volunteers to understand their role and contribution to the organisation and, for those workers looking to gain skills and experience relevant to paid work, they may appreciate a formal contract involving training, together with feedback on performance. All categories of volunteers, whether delivering services directly to service users or as trustees, require training and monitoring. In some cases this needs to be formal, perhaps paying for a volunteer to attend a training course but in others, their colleagues may provide on-the-job training and assistance. Both of these approaches place a demand on resources. Furthermore, as unpaid workers' motivation is not based on financial reward, it is important to ensure that their work is rewarding and interesting in order to maintain motivation and fulfil an exchange relationship (Willis, 1992). Elements such as variety in tasks, creativity, learning, personal and skills development, autonomy, feelings of accomplishment and belonging, help provide a stimulating working environment.

Conclusion

Volunteers often play a crucial role in providing care services and as part of the ideology of the organisations and although they are unpaid, they do have hidden costs for organisations (Leat, 1993). Recruitment, training and management of unpaid workers have financial costs and make demands on paid staff's time. Thus, it is crucial that full consideration is given to the role of volunteers and why and where their contribution is most useful. Furthermore, managers need to understand the different motivations of unpaid workers and the nature of the exchange relationship in order to manage sensitively.

REFERENCES

Cornforth, C. (2001) *Recent Trends in Charity Governance and Trusteeship*, London, NCVO.

Davis Smith, J. and Heath, R. (1992) *Volunteering and Society: Principles and Practice*, London, Bedford Square Press.

Handy, C. (1988) *Understanding Voluntary Organisations*, London, Penguin.

Hornby, S. and Atkins, J. (2000) *Collaborative Care. Interprofessional, Inter-agency and Interpersonal*, Oxford, Blackwell.

Hudson, M. (1995) *Managing Without Profit: Managing Third Sector Organisations*, London, Penguin.

Institute for Volunteering Research (2001) *1997 National Survey of Volunteering in the UK*. www.ivr.org.uk/nationalsurvey.htm (accessed 7.11.01)

Leat, D. (1993) *Managing Across Sectors: Similarities and Differences Between For-Profit and Voluntary Non-Profit Organisations*, London, City University Business School.

Locke, M., Begum, N. and Robson, P. (2002) 'Service Users and Charity Governance', in Cornforth, C. (ed.) *The Governance of Public and Non-Profit Organisations: What Boards Do*, London, Routledge.

Reading, S. (n.d.) *Voluntary Service*. Document issued to WRVS volunteers.

Toynbee, P. (2001) 'Local Involvement – That's the New Prescription', The *Guardian*, 12 January, p. 18.

Wardell, F., Wishman, J. and Whalley, L.J. (2000) 'Who Volunteers?', *British Journal of Social Work*, 30, 227–48.

Whelan, F. (1999) *Involuntary Action. How Voluntary is the 'Voluntary' Sector?* London, IEA Health and Welfare Unit.

Willis, E. (1992) 'Managing Volunteers', in Batsleer, J., Cornforth, C. and Paton, R. (eds) *Issues in Voluntary and Non-profit Management*, Addison-Wesley.

EIGHT

WHISTLEBLOWING: PUBLIC CONCERN AT WORK

Philip Ells and Guy Dehn

Source: *The Law and Social Work: Contemporary Issues for Practice*, Cull, L.-A. and Roach, J. (eds), Buckingham, Palgrave/Open University, 2001.

Public Concern at Work is an independent charity that has been recognised by the UK government, the European Commission and the Organization for Economic Co-operation and Development as a leading authority on public interest whistleblowing. It has three key activities:

1   It runs a free legal helpline for people concerned about serious malpractice in the workplace.
2   It offers professional and practical help to organisations on how to encourage responsibility and accountability in the workplace.
3   It conducts research and informs developments in public policy.

Since its launch in 1993, Public Concern at Work has helped over 2000 people who have been concerned about serious malpractice at work. Its charitable remit means that the charity cannot deal with private grievances or dispute but only with matters that affect the wider public interest. Examples of these are fraud, public danger and abuse in care.

The free, confidential advice service is most useful for people at work who are not sure whether or how to 'blow the whistle'. In these cases, the approach of the charity is that, wherever possible, the people in charge of the organisation should have a chance to investigate the matter. This is usually the quickest and most effective way to remove any danger of malpractice and also the way that avoids, removes or reduces any risk to a client. Inevitably, it is sometimes necessary for the matter to be raised outside.

Building on this approach to whistleblowing, the charity was closely involved in the scope and detail of the Public Interest Disclosure Act 1998. A summary of this important new legislation is provided in this article...

When the idea of an independent resource centre on whistleblowing was first discussed in 1990, the issue was seen almost invariably in a hostile light. The term was most frequently used to describe public officials who had paid a heavy penalty for leaking information, usually anonymously to the media. Whistleblowers were presented, if not as villains, then as loners and losers. For this reason, there was some initial scepticism about the need for or role of a charitable organisation in this area.

Events conspired to give the charity a receptive audience. The background to the legislation lies in the major disasters and scandals of the last decade of the twentieth century, such as the ferry disaster at Zeebrugge,[1] the rail crash at Clapham Junction,[2] the collapse of the Bank of Credit and Commerce International[3] and the Arms to Iraq scandal.[4] Almost every official inquiry has shown that workers had been aware of the danger but either had been too scared to sound the alarm or had raised the matter with the wrong person or in the wrong way. This communication breakdown cost hundreds of lives, damaged thousands of livelihoods, lost tens of thousands of jobs and undermined public confidence in the organisations on which we all depend. Lyme Bay,[5] Barings,[6] Bristol Royal Infirmary[7] and numerous incidents of abuse in care have reinforced our essential message that misconduct would not be deterred and accountability could not work in practice while people felt that they had little choice but to remain silent. At the same time, individual cases, such as those of Chris Chapman,[8] Graham Pink,[9] Andy Millar[10] and Paul van Buitenen,[11] highlighted the plight of those who did blow the whistle.

Soon after the charity's launch in 1993, the Audit Commission[12] was quick to understand the relevance of the message of the charity and to endorse its work in the context of probity in local government. Even before the launch, the European Commission and Parliament had asked it to report on the role of whistleblowers in controlling financial malpractice in Europe.[13] Within its first year, a number of leading employers also offered their support, some having learnt, from bitter experience, the cost of a culture in which their employees had minded their own business.

The media, while disappointed that the cases the legal helpline handled were confidential, proved invaluable in promoting the message and publicising the charity's work. Several editorial endorsements ensured that the issue received the attention of opinion-formers. Beyond this welcome support, the fact that *The Times* helped to fund the successful legal claim of the British Biotech whistleblower is an important development in the attitude of the media toward those who make public interest disclosures.[14]

The most significant endorsement of the charity's work came in 1995 from the Committee on Standards in Public Life,[15] which accepted Public

Concern at Work's view that unless staff thought it safe and acceptable to raise concerns about misconduct internally, the probable result was that they would stay silent or leak the information. It was this culture which had provided fertile grounds for the birth of sleaze, in which the perception of possible misconduct appeared to justify as much – if not more – attention as proven malpractice. The Committee recommended that public bodies:

> institute codes of practice on whistleblowing, appropriate to their circumstances, which would enable concerns to be raised confidentially inside, and if necessary, outside the organisation.[16]

Key aspects of these procedures, endorsed by the Committee on Standards in Public Life, are:

- a clear statement that malpractice is taken seriously in the organisation
- respect, if they wish it, for the confidentiality of those staff raising concerns
- the opportunity to raise concerns outside the line management structure
- access to independent advice
- an indication of the proper way in which concerns may be raised outside the organisation if necessary
- penalties for maliciously making false allegations.

Public Interest Disclosure Act 1999

The Public Interest Disclosure Act came into force in Great Britain on 2 July 1999 and in Northern Ireland on 31 October 1999. The legislation has been described by American campaigners as the most far-reaching whistleblower protection law in the world. In the House of Lords, Lord Nolan, one of the most senior judges, praised it as 'skilfully achieving the essential but delicate balance between the public interest and the interests of employers'.

By setting out a clear and simple framework for raising genuine concerns about malpractice, and by guaranteeing full protection to workers who raise such issues, the Act addresses this issue in a constructive and effective way. While the legislation readily acknowledges that concerns about malpractice are best raised and addressed in the workplace, it also recognises the role that regulatory authorities and outside bodies – including the media – can and do play in deterring and detecting serious malpractice. The Act signals a break from a culture in which inertia, secrecy and silence have allowed crime, negligence and misconduct to go unchallenged, all too often with devastating consequences for the individuals and organisations involved. It means that ordinary, decent people will be less likely to turn a blind eye to wrongdoing and more likely to do the right thing. The legislation is now being used as a benchmark against which developments in Europe and elsewhere will be judged.

The Act sets out a clear and simple framework to promote responsible whistleblowing by:

- reassuring workers that silence is not the only safe option
- providing strong protection for workers who raise concerns internally
- reinforcing and protecting the right to report concerns to key regulators
- protecting more public disclosures provided that there is a valid reason for going wider and that the particular disclosure was reasonable
- helping to ensure that organisations respond by addressing the message rather than the messenger and resist the temptation to cover up serious malpractice.

Scheme of the Act

The provisions are inserted into the Employment Rights Act 1996. The scheme of the Act is to provide protection to workers who make a 'protected disclosure'. The Act enables employees who make a protected disclosure to disclose information, confidential or otherwise:

- internally
- to prescribed regulators
- to a wider audience, usually indicating the media.

Workers who are victimised or dismissed for making a protected disclosure will be able to make a claim in an employment tribunal.

Individuals covered

In addition to employees, the Act covers agency staff, contractors, homeworkers, trainees and everyone who works in the NHS. The usual employment law restrictions on the minimum length of service and age do not apply here. The Act does not currently cover the genuinely self-employed, volunteers, the intelligence services, the army or police officers.

Malpractice

Under the Act, a protected disclosure is defined as 'any disclosure of information which, in the reasonable belief of the worker making the disclosure, tends to show one or more of the following:

a   that a criminal offence has been committed, is being committed or is likely to be committed

b   that a person has failed, is failing or is likely to fail to comply with any legal obligation to which he is subject

c   that a miscarriage of justice has occurred, is occurring or is likely to occur

d   that the health or safety of any individual has been, is being or is likely to be endangered

e   that the environment has been, is being or is likely to be damaged, or

f   that information tending to show any matter falling within any one of the preceding paragraphs has been, is being or is likely to be deliberately concealed (s.43B (1))

The range of information capable of constituting a protected disclosure is extremely wide, applying to most malpractice.

Reasonable belief

The requirement that the worker has a 'reasonable belief' means that the belief need not be correct but only that the worker held the belief and it was reasonable for him or her to do so. Accordingly, it would still be a protected disclosure if the worker reasonably but mistakenly believed that a specified malpractice was occurring. The Act confirms that workers may safely seek legal advice on any concerns that they have with regard to malpractice.

The Act protects disclosures made in *good faith* to bodies such as the Health and Safety Executive,[17] the Inland Revenue,[18] Customs and Excise[19] (for sanctions controls) and the Financial Services Authority,[20] where the whistleblower *reasonably believes that the information and any allegation in it are substantially true*. At the time of writing, in the care field, the SSI is not a prescribed regulator.

Wider disclosures: (1) good faith, (2) reasonable belief, (3) the trigger to go wider, and (4) reasonable in all the circumstances

Wider disclosures (for example to the police, the media, MPs, pressure groups and non-prescribed regulators) are protected if, in addition to the tests for regulatory disclosures (good faith, reasonable belief and reasonable belief that the allegation is substantially true), there is a specific trigger for the whistleblower to go wider *and* the disclosures are reasonable in all the circumstances. The whistleblower is not protected if the wider disclosure is made for personal gain.

For wider disclosures only, whistleblowers must satisfy one of the following tests. They must have:

a   reasonably believed they would be victimised if they raised the matter internally or with a prescribed regulator;

b   reasonably believed that a cover-up was likely and there was no pre-
    scribed regulator;
c   already raised the matter internally or with a prescribed regulator.

When considering the category of 'reasonable in the circumstances', the
employment tribunal is, in deciding the reasonableness of the disclosure,
directed under the provisions of the Act to consider, among other factors:

■ the identity of the person to whom it was made
■ the seriousness of the concern
■ whether the risk or danger remains
■ whether the disclosure breached a duty of confidence that the employer
  owed a third party
■ where the concern had first been raised with the employer or a prescribed regulator, the reasonableness of his or her response (which will
  be particularly relevant)
■ if the concern had first been raised with the employer, whether any
  whistleblowing policy in the organisation was or should have been
  used. (This means that it is not enough just to have a whistleblowing
  policy. Concerns that are reported must be investigated and action
  taken as appropriate.)

Where the concern is exceptionally serious, the Act provides a further
safety valve for workers who make a wider disclosure without having
satisfied the normal conditions of raising the matter internally or with a
prescribed regulator. This is in practice likely to apply only when, for
example, a worker is genuinely concerned that a child is being sexually
abused and that there is no time to waste, thus immediately reporting the
matter to the police. [. . .]

The publication in February 2000 of *Lost in Care*, the Waterhouse
Report into Child Abuse in North Wales (DoH/Welsh Office, 2000), reinforces [the importance of clear procedures]. The investigation was initiated
by Alison Taylor, a care worker who had sought repeatedly but unsuccess-
fully to blow the whistle internally and to the appropriate authorities.
The report was a vindication of Mrs Taylor and led to recommendations
that:

(8) Every local authority should establish and implement conscien-
    tiously clear whistleblowing procedures enabling members of staff
    to make complaints and raise matters of concern affecting the
    treatment or welfare of looked after children without threats or
    fear of reprisals in any form.

                                                    (DoH/Welsh Office, 2000)

Whistleblowing policies assisted by the new legislation are therefore now recognised as an important tool in combating abuse.

Practical implications for health and care sectors

In the light of these developments, health and care providers would be well advised to consider the following:

- Employers should make it clear that it is both safe and acceptable for workers to raise any concern that they may have about misconduct or malpractice in the organisation.
- When a worker raises a concern about a specified malpractice, every effort should be made to ensure that the employer responds to the message rather than shoots the messenger.
- Employers ought to recognise that it is in their own interests to introduce effective whistleblowing procedures. This will help both parties to separate the message from the messenger.
- Employers should decide upon a person in the organisation to whom confidential disclosure can be made. This person must have the authority and determination to act if concerns are not raised with – or properly dealt with – by immediate line management.
- When a protected disclosure has been made, employers should take all reasonable steps to try to ensure that no colleague, manager or other person under its control victimises the whistleblower.
- In-house legal advisers should be directed to review confidentiality clauses in contracts of employment and in severance agreements when the working relationship has terminated.
- Although requiring a higher level of proof than internal whistleblowing, disclosure to a prescribed regulator is protected, whether or not the concern had first been raised internally. When workers reasonably believe that they will be victimised if they go to a prescribed regulator, they will be entitled to protection under the Act if they make a wider, public disclosure. Accordingly, employers should make it clear that reporting concerns to a prescribed regulator is acceptable.
- Anything that might be construed as an attempt to suppress evidence of malpractice is now particularly inadvisable since (a) reasonable suspicion of a 'cover-up' would itself provide a basis for a protected disclosure; (b) a disclosure to the media is more likely to be protected; and (c) there is a much reduced scope for containing any damage by a private settlement with a confidentiality clause.
- Anonymous whistleblowing may not afford any protection because an employment tribunal must be satisfied that the employer believed that the whistleblower made the disclosure and victimised him or her because of it.

. . .

There is growing recognition that whistleblowing needs to be encouraged as best practice not only to comply with the provisions of the Act, but also as a means of establishing a change in the culture of organisations. For this change to occur, it is essential that a lead is given from the top, that responsible whistleblowing is promoted and that management genuinely appears to address the issue. In England and Wales, all NHS trusts have purchased Public Concern at Work's toolkit on whistleblowing. The toolkit provides a means of devising and implementing a whistleblowing policy.

The existence of legislation protecting whistleblowers is a radical shift away from the old perceptions of whistleblowers being labelled sneaks or telltales. It is early days in terms of the legislation, but the imperative must now be for employers generally to encourage and promote whistleblowing. [. . .]

Raising it internally – defusing the situation

Where workers reasonably suspect malpractice (including physical abuse) they will be protected from victimisation if they raise the matter with their employer in good faith.

Case study

Jane worked as a day care assistant at a private rest home. She had been there for eight months and worked happily with 20 other staff looking after the elderly residents. The only downside to the job was one of her colleagues, Mary, who was abusive to the residents and bullied the staff.

Mary was particularly unpleasant to two residents: she would startle them from behind and push them around. On one occasion, Jane saw Mary bend one of their thumbs back. When Jane asked Mary what she was doing, Mary said that she had been given permission to do this. Jane raised the matter with the home's owner; he said he would sort it out and told Jane to keep on smiling.

A few weeks later, some of Jane's colleagues told her that they had seen Mary hit one of the residents and that they had reported the matter to the owner. Mary nevertheless carried on working normally, and nothing seemed to happen. Thus, while Jane liked the owner of the home, she thought that it would be futile to raise the matter with him again. Jane knew that the local authority inspectors would be visiting the home soon and decided to mention her concerns directly to them.

When the inspector came, Jane mentioned the matter. The inspector asked whether the colleagues who had seen Mary hit the resident would give a statement. Jane discussed this with them, and the colleagues contacted the inspector. When the inspector had all the evidence, he wrote to the home and said that the matter was so serious that he was referring the incident to the police.

Mary was suspended, but Jane was suspended too in case her presence at work hindered the investigation. Jane was told she could not talk to anyone about the suspected misconduct or about her suspension. She was very upset because she thought she had done nothing wrong. Two weeks later, she got a letter at home telling her she was to return to work the following week. The letter also said that she was to receive a written warning: she had disclosed confidential information and had damaged the reputation of the home. Jane thought this was a prelude to her being sacked, and contacted Public Concern at Work.

A legal adviser discussed the matter with Jane over the telephone and assured her she had done nothing wrong. As it was clear that she liked the home and did not want to lose her job, she was advised to try to defuse the situation rather than assert her legal rights or have the charity write a lawyer's letter. With the assistance of a legal adviser, Jane drafted a letter to send to the owner in which she apologised for any inconvenience she had caused. Jane also explained that she had tried to do the right thing and hoped that the owner would in time recognise that Jane had been protecting rather than undermining the reputation of the home. She also pointed out that she herself had not called in the police and stressed how much she liked working at the home. The letter worked. The written warning was withdrawn, and the owner, residents and colleagues welcomed Jane back into the home.

[. . .]

NOTES

1   The ferry sank, and 194 people died, because it had been sailing with its bow doors open. The inquiry found that staff had on five previous occasions reported that this was happening, but their concerns had got lost at the level of middle management.

2   The inquiry found that a supervisor had noticed the loose wiring in the junction box a couple of months earlier but said nothing as 'he did not want to rock the boat'; 35 passengers died.

3   The inquiry into the £2 billion collapse found there had been an autocratic environment at The Bank of Credit and Commerce International in which no one was prepared to speak up. The only employee who had was an internal auditor who was made redundant.

4 An employee at Matrix Churchill had written to the Foreign Secretary warning that munitions equipment was being exported to Iraq. Although this letter was ignored by civil servants for a number of years, it was a fear that the whistle-blower would contact the press during the prosecution of the company for breaching the arms embargo that caused the Deputy Prime Minister to refuse to suppress evidence that the government had been aware of the suspect exports.

5 Four schoolchildren drowned when a school canoeing trip went badly wrong. One of the instructors at the centre had written to the managing director weeks before the tragedy warning that 'You should have a careful look at your standards of safety. Otherwise you might find yourself trying to explain why someone's son or daughter will not be coming home.' Because he had ignored this graphic warning, the Managing Director was jailed for two years for corporate manslaughter.

6 The official regulator banned one of the senior managers at Barings Bank from future work as he had been aware of the risk inherent in Nick Leeson's activities. Although the manager said that he had expressed his fears, the regulator found that he had failed to blow the whistle either loudly or clearly.

7 A consultant anaesthetist, Steven Bolsin, was victimised after raising concerns about the techniques of surgeons working on children with heart complaints. An inquiry into the deaths of 29 children found that the standard of care at the hospital was inadequate.

8 Chris Chapman was a biochemist who was made redundant shortly after raising his concern about misconduct in the area of medical research.

9 Graham Pink was a nurse who challenged understaffing in geriatric wards, leading to the neglect of and danger to the patients. On going to the media, he was suspended and later dismissed.

10 Dr Millar was sacked as head of clinical trials for British Biotech after he raised his concerns about the efficacy of key drug developments.

11 The European Commission internal auditor whose disclosure of financial irregularities led to the resignation of the European Commission in March 1999.

12 Appoints auditors to all local authorities and NHS bodies in England and Wales, as well as addressing issues of financial conduct and value for money in these services.

13 First published in 1996 by Public Concern at Work as an analysis of the laws and practices in Europe that affect attitudes toward whistleblowing, fraud and the European Union.

14 Times Newspapers and the British Medical Association helped to finance the cost of Dr Millar's successful legal defence in an action for breach of confidence.

15 Cm 3270-1 (May 1995). The Committee was set up to examine current concerns about the standards of conduct of all holders of public office, including arrangements relating to financial and commercial activities, and to make recommendations on any change in present arrangements that might be required to ensure the highest standards of propriety in public life.

16 ibid., Recommendation 2.

17 Aims to ensure that risks to people's health and safety from work activities are properly controlled.

18 Responsible, under the overall direction of Treasury Ministers, for the efficient administration of taxes.
19 Deals with VAT (Sales tax). Enforces export sanctions, including arms embargoes.
20 Responsible for the supervision of banks and the wholesale money market regime.

REFERENCE

Department of Health/Welsh Office (2000) *Lost in Care: Report of the tribunal of the inquiry into the abuse of children in care in the former county council areas of Gwynedd and Clwyd since 1974*. London: The Stationery Office.

NINE

MANAGING LOSS IN CARE HOMES

Jeanne Samson Katz

This reading explores the challenges managers face in coping with loss in care homes for older people. It focuses on how, following the death of a resident, managers can ensure that the home continues to run smoothly; and can put in place strategies for maintaining the equilibrium of surviving residents; and support care staff in coping with loss. Much of the evidence for this reading is based on two Department of Health funded research projects undertaken between 1995 and 2000 (Sidell *et al.*, 1997; Katz *et al.*, 2000a).

Background

Substantial numbers of older people die in residential settings in the United Kingdom. Exact figures are hard to come by because of the methods of collecting mortality statistics, but it is estimated that more than 20 per cent of people over the age of 80 die in care home settings (Office for National Statistics, 1998) and a higher percentage of those over the age of 84 (Peace *et al.*, 1997). Death is a frequent occurrence in care homes and this pattern is well established: over 20 years ago Clough (1981) suggested that about a third of residents die annually in residential care. This means that care staff and other residents are repeatedly confronting death and managers are having to deal not only with the practical implications of managing a death, but also with the emotional repercussions on themselves, their staff, other residents (Clarke, 1996; Scrutton, 1996) and relatives of deceased residents.

Until the introduction of National Minimum Care Standards for care homes, which includes a standard for registered managers which specifies ensuring that significant life events are managed effectively (Department of Health, 2001), there was little evidence that loss and bereavement featured high on the training agenda. In their study of care homes, Dalley and Denniss (2001) found that loss and bereavement were taught in only 3 per cent and communication skills in only 2 per cent of the homes providing basic training for care assistants. In contrast, food hygiene was taught in 34 per cent of these homes. Although a substantial minority of homes have some practical instructions for immediate action following a death (Sidell *et al.*, 1997), there was little guidance provided on how to deal with the emotional implications of bereavement for staff and surviving residents (Centre for Policy on Ageing, 1995; Sidell *et al.*, 1997). This reading will primarily examine how managers describe how they succeed in containing the emotional ramifications of bereavement and loss.

Loss and ill-health

Care staff develop close relationships with residents, and often see themselves as surrogate family (Katz *et al.*, 2000b). Therefore they experience real grief when a resident dies. There is much evidence which suggests that regardless of the cause of death, the bereaved person may experience physical and/or mental ill-health (see, for instance, Katz, 2002). Not only can ill-health be a consequence of bereavement, but bereavement could indirectly lead to behaviours which in themselves create damage to health, such as increased alcohol consumption (Stroebe and Stroebe, 1993). It might be hypothesised that drug misuse is a risk for the younger age group. It is important to note that in many homes, carers are young women with little exposure to death in their own families. For some, this is their first experience of death and they are often unprepared for their own reactions (Katz *et al.*, 2000b).

Physical responses to bereavement may arise partly from exhaustion following an intensive period of caring for the dying person. These range from general debility (which includes increased susceptibility to common infections or other diseases) to increased levels of mortality in bereaved people. Common symptoms include fatigue, or changes in sleep patterns – for example, insomnia. Less usual symptoms include various kinds of physical discomfort, such as headaches, chest discomfort or musculo-skeletal pain.

Care homes are notoriously understaffed and staff absence through sickness is a source of great stress for managers. It is therefore very relevant to enable managers to acquire skills in coping with staff distress following a resident's death.

What happens when someone dies

Most care homes follow similar procedures when a resident is believed to have died. The carer who discovers the body either calls the manager (if on duty) or another colleague to check that the resident is dead. A cursory check usually takes place:

> What I normally do is check the pupils, listen to the chest and that is it.
>
> (Manager, voluntary nursing home 45)

Both the location of death and the time of the day have implications for managing the home. Dealing with the body of the deceased is most problematic in sudden deaths. When a resident dies in a public area, care staff have to decide whether to move the body or close the area to other residents. Where the resident has not been seen for some time by a doctor, the coroner or police may need to be informed and therefore moving the body may be problematic. However, residents usually die in their own rooms and they remain there until their bodies are removed from the home. The immediate tasks for the most senior person on duty are to call the GP to certify death, then to notify relatives and, finally, call the funeral directors.

Freeing the home manager to undertake these time-consuming tasks has knock-on effects on the normal life of the home. Thus death can disrupt meal times, constrain free movement for other residents and reduce the number of staff available to undertake routine tasks. For example, the doctor will need to be accompanied to the body, as will the funeral directors. Some homes, particularly those with religious affiliations, will prioritise caring for the deceased and will assign a staff member to sit with the body. However, staffing constraints rarely permit this in most homes.

Caring for other residents

Managers assumed that residents accept death both for themselves and for their peers (Sidell *et al.*, 1997). This resembles the findings of Moss and Moss (1996) who suggest that societal ageism does not recognise the bereavement needs of older people. Yet, despite a firm belief that residents accepted death, managers maintained that residents did not want to talk about it:

> I think we are still dealing with a group of people who feel that death is something that is not going to happen to them. It is not discussed. It's all behind closed doors. I mean, when you think about it, it is

really only in the last fifteen years that people talk openly about death.
Death was something you whispered about.

> (Manager, voluntary residential home 46)

This assumption that residents did not want to talk about death often
meant that despite this being a question on the admission form, managers
rarely ascertained residents' disposal wishes, and this in itself created stress
for them and for relatives immediately following a death.

Managers' views that residents should be shielded from death included
protecting residents from seeing the removal of bodies. This would reinforce residents':

> awareness of their own frailty – you have to be aware of the residents'
> needs, you could so easily have the trauma of one trigger the trauma
> in another.
>
> (Manager, voluntary residential home 47)

Not only might the visibility of bodies being removed reinforce residents'
awareness that they were in 'God's waiting room' (Manager, nursing
home, 49) but the manner in which bodies were removed might upset
residents as much as it did managers:

> I won't say to residents, 'Go away, a coffin's coming past' or 'a body's
> coming past.' But neither will I invite them to be there because I think
> it matters to them to know that they will be going out in a dignified
> way and a golf bag is not [dignified].

Consequently most bodies were removed in a clandestine manner, usually
via a back door. Until the funeral director arrives, the body is usually left
in bed as 'life-like' as possible, or in religious homes might be placed in the
chapel. Managers did not usually offer other residents the opportunity to
view the body, but if asked did not refuse access:

> Those who wanted to had already been in to see her. The majority of
> them no, they would rather stay out of the way.
>
> (Manager, home 35)

Following a death, managers have to decide whether, how and when to inform the other people residing in the home. Lack of communication often leads to a sense of insecurity in the remaining resident population, so informing them can be urgent and might require considerable staff time. The manager of a voluntary residential home explained their procedures:

> If it's in the daytime, they can be aware that someone has been ill when they see doctors come rushing in, [and] they tend to fear the worst anyway, so they can half understand and appreciate what is happening. If there is a relative [of the deceased] we see that they are ok and leave a member of staff with them, and whoever is in charge that day will go around all the other residents and tell them in their own rooms. We go round the rooms individually – it's the safest way. If anyone is upset then they will usually fetch another member of staff to stay with them while they go on to the next. If something happened when we are in between meals, it would be important to make sure that everyone knows before they come down so that they are all aware and you don't have everyone sitting down for tea and announce a death. That is not good practice from a caring point of view and also from a practical point of view.
>
> (Manager, home 47)

When death occurs at night, residents are usually not informed until the morning, as it is assumed that this knowledge might affect their sleep. Some managers inform residents about funeral arrangements and involve them if they so wish. However, residents' attendance at funerals is very rare.

Managers may find themselves in a counselling role (Clarke, 1996) facilitating residents' questions about the death. Their questions echo those of family members and care staff – was the death pain free, was the resident alone, did the resident appear peaceful?

Informing relatives

The most senior person on duty (usually the manager) was responsible for informing relatives that a resident is failing. In some homes, relatives were present at the death – in religious homes, carers endeavoured to sit with relatives wherever possible. Where relatives live nearby, they were encouraged to come to the home before the resident was moved. When a death is predicted and the relatives do not want to be present, the time of notifying them is sometimes negotiated in advance – for example, not to call relatives at night. A few home managers recalled going to relatives' homes themselves to break the news.

Managers provide information for relatives about death registration and funeral arrangements. Communicating with relatives who have not had much to do with residents when in the home can pose difficulties, partly because managers and staff may feel resentful that they did not pay enough attention to residents during their lifetime. In most cases, the next time that home staff saw relatives was either at the funeral or when they came to collect the belongings of the deceased. Dealing with the relatives' emotions can be a pressure for managers – several managers, even trained nurses, noted that they had not been trained to deal with relatives' emotions, nor to counsel them. They suggested that at times they floundered in this task.

Supporting staff

Managers endeavoured to minimise disruption of routines when a resident was dying or a death had occurred. As noted above, their goal was to maintain the equilibrium of the home, as surviving residents were seen to respond unfavourably to anxiety and rushing around of staff. Inevitably the presence of a dying resident increased pressure of work for care staff. Staffing levels rarely took into account the expectation that residents would need intensive caring and therefore all other jobs needed to be squeezed in order to create the space to care for a dying person. Popping in regularly to check on or turn a dying resident, negotiating with GPs, community nurses and relatives were all time-consuming tasks and placed additional pressure on what, for most homes, was an already stretched workforce.

Managers therefore grapple with the dilemma of ensuring that their staff can address the needs of all the residents at the same time as being supported practically and emotionally. They noted (Sidell *et al.*, 1997) that at different points in the dying and death trajectory staff needed different types of support. This may entail reducing the workload to free a carer to provide one-on-one care to the dying person, or freeing up another member of staff to help with turning, bathing, administering pain control or to talk to distressed relatives.

Two primary reasons were suggested for supporting staff around a bereavement (Katz *et al.*, 2000b). First, to acknowledge the carers' loss, and, second, to enable them to continue with their other tasks. Three critical stages influence the functioning of carers following a resident's death. The first relates to how they find out about the death, as this indicates the strength of the network within the home. The second concerns the way in which managers directly support staff. The third explores the opportunity for staff to bid farewell to deceased residents and move on from their bereavement.

Informing staff about a death

Carers' experience of bereavement is influenced by the manner in which they discover that the resident has died. Most managers interviewed in Sidell *et al.*'s 1997 study said that carers were instructed not to notify their off-duty colleagues. The reasons given for this related to a) cost of calling, b) time this would take away from work duties, and c) the imposition this would place on the private lives of carers. Despite this, it was apparent that this did not always reflect the reality of what happened or the wishes of the carers. Off-duty staff sometimes phoned in to enquire about an ailing resident. Some off-duty care workers were notified because a) they had requested this, or b) the manager believed that the particular carer was vulnerable, or c) was seen to be especially close to the dying person or relatives.

Regardless of the manager's instructions, there was sometimes a spontaneous and unofficial chain which operated to notify other care workers. This reduced both the cost and the burden and enabled close friends to inform and comfort each other:

> On the day it happens we divide the staff up and we ring, all of us that are on, we say well I'll tell so and so. We wouldn't want anybody to come in and find that that had happened...

Indeed many carers told the researchers that they preferred to know if someone had died in order to prepare themselves before reporting for duty. Yet the majority of carers find out about a resident's death when they are next on duty through meeting a colleague, looking in the diary or notice board, at a meeting or, the worst case scenario, finding a new resident in the bed of the deceased. Establishing the wishes of a carer in relation to being informed, in the same way as asking a relative, might be seen as good practice for managers.

Acknowledging carers' bereavement needs

Managers welcomed the opportunity to discuss their concerns about supporting themselves and their staff in relation to loss. Most did not feel sufficiently skilled in preparing staff for a death or addressing their emotional needs thereafter. Although about half the managers said they offered support to their staff, most felt inadequate in this role:

> I never feel they get that much support. They should but they don't. It is just time and we talk about it but you can't sit and listen. Time is so

expensive and such a luxury. We find over the months, things come out which is probably not the way it should be at all, but we sit down at report [daily meeting to discuss residents].

(Manager, home 24)

The reasons for their feelings of inadequacy related to their perceptions of their poor counselling skills as a result of little or no training; the chronic state of understaffing which meant little opportunity for one-on-one support with a carer and the burden of their other responsibilities following a death.

The most inexperienced carers needed particular attention:

I find it's the junior staff that usually get most distressed and usually they are comforted by a senior member of staff; they are usually asked if they would like to see the body as well, so if they are on duty in the morning, they would come in and we would go in with them if they wanted, but there is no support offered, it's literally the staff comforting each other.

(Manager, home 15)

The importance of feeling and expressing emotions was noted by several managers:

I always tell them that the day they don't cry is when they don't work here, because they have got to care or they wouldn't enjoy it . . .

(Manager, home 23)

Managers thus set the tone regarding what constitutes acceptable demonstrations of emotion by carers.

In addition to having permission to demonstrate emotions, managers suggested that carers require opportunities to talk to their superiors and their peers about the deceased resident. Like surviving residents, carers need to rehearse the events surrounding the death. Some carers, however, found it difficult to talk about their feelings and this needs to be respected.

Carers themselves recognised that after their cry and their verbal post-mortem on the resident's death and their life in the home, they had to leave them behind and get on with the task at hand. This was particularly difficult after several deaths in succession when a tension emerged between having to maintain what carers saw as an appropriate demeanour, and feeling enabled to express their feelings and getting upset, even in front of relatives.

Good practice would therefore include managers endeavouring where possible to set up structured opportunities for bereaved carers to debrief to more senior staff.

Saying goodbye to residents

Only a few homes encouraged staff on duty to bid farewell to deceased residents. Yet most homes sent representatives to residents' funerals; about 40 per cent of home managers saw it as their duty to attend funerals themselves. Where geographically possible, home staff strove to go to funerals, viewing this as the end point of their caring for that resident. Many carers went even when off duty, and were rarely financially compensated. As attending funerals appears to be so central to carers' jobs, managers should endeavour to facilitate this and, where possible, compensate them for going in their private time.

Conclusion

Managers of care homes for older people encounter residents' deaths frequently, yet can find it difficult to support surviving residents, relatives and their own staff in their bereavement. Care homes become surrogate domestic environments for residents and, consequently, their carers experience grief when residents die. Managers, therefore, have the dual burden of coping with their own feelings of loss and of frustration in not always being able to provide their staff with what they see as adequate support. Managers working in homes with good staffing levels, and where their job description includes ongoing professional development, will have the best chance of feeling competent in managing loss.

REFERENCES

Centre for Policy on Ageing (1995) *A Better Home Life*, London, CPA.

Clarke, J. (1996) 'After a Death in Sheltered Housing: the Warden's Job', *Bereavement Care*, 15, 3, 30–1.

Clough, R. (1981) *Old Age Homes*, London, Allen and Unwin.

Counsel and Care (1995) *Last Rights*, London, Counsel and Care.

Dalley, G. and Denniss, M. (2001) *Trained to Care? Investigating the Skills and Competencies of Care Assistants in Homes for Older People*, London, Centre for Policy on Ageing.

Department of Health (2001) *Care Homes for Older People. National Minimum Standards. Care Standards Act 2000*, Norwich, the Stationery Office.

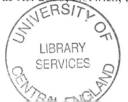

Katz, J. (2002) 'Health and Loss', in Thompson, N. (ed.), *Loss and Grief: A Guide for Human Services Practitioners*, Routledge.

Katz, J.S., Sidell, M. and Komaromy, C. (2000a) *Investigating the Training Needs of Staff in Residential and Nursing Homes,* research report to the Department of Health.

Katz, J.S., Sidell, M. and Komaromy, C. (2000b) 'Death in Homes: Bereavement Needs of Residents, Relatives and Staff', *International Journal of Palliative Nursing*, 6, 6, 274–9.

Moss, M. and Moss, S. (1996) 'The Impact of Family Deaths on Older People', *Bereavement Care*, 15, 3, 26–7.

Office for National Statistics (1998) *Social Trends*, 28, London, HMSO.

Peace, S., Kellaher, L. and Willcocks, D. (1997) *Re-evaluating Residential Care*, Birmingham, Open University Press.

Scrutton, S. (1996) 'What Can You Expect, My Dear, At My Age?', *Bereavement Care*, 15, 3, 28–9.

Sidell, M. (1995) *Health in Old Age, Myth, Mystery and Management*, Buckingham, Open University Press.

Sidell, M., Katz, J.S. and Komaromy, C. (1997) *Death and Dying in Residential and Nursing Homes for Older People*, Report to the Department of Health.

Stroebe, M. and Stroebe, W. (1993) 'The Mortality of Bereavement: a Review', in Stroebe, M., Stroebe, W. and Hanson, R. (eds), *Handbook of Bereavement: Theory, Research and Intervention*, Cambridge, Cambridge University Press.

TEN

MANAGERS' TALK

Deborah Tannen

Source: *Talking From 9 to 5: How Women's and Men's Conversational Styles Affect Who Gets Heard, Who Gets Credit, and What Gets Done at Work*, London, Virago, 1995.

Amy was a manager with a problem: She had just read a final report written by Donald, and she felt it was woefully inadequate. She faced the unsavory task of telling him to do it over. When she met with Donald, she made sure to soften the blow by beginning with praise, telling him everything about his report that was good. Then she went on to explain what was lacking and what needed to be done to make it acceptable. She was pleased with the diplomatic way she had managed to deliver the bad news. Thanks to her thoughtfulness in starting with praise, Donald was able to listen to the criticism and seemed to understand what was needed. But when the revised report appeared on her desk, Amy was shocked. Donald had made only minor, superficial changes, and none of the necessary ones. The next meeting with him did not go well. He was incensed that she was now telling him his report was not acceptable and accused her of having misled him. "You told me before it was fine," he protested.

Amy thought she had been diplomatic; Donald thought she had been dishonest. The praise she intended to soften the message "This is unacceptable" sounded to him like the message itself: "This is fine." So what she regarded as the main point – the needed changes – came across to him as optional suggestions, because he had already registered her praise as the main point. She felt he hadn't listened to her. He thought she had changed her mind and was making him pay the price. [. . .]

I believe this was one of innumerable misunderstandings caused by differences in conversational style. Amy delivered the criticism in a way that seemed to her self-evidently considerate, a way she would have preferred to receive criticism herself; taking into account the other person's feelings, making sure he knew that her ultimate negative assessment of his report didn't mean she had no appreciation of his abilities. She offered the praise as a sweetener to help the nasty-tasting news go down. But Donald didn't expect criticism to be delivered in that way, so he mistook the praise as her overall assessment rather than a preamble to it.

This conversation could have taken place between two women or two men. But I do not think it is a coincidence that it occurred between a man and a woman. [...] Differing rituals typify women and men (although, of course, not all individual men and women behave in ways that are typical). Conversational rituals common among men often involve using opposition such as banter, joking, teasing, and playful put-downs, and expending effort to avoid the one-down position in the interaction. Conversational rituals common among women are often ways of maintaining an appearance of equality, taking into account the effect of the exchange on the other person, and expending effort to downplay the speakers' authority so they can get the job done without flexing their muscles in an obvious way.

When everyone present is familiar with these conventions, they work well. But when ways of speaking are not recognized as conventions, they are taken literally, with negative results on both sides. Men whose oppositional strategies are interpreted literally may be seen as hostile when they are not, and their efforts to ensure that they avoid appearing one-down may be taken as arrogance. When women use conversational strategies designed to avoid appearing boastful and to take the other person's feelings into account, they may be seen as less confident and competent than they really are. As a result, both women and men often feel they are not getting sufficient credit for what they have done, are not being listened to, are not getting ahead as fast as they should.

When I talk about women's and men's characteristic ways of speaking, I always emphasize that both styles make sense and are equally valid in themselves, though the difference in styles may cause trouble in interaction.

[...] A woman who headed a regional sales team had to confront her boss. He had taken to assigning special projects in a neighboring district to one of the men on her team, who would announce to her that he could not do what she had asked of him because he had to complete a project for her boss – a higher authority she could not argue with. She geared herself up and explained to her boss that when he gives assignments directly to someone who reports to her, it makes it difficult for her team to meet its goals. She cannot depend on that employee's work to fit into the plan she has set for her team. Her boss agreed that she had a point. Satisfied, she said, "So you'll tell him to check with me before he takes on something for you?" At this her boss balked: "I can't tell him to ask Mommy for permission."

Perhaps this women would have done better to say, "So please check with me before giving him projects that will take him away from my team." But what is interesting here is the image that sprang to her boss's mind when she put it the way she did: Checking with a superior – a gesture that should be a matter of course in a work situation – was reframed as a humiliating and inappropriate one, "asking Mommy for permission." The prospect of a man checking with a woman before doing something brought to her boss's mind the scenario of a child supplicant, because a mother is one of the few images we have of female authority – whereas men in authority are as likely to suggest a military commander or a sports coach or captain (in itself modeled on the military metaphor) as a father.

This is not to say that there are no negative stereotypes of men in authority. If a man has a particular characteristic that is noticeable in our culture, he may invoke stereotypes that can be used (often unfairly) to characterize him. If he is short and authoritarian, for example, he may be called "a little Napoleon" – again, a military figure. But simply being male in a position of authority alone does not invoke stereotypes, whereas simply being female in such a position can call to mind stereotypical images of women, including, prominently, that of mother. [. . .]

When I heard the same remark twice in one week about two different women, I knew there was something going on. "Before I came to work for Ann," a man who reports to her told me, "everybody warned me to watch out. They called her the dragon lady. But I don't know what they were talking about. I've always found her great to work with." A few days later, a woman at another company commented about the woman she works for, "I've heard people call Marie the dragon lady. But I've never seen anything to justify that. She's the best boss I've ever worked for." I wondered, Why the dragon lady? Not only was there nothing dragonlike about either Ann or Marie, but they were as different from one another as could be, in age, temperament, and personal style. The only thing they had in common was the "lady" part. Being women highly placed in their organizations seems to have caused people to look at them through conventional images of women in positions of authority. Our culture gives us a whole menagerie of stereotypical images of women: schoolmarm, head nurse, headmistress, doting mother, cruel stepmother, dragon lady, catwoman, witch, bitch. [. . .]

Newsweek's review of Margaret Thatcher's memoir about her years as British prime minister began this way:

> For 11½ years, Margaret Thatcher presided over the British government like a strong-minded headmistress. She reshaped the economy, broke the unions and starched up Britain's languid posture in world affairs. Through it all, she thoroughly dominated the "wets" in her own cabinet, clobbering them with a metaphorical handbag whenever they showed too little spine in the defense of conservative ideology – or too much in opposing her will.

Images of authority come drenched in gender. Even when describing situations that have nothing to do with gender – for example, shoring up

Britain's "posture in world affairs" – by choosing the verb "starched up," the writer indirectly evoked a housewife doing the laundry, if not a head nurse stiff in a starched uniform. The image of Thatcher "clobbering them with her metaphorical handbag" undercuts the force of her actions, even as it gives her credit for attacking her opponents. A woman clobbering men with her handbag is an object of laughter, not fear or admiration.

Part of the reason images of women in positions of authority are marked by their gender is that the very notion of authority is associated with maleness. This can result simply from appearance. Anyone who is taller, more heftily built, with a lower-pitched, more sonorous voice, begins with culturally recognizable markers of authority, whereas anyone who is shorter, slighter, with a higher-pitched voice begins with a disadvantage in this respect. [. . .]

When I asked people for their impressions of the men and women they worked with and for, I noticed a pattern: When they commented on women in managerial positions – but never when they commented on men – people often said, "She's abrasive," or, just as often, "She's not abrasive," "not aggressive," or "has a soft touch." It is one thing to describe how you think someone is – "abrasive," "aggressive," and so on. But why would people mention what someone is not? It makes sense only against the expectation that the person would be that way. So it seems that when a woman is in a high position, there is an expectation that she will be unfeminine, negative, or worse. When she isn't, it is perceived as worth mentioning. And these prevalent images ambush professional women as they seek to maintain their careers as well as their personal lives – and their femininity. [. . .]

Individuals in positions of authority are judged by how they enact that authority. This poses a particular challenge for women. The ways women are expected to talk – and many (not all) women do talk – are at odds with images of authority. Women are expected to hedge their beliefs as opinions, to seek opinions and advice from others, to be "polite" in their requests. If a woman talks this way, she is seen as lacking in authority. But if she talks with certainty, makes bold statements of fact rather than hedged statements of opinion, interrupts others, goes on at length, and speaks in a declamatory and aggressive manner, she will be disliked. [. . .]

When I talked to people about their work lives, I asked them, among other things, what they think management is all about, and what makes a good manager or a poor one. When I put these question to women in positions of authority, one of the most frequent statements they offered to explain what makes them good managers is that they do *not* act like an authority figure – insofar as an authority figure is thought to be authoritarian. They told me that they don't lord it over subordinates, don't act as though they are better than those who report to them. I began to wonder why women in authority are so concerned not to appear authoritarian – not to appear as if they think they are superior or are putting themselves in a one-up position, even though that is exactly the position they are in. [. . .]

Women downplay their authority while exercising it. It seems that creating their demeanor in a position of authority is yet another conversational ritual growing out of the goal of keeping everyone on an equal footing, at least insofar as appearances are concerned. This doesn't mean that women or men who speak this way really think everyone is equal; it means they have to do a certain amount of conversational work to make sure they maintain the proper demeanor – to fit their sense of what makes a good person, which entails not seeming to parade their higher status. If they have to tell others what to do, give information, and correct errors – all of which they will have to do on the job, especially if they are in a position of authority – they will expend effort to assure others that they are not pulling rank, not trying to capitalize on or rub in their one-up position. In contrast, since men's characteristic rituals have grown out of the assumption that all relationships are inherently hierarchical, it is not surprising that many of them either see less reason to downplay their authority or see more reason to call attention to it – to ward off inevitable challenges.

Choices of ways of speaking that highlight or downplay authority are not deliberate decisions that are thought through with each utterance but are rather habitual phrasings learned over time that become automatic, seemingly self-evidently appropriate ways to say what you mean.

I cannot emphasize enough that the appearance of equality I am referring to is ritual, not literal. I am not implying that individual women doubt their superior position in the hierarchy. [. . .]

Those whose characteristic conversation rituals place less value on denying hierarchy (including many men) may find women's protests that they treat others as equals to be hypocritical. Accusations of hypocrisy are often a sign that cultural differences are at work; it is the universal impression one gets from observing those whose rituals are unfamiliar. "Hypocrisy" is acting in a way that is not a sincere reflection of how you feel. In other words, the way it seems "natural" to talk and the way you see someone talking don't match up. Though this could certainly be the result of true hypocrisy – putting on an act for some ulterior motive – it is also the unavoidable impression made when people have different ideas of how it is "natural" to talk, given a particular context and set of emotions.

Another liability for women in authority is that if they do not talk in ways that highlight the power of their position, they are more vulnerable to challenges to it. Like many conversational rituals common among women, talking as if "we're all equals" but still expecting to receive the respect appropriate to the higher-status position depends on the participation of the other person to respect that position. The president of a women's college had a long and difficult meeting with a student who protested her choice of commencement speaker. Finally, the president said, "What it comes down to is that you don't accept my right to make this decision, after considering your point of view and everyone else's." The student thought about it and agreed. "When I see you on campus after hours dressed informally, I forget about your position," she said. "If you were an older white man, it would be easier." In addition to dressing informally when she went to her office evenings and weekends, the president probably also spoke in ways that did not continually create a stance of authority, and this no doubt contributed to the student's forgetting the power of her position.

Saving face is a two-person job

Part of the reason that many women in positions of authority speak in ways that downplay rather than emphasize the power of their position is simply an expression of the ethics characteristic of many women's conversational rituals . . .: the desire to restore balance to a conversation and take into account the effect of one's words on the other person. Whereas one might expect the person in the subordinate position to take more care about not offending a boss, research has found that women in superior positions often take more care to avoid offending when talking to subordinates than to superiors. [. . .]

An example of this way of talking comes from my own tape recordings of office talk. A woman I will call Marge, who heads a division, noticed that her secretary had made a mistake in a list of office assignments:

MARGE: Oh, but you've still got Mitch and Evan in the same office, you know!
SECRETARY: Are you *kidding*? Oh, darn.
MARGE: [Laughing] You know, it's *hard* to do things around here, isn't it, with all these people coming in!

Although she told the secretary directly that she had made a mistake, Marge hastened to soften the criticism by providing a reason for why she might have made the mistake – and by laughing, to show that it was not a serious error and there were no hard feelings.

Marge spoke in a way that saved face for her secretary. Though it might seem that saving face is primarily something one does for oneself, saving face works especially well if two people do it for each other, as often occurs in ritual exchanges characteristic of women's conversation. And this highlights the importance not only of how you speak, but how others speak to you. [. . .]

Same words, different reactions

Studies showing that we tend to react differently to the same way of speaking if we think the speech is coming from different speakers help explain why women and men can get very different reactions even if they speak the same way. When people told me about men who had "strictly business" or "no-nonsense" styles, they simply said, "He's a strictly business type," or they referred to his profession: "He's a typical accountant." But when they were commenting on the same style in a woman, I frequently heard, "She's got a pseudomasculine style." Because this style was expected of and associated with men, women who adopted it were seen not as trying to be efficient, competent, and businesslike, but as trying to be like men.

One man I interviewed mentioned the same characteristic – directness – in talking about three people in his company. But it was a complaint in the case of the two women and a compliment when applied to the man. About one woman he said:

> Well, her style was very direct. I think very direct and abrupt. Because that was one of the criticisms I had of her ... was a, somewhat of a lack of tact. Because she could make statements which were right, but not tactfully made. And she tended to upset – or ruffle some feathers.

At another point in the interview, he said he didn't like working with a particular woman because her failure to engage in small talk made her seem too direct: "It was more, 'Okay, here's the question, here's the answer. That's the story.' No small talk." I asked, "Do you think she also had a very direct style?" He answered,

> Yes. Yes, she was very direct too. Very much. Here's the task at hand, here's what needs to be done. Okay, we're done. There wasn't a lot of side stuff.

And yet, in telling me why he particularly admired a man he worked with, he mentioned the same quality – directness:

> And I had a great deal of admiration for him. I think he's direct, he's aggressive, he's very intelligent. . . . On the other hand, he does carry a big hammer! And if he needs to, he'll use it and you'll get squashed!

I have no way of knowing whether the people this man was referring to really did talk in the same way. No doubt there were many aspects of their styles and personalities that were different. But it is clear that the quality of directness made a different impression on him when it was used by the man and by the two women.

Another facet of this dynamic is that individuals within a culture may be punished by others if they do not conform to expectations for their sex. Anne Statham (1987) notes in her study of male and female managers that individuals of both sexes who departed from the norms for their own sex were viewed negatively by subordinates of the same sex. A male manager whose style approximated those of the women was seen as "fairly meek" and "weak" by men who worked for him, though he was highly praised by women subordinates. A woman manager whose style was more like those of the men in the study was criticized for neglect by a woman who reported to her (she "never shows any personal interest in me ... has only asked me to lunch once") and by her secretary for having "superior airs." The woman herself felt that women subordinates resisted accepting decisions she made independently. [. . .]

What's a woman to do?

All this means that women in positions of authority face a special challenge. Our expectations for how a person in authority should behave are at odds with our expectations for how a woman should behave. If a woman talks in ways expected of women, she is more likely to be liked than respected. If she talks in ways expected of men, she is more likely to be respected than liked. It is particularly ironic that the risk of losing likability is greater for women in authority, since evidence indicates that so many women care so much about whether or not they are liked.

Many of the constraints I have discussed apply equally to women and men. A man who quietly does a good job but is not good at letting others know about the job he is doing may go unrecognized. And there are many men who for reasons of cultural background, upbringing, or personality are not comfortable "blowing their own horn," not good at speaking up at meetings, too succinct and understated to command attention But their situations are really not the same, because if such men were to take assertiveness training and alter their styles, they would enhance not only their chances for success. Everything they did to enhance their assertiveness at work would also enhance their masculinity, in others' eyes. But a woman is in a double bind. Everything she does to enhance her assertiveness risks undercutting her femininity, in the eyes of others. And everything she does to fit expectations of how a woman should talk risks undercutting the impression of competence that she makes. [. . .]

REFERENCE

Statham, Anne (1987) "The Gender Model Revisited: Differences in the Management Styles of Men and Women." *Sex Roles* 16: 7.409–29.

ELEVEN

WHAT DO WE WANT FROM SOCIAL CARE MANAGERS? ASPIRATIONS AND REALITIES

Jeanette Henderson and Janet Seden

Introduction

Writing in *Community Care*, Frances Rickford suggests that managers are 'first in line for blame ... but not always first in line for training' (Rickford, 2000). There is a growing realisation that effective services require managers to be better at what they do and better equipped to do it. Many frontline managers have no management training. It may also be argued that some management training does not equip them for the challenges of delivering social care in current contexts:

> The transition from practitioner to frontline manager is probably the most difficult career transition in social services – people struggle with how to do the job and we would strongly argue for formal pathways.
>
> (Kearney, 1999)

However, a manager we spoke with who had both a social work and a management qualification commented that:

> No training or qualification could have prepared me for the management role I undertook.
>
> (Frontline manager)

This reading is drawn from research we conducted to identify the day-to-day challenges managers – and to some extent their organisations and agencies – face under the constant pressure to deliver services according to standards and frameworks developed by central government. There is little in the way of management training in the Diploma in Social Work (DipSW), a small amount in community work education and none in nurse education. Management qualifications seek to apply traditional management models to social care settings. This misses the complexity of managing in social care. A discourse of customer care, for example, does not fit easily with service users who are compelled to receive services in child protection or mental health.

Research method

Over a nine-month period, we undertook a series of 26 individual and four group interviews with managers, practitioners and users of services in a range of local authority, voluntary sector and private agencies to consider the tasks and roles of frontline managers. In addition, we obtained job vacancy particulars from advertisements reflecting a wide range of social care settings.

We argue that what employers want from managers is that they manage the dilemmas, constraints and challenges which face them, with limited opportunity to become the well-qualified, professionally developed people aspired to in job descriptions and person specifications. In other words, they may be nicely set up for blame and certainly are operating in a situation of meeting conflicting requirements with little opportunity for the professional development of themselves or others. Becoming a manager is a steep learning curve:

> The transition to management was de-skilling in the sense that I came to a new unit [. . .] I needed to build up networks, but was seen as the manager, who is the ultimate boss, and yet I felt completely out of my depth when the staff were talking about a family or child who they knew well, but where I couldn't even picture them in my head. You are supposed to be organising the whole unit, but you don't yet know about your staff's skills, abilities, histories or strengths, and that's hard.
>
> (Frontline manager)

Great Expectations: A survey of 40 job descriptions and person specifications for frontline management posts

Over a two-month period, we obtained details of 40 jobs. These were selected to represent the diversity of frontline management posts in social care and were in the salary range of £12,000–£30,000. They included health-based, local authority and voluntary sector fieldwork, project and residential management positions.

When asking for qualifications, employers mostly sought professional and task-related qualifications. There was little evidence of employers prioritising management expertise rather than professionally defined skills, abilities and experience. To manage in social care, applicants need above all to have demonstrated they are able to do the job. In our sample of 40 job descriptions only three posts required a management qualification as essential, although ten listed it as desirable.

More important was proven experience of managing. Experience was essential for 22 posts, ranging from one year to unspecified amounts of time. This range largely reflected the seniority of the management position advertised (the more senior the post, the more experience requested). It also demonstrated the pragmatism of employer expectations and their knowledge that few candidates with professional and management qualifications would be forthcoming from the bank of people who have 'acted up', deputised or gained hands-on management experience and who might well be looking for management posts.

For most posts the list of main roles and responsibilities was extensive. What employers want frontline social care managers to do is to access, account, act, adhere to policies, analyse, arrange, assess, assist, advise, budget, chair meetings, coach, commit, communicate, consult, contribute, co-ordinate, delegate, decide, deliver, demonstrate, deploy, deputise, develop, discipline, ensure, establish, evaluate, facilitate, gather, grasp, identify, induct, influence, initiate, instigate, integrate, join-up, lead, liaise, maintain, monitor, motivate, negotiate, network, organise, oversee, participate, plan, prepare, present, prioritise, produce, promote, purchase, provide, pro-act, provide, record, recruit, resolve, be responsible, review, supervise, support, teach, think, train, undertake training, work and write.

It may be argued from these examples, that when employers write job descriptions and person specifications and advertise to recruit a social care manager, they are not sure that potential candidates will have management qualifications and training. However, they require that new managers be:

strategic: 'develop strategies, systems and procedures to meet the overall objectives'.

operational: 'ensure that the care services are effectively managed and adhere to departmental objectives to resolve operational problems'.

professional: 'take responsibility for managing all domestic and ancillary staff which includes their induction, supervision, training and development and appraisal. Ensuring staff are empowered, consulted and involved in decision-making and effective supportive, corrective or disciplinary action is taken'.

Hard Times: frontline manager group and individual interviews

We chose to explore the experiences of managers from three different, but interrelated, viewpoints. The geographical focus of the locality-based consultation sessions is in line with moves towards partnership working in specific localities required by various documents (Department of Health, 1999, 2000). Single agency groups were structured according to a participant's role in the organisation to give an indication of perceptions and expectations of frontline managers from various places within the same organisation. Lawler and Hearn (1997) consider management from the perspectives of senior managers in social services, Balloch *et al.* (1998) looked at a range of views within agencies. This study seeks to make comparisons within and between agencies and settings. So, in the single agency sessions, participants were split into middle manager, frontline manager and practitioner groups.

Workshops were held in three organisations. The first had integrated adult social work and health services several years ago, the second was moving towards integration in two areas – mental health and learning disabilities (as well as planning for joint review). The third workshop was held with managers, practitioners and service users selected on a regional basis to represent local authority, voluntary and private agencies. The final strand of the fieldwork was a series of in-depth, semi-structured interviews with managers from social services and voluntary sector organisations.

The similarities between groups was marked. One theme echoed through the workshops and interviews very clearly indeed. The role of the manager in social care is in a state of change and confusion with a plethora of policies and procedures, but no real recognition of the day-to-day management challenges of implementing policy and procedural changes – the lived realities for managers. We draw out some of those day-to-day challenges and dilemmas for managers – and the people with whom they work. We have structured our discussion around the areas identified by the participants as central to their experience – the operational, strategic and professional aspects of management.

Operational

There is a strong tension between the operational aspects of the management role and the frontline manager's involvement in strategic developments and decision-making. On the one hand, frontline managers focused on the operational component of their management role – the day-to-day support and supervision, work allocation, developmental and enabling role working with team members. On the other hand, middle managers recognised the difficulties faced by frontline managers, but saw the strategic aspects of the frontline manager task as priority:

> I've just appointed two temporary team managers [in child protection] to cover for people who aren't there. I would love to have said to those two people, you just concentrate on looking after those teams for the next 3/6 months. If I did that I had to decide who was going to take on our statutory function in the Education Action Zones, the Sure Start initiative, the Health Improvement Group and pick up the chair of the Parenting Skills strategy group [...] There's just four things I had to allocate to those two people in the first few weeks. And they're not things I could say, 'That's not a priority at the moment'.
>
> (Middle manager, social services)

The operational challenge of managing multi-disciplinary teams was seen as linking all aspects of the management role. Implementing the changes at an operational level held profound challenges for frontline managers:

> You've got to allow people to maintain their own professional identity but at the same time to manage them and that's a very difficult balance [...] otherwise there's no point in having a multi-disciplinary team.
>
> (Frontline manager, social services)

Participants referred frequently to the frontline manager as a bridge or translator. This was seen as a central operational role, although we argue that it crosses into strategic and professional arenas. The manager communicates with and mediates between groups and individuals about policies, practices and strategies that are often very new to the manager him/herself.

The importance of communication and relationships was stressed by service users who thought that the more distant from practice a manager becomes, the less the manager was aware of the very real effects of decisions. Practitioners also felt that managers were becoming more remote and removed from the day-to-day work of the team. Managers were often away from the office on 'strategic business', unavailable to deal with many of their operational or team demands:

> Time management is difficult, because you have to be out of the build-ing sometimes up to half the week at meetings, manager's days and other projects that you are working on and it's difficult to keep up to speed with what's happening in the unit.
>
> (Frontline manager)

Decision-making was identified as another important operational task. Some practitioners felt that managers were not always able to make diffi-cult decisions:

> Managers don't like making difficult decisions – I think they often run away from it and that frightens the life out of me.
>
> (Social worker)

Managers saw the complexity of their decisions:

> All of a sudden people come to you for a decision, and you have to stand by it and think of the long-term effects of it. If I make this judge-ment it will mean certain things, but if I do the other thing there are different implications. I have to try and look at everyone's needs and think of the welfare of staff and users.

Strategic

While frontline managers identify operational issues as their priority, middle managers consider that the frontline manager has crucial local knowledge that is vital in strategic planning. Frontline managers feel over-whelmed by so many policy initiatives over which they have no control or influence and by the development of procedures and standards that do not take implementation time into account. New policies and procedures appear from national government and from City or County Hall at a frightening pace. Managers do not have time to consolidate the informa-tion or practice with their partners and teams before the next new pro-cedure comes along.

Although some authorities have focused on time management courses the problem, however, appears to be a finite amount of time with an infinite amount of expectations that no amount of training will address. Clarity about role may help in this respect:

> It isn't actually fair to say to people, 'If you're going to be a team manager simply be the manager of a team'. Maybe we're saying we can't do that. What we are doing is recruiting people to manage operational, day-to-day demands in a busy social work team and at the same time be involved in the development of services within their locality in partnership with other agencies and the wider department. We shouldn't suggest to people that it's anything else but that.
>
> (Middle manager)

Another middle manager pointed to the implications of:

> Management styles, management speak, competencies and inspection are influential – things can get very mechanical.

Again we have the manager as translator, this time in a strategic sense – between the wider department and team members, between policy and practice and between people from different agencies and backgrounds.

A barrier to developing effective strategic partnerships was identified as a lack of real delegated power to managers. Decision-making is important in partnership working but there may be constraints in this area:

> We may go to a meeting with health managers and come away having to get authorisation to do something which health managers could give approval to on the spot. So you have people trying to develop partnerships but feel they don't have equal levels of authority.
>
> (Middle manager)

The challenges of developing partnership working and the cultural changes and challenges this involves are complex and time consuming. There is a lack of understanding within other organisations and agencies about the nature of social services and this adds to the difficulties for managers.

Professional

This is an area of some anxiety for frontline managers and practitioners – especially in adult services – although less so for middle managers. Moves towards integration of health and social work teams and the development of multi-disciplinary teams within some specialisms brought the issue to the fore for many participants:

> It can cause quite a bit of resentment being managed by someone who is not of your profession.
>
> (Practitioner)

However, others felt

> Having a multi-disciplinary team gives us the right skills mix and the ability to talk to other agencies in the right language as well. It makes a difference.
>
> (Children's home manager)

Teams developed without a professional identity and practitioners were concerned that their own professional identity was being diluted. As a result of service integration, one social worker we spoke with had joined BASW (British Association of Social Workers) and a nurse had become involved with a nurses action group fighting to preserve their professional identity. Both people said that they would not have joined profession-specific groups prior to integration.

Managers increasingly need to direct team members' attention away from their professional backgrounds towards a single system of care management and planning. As a result managers may find themselves torn between their own practice and professional background and organisational and policy requirements and expectations. Both practitioners and managers find the role of translator between people and agencies challenging, especially in relation to language in multi-disciplinary teams:

> There isn't a shared language – a vocabulary to express what I had been trained to express in the way I had been trained to express it [. . .] over time I don't think it's changed. I think I've got more used to it and can accommodate it more perhaps.
>
> (Practitioner)

> Managing multi-disciplinary teams is a big threat because you don't have understanding of their professional expertise or language.
>
> (Frontline manager)

For a management post, a background in social care was seen as essential by service users and managers alike, although experience of a particular specialism such as learning disabilities or mental health was not as important. When it came to the move from practitioner to manager, participants felt there was little in the way of preparation or support. There are more opportunities for staff to take part in development and project work – as a form of preparation for possible future management roles – but at some cost for remaining team members who must then take on extra work. Management development programmes are often only available after someone has taken a post as a frontline manager.

Bleak House?

In the Syrett et al. (1997) study, participants felt that managers did not see the real issues for practitioners and service users. Our research shows that managers see the operational issues all too clearly but feel unable to respond because of strategic demands on their time. The tension between operational and strategic functions discussed above is being addressed by several organisations through the introduction of senior practitioner posts to oversee many of the day-to-day operational matters within teams. In some cases this includes the very areas of management that attracted frontline managers to the role in the first place – staff supervision and support, workload allocation and day-to-day team maintenance. On the one hand this is seen as an essential support for frontline managers and as an opportunity for staff to gain some experience of managerial roles. On the other hand it may also serve further to distance a manager from his/her staff and may place the senior practitioner in an invidious position of being neither practitioner nor manager.

Some middle managers recognise the difference between what they did as new managers and what managers now undertake. However, they continue to look at the frontline manager job in terms of skills rather than look at the job itself. This would seem to support Lawler and Hearn's (1997) finding that senior managers saw their own social work experience as giving them credibility with staff, but having little or no relevance otherwise. The focus of middle managers in our study was clearly on the centrality of the strategic function of management. Middle managers spoke rather grandly about the role of the manager being to 'prioritise in the light of changing demands' but not about the reality of doing so when the needs of practitioner and department are in competition or when strategic aims clash with operational realities.

Frontline managers are pivotal in ensuring client, worker, departmental and governmental needs are met. This may feel overwhelming especially as expectations on frontline managers continue to grow. As one manager commented, the fast pace and overwhelming amounts of change are such that 'we are making our own histories'. Delegation has implications for team members who may feel pressure to accept extra work in an attempt to support the team manager, and prioritisation is difficult when, as one participant noted, 'they're all priorities'. This manager went on to say that a member of her team 'shouldn't have to say she feels sorry for me'. Our research has indicated that the lived realities of frontline managers in social care are taking place in 'Hard Times' indeed. The 'Great Expectations' of managerial discourse are able as Clarke (1998) argues, to claim the moral high ground of quality and efficiency. None of the participants in our study disputed the importance of improving the quality of social care. What they argued for was a closer relationship between the aspiration and the reality.

REFERENCES

Balloch, S., McLean, J. and Fisher, M. (eds) (1998) *Social Services: Working Under Pressure*, Bristol, The Policy Press.

Clarke, J. (1998) 'Thriving on Chaos? Managerialism and Social Welfare', in Carter, J. (ed.) *Postmodernity and the Fragmentation of Welfare*, London, Routledge.

Department of Health (1999) *The Relationship Between Health and Social Services*, Cm 4320.

Department of Health (2000) *Implementation of Health Act: Partnership Arrangements*, HSC 2000/010: LAC (2000)9.

Kearney, P. (1999) *Managing Practice: Report on the Management of Practice Expertise Project*, London, NISW.

Lawler, J. and Hearn, J. (1997) 'The Managers of Social Work: the Experiences and Identifications of Third Tier Social Services Managers and the Implications for Future Practice', *British Journal of Social Work*, 27, 191–218.

Rickford, F. (2000) 'First in Line for Blame', *Community Care*, 20–1, 3–9 August 2000.

Syrett, V., Jones, M. and Sercombe, N. (1997) 'Implementing Community Care: the Congruence of Manager and Practitioner Cultures', *Social Work and Social Sciences Review*, 7, 3, 154–69.

TWELVE

MESSAGES FOR MANAGERS: THE DILEMMAS OF MEANS TESTING

Greta Bradley, Bridget Penhale and Jill Manthorpe

Introduction

In the 1990s, social care services became increasingly targeted on those most in need through a process of rationing using eligibility criteria and the development of other gate-keeping mechanisms (Means and Smith, 1998). This triggered new structures to embrace the private sector and the contract culture. A change of government in 1997 did not derail such developments (for example, Department of Health, 1998).

The continuing emphasis on modernisation means social services departments are likely to experience further upheavals in terms of management and inter-agency scrutiny in health and social care. However the new landscape is drawn, management structures will need to be in place which promote transparent decision-making based on accessible procedures. Such structures need to respond to external and internal quality controls. In this reading we draw on a recent research study on the subject of charging older people for long-term care to illustrate the challenges facing managers in social services departments (SSDs). These include ongoing deliberations about the future of long-term care (Sutherland, 1999). Indeed, this world is not static; new rules and guidance are frequently introduced and updated. We do not yet know how the Single Assessment Process introduced in April 2002 will operate within an already complicated charging system. Means testing remains central to the funding and rationing of this revised system and this presents managers with significant challenges in operating the system fairly and justly.

The research

This study, funded by the Nuffield Foundation, examined the views of care managers, their managers and local politicians in five SSDs about the principles and processes of financial assessment and charging of older people actively considering residential and nursing home care. We compared these views with those of independent legal practitioners, working in the same localities, who could be involved in giving advice to older people. The study focused on perceived ethical dilemmas, possible conflicts of interest and the extent to which attitudes, policies and expressed practices could affect the fairness of the charging system.

Fieldwork took place between December 1998 and January 2000, using both quantitative and qualitative research methods. Postal questionnaires were sent to all care managers in each authority and we interviewed 28 independent legal practitioners and 64 professionals from the five social services departments. Those in the latter group were predominantly care managers and in each authority we also interviewed a fixed number of team managers (10), financial officers (8), legal advisers (5), senior managers (5) and Chairs of Social Services Committees (5). Throughout this chapter we indicate when findings are taken from the questionnaire data or from interviews (for further details of the study, see Bradley *et al.*, 2000) and concentrate here on managerial perspectives.

Consider quality and equity

Some writers draw a sharp distinction between managers whose values are 'rooted in social work' and those who are 'general professional managers with values rooted in managerialism' (O'Sullivan, 1999: 36). This difference implies that the two sets of values are at odds and that care managers may need to set themselves in opposition to managerial perspectives. In practice, we found that this distinction was not so clear in attitudes towards charging. Managers at middle levels of social service hierarchies voiced similar views to those working directly with service users. Managers could see difficulties in applying a means tested system at individual level and also as a means of maximising the department's resources.

Staff working in finance sections also set the principle of equity as important in their discussions of paying for services. This principle has been taken up at national level in respect of variation in levels of charges and in the means of calculation. The government has begun to address these concerns (see Audit Commission, 2000), although the ironing out of such variations has been more focused on domiciliary, day care and respite payments rather than the national threshold figures set by central government under Charging for Residential Accommodation Guide (CRAG). Nonetheless, the issue of equity arose in respect of decisions made at senior level about pursuit of non-payment or decisions about gifts or forms of estate planning. For many managers issues of access were tempered by their knowledge of the 'financial facts of life'. They referred to problems that would arise if 'generous' or lenient understanding was given to some individuals, which might result in others receiving less or no service.

In interviews with managers and their staff, knowledge of the system of charging was variable, with little evidence of a clear and transparent application of national legislation, rules and guidance. Whilst many were familiar with basic facts such as the charging thresholds, few had a sound grasp of the relevant legislation and guidelines as outlined in Health and Social Services and Social Security Adjudications Act 1983, and CRAG. Criticism of the latter by managers suggested that it had been written to inform and steer directors of social services, legal advisers and finance officers rather than being a useful guide for practitioners and their line managers. Those managers who were more familiar with CRAG were split in their views; some described it as 'straightforward' and 'formula driven' whilst others could see 'loopholes' particularly when dealing with people suspected of charge avoidance. Whilst some professionals thought that a set of principles and procedures were in place to pursue charges, a minority felt that the charging policy did not work in practice. As one local authority legal adviser explained:

> It does not work as we don't enforce it properly . . . it looks fair on the face of it, but not everyone [who should pay] pays, so charges are raised for those who do . . . the charging routes, regimes and enforcement provisions are there, but it's a wishy-washy approach and we do not drive to recover charges.

Within this uncertainty, it is likely that some managers find themselves in some difficulty in giving the correct local policy steer to practitioners. The position of managers as 'piggy in the middle' has been compounded in this complex area of charging.

Monitoring what is going on

At first glance the national rules and regulations on charging for long-term care are neither open to interpretation nor to the exercise of discretion. From the research this proved not to be the case.

Four of the five authorities had guidelines on financial assessment for practitioners. Nonetheless, in two authorities, many care managers said that there was a 'lack of written procedures' and a lack of direction at senior level on how best to implement them. In these authorities, care managers did not seem comfortable with the information manuals provided to them, as the following quotation illustrates:

> No-one knows where the guidelines come from. I don't like this. My profession is supposed to be open and honest and that isn't.

In two other local authorities most care managers interviewed said that the directives were clear, but some were unclear of the legislative framework and administrative context and this added to the uncertainty of their work.

In those authorities where care managers were responsible for checking the details of bank accounts, 75 per cent of survey respondents reported that they carried out this task, whilst 22 per cent said they did not. There was diversity between authorities; 38 per cent of care managers from one authority stated that they did not check bank account details compared to 5 per cent in another. In this latter authority, a team manager had stated that 'jobs would be on the line' in situations where staff did not fully examine financial details.

From one interpretation of fairness and equity, it is important that practitioners follow the rules, that managers know what is going on in their own teams and that there is consistency of approach within and between authorities. It is helpful if managers are informed about practitioners' perceptions of guidance and procedures and the effect these may have on the way the system is operated. Monitoring by managers is a key means of obtaining relevant information about current practices. From our research, a commonly held view was that 'monitoring happens naturally' rather than formally. That which occurs is normally done on an *ad hoc* basis. Team managers confirmed that practices within their teams were inconsistent. A typical response from one team manager was:

> ...there is inconsistency ... we don't apply the rules rigorously ... there is no formal checking ... we just accept the information we are given. We don't want to be financial police.

In four of the SSDs we found some discrepancy between care managers' views on the guidelines and those of senior staff. Senior managers, particularly from two areas, thought that guidelines were clear, even if they were given as verbal guidance. Finance staff were also more likely to take the view that processes were clear, and that there was 'no discretion at the beginning of the [financial assessment] process when care managers are involved'. Similarly, Chairs of Social Services Committees held the view that they expected care managers to carry out this functional activity, regarding them, as one Chair remarked, as 'foot soldiers with no discretion and [who] should follow the set criteria'.

Use of discretion

We found discretion when implementing the charging policy exercised at all levels. Why professionals, from care managers to legal advisers to senior managers, exercise discretion when there is no apparent remit again raises questions of equity and legality, and the need to make systems work in a social and political context.

Common explanations given for the use of discretion were lack of clear guidelines, little ongoing training, uncertainty of role and general lack of communication about dealing with complex cases throughout the department. Some care managers were genuinely uncertain whether they should or would report evidence of charge avoidance and some admitted using their own judgement and personal professional values in their decision-making.

In the interviews with team managers, we catalogued a range of examples of ways in which discretion was exercised and managed. Some team managers assumed they had the power to decide on the type and amount of information care managers should give to service users. The approach, however, was not consistent within or between authorities. For example, one team manager had instructed staff to give service users a 'letter on the benefits loophole' and Age Concern leaflets, whilst other managers at the same level in the same authority did not. In another example, a team manager decided not to inform the finance section that a service user had given her adult child £1500 for a holiday shortly before she was admitted into a residential home. The team manager said that she felt 'justified' since 'the service user was a very independent lady and had not used the services before so I ignored it'. Others said that they would always report suspicious cases of charge avoidance and would 'do it by the book'.

Sometimes managers were not pleased by the outcome of cases that they had referred to senior levels and this affected their views on the fairness of the system. For example, a team manager said that he had reported a daughter of suspected charge avoidance, since shortly after her mother was admitted to residential care, the daughter had decided she should have a gift of £5000 for her 50th birthday. The team manager said, 'the local authority did not back me up and I felt peed off!' Other team managers gave similar examples of this happening to care managers; as one reflected, 'the ground-staff sometimes feel let down'. A second described the process as 'we start hard and finish soft', meaning that the perception was that the agency operated rigorous gate-keeping activities at the outset but that ultimately little action was taken by the authority against people who allegedly avoided charges. It was widely believed by managers that the 'soft' approach was the result of political factors. As one team manager commented:

> The authority is paranoid about publicity ... as a team manager if I say something controversial it may antagonise members and my job could be at risk ... they are just disinterested in pursuing, as they do not want to be seen to be harassing people.

Additionally, our study showed that some senior managers exercised discretion quite openly and systematically, whilst others used more covert methods. It appeared that those senior managers, who were some years away from practice experience, were more likely to set the picture in a political context and referred more readily to the department's difficulty in balancing budgets.

The political dimension of this mainly relaxed or covert policy steer was heard from the Chairs of Social Services Committees. Irrespective of political affiliation, in interview, Chairs said that they were sympathetic to older people who could 'lose their assets' to pay for care. Generally the instruction given to managers was 'don't bring this to my attention, just manage it'.

The use of discretion in particular areas of financial assessment was variable and inconsistent at most levels within the authorities. From our data, it proved difficult to locate consistent practice in any one authority. Much appeared to depend on the perceived competence and knowledge of the care manager. Some care managers accepted that their particular approach was marked by inconsistency. As one care manager commented:

> The guidelines tell us we should advise clients to seek independent advice ... However, I have crossed the line occasionally and given direct advice ... I've told my line manager and he says 'you're an officer of the authority and shouldn't do this'. But he needs to understand that we are there for the client.

This type of anxiety and the practice that underlies it are clearly of importance to quality control and the tasks of managers.

Managing public relations and communications?

One of the indicators of an equitable and fair system could be the provision of consistent and transparent information to service users. We found little concrete evidence of this. There was little clarity about the amount of advice that should be provided. The main question centred on what was appropriate, particularly with regard to advice, which could help to protect assets. Senior managers thought that, although the area was problematic, the policy steer was clear. One senior manager, reflecting on the responsibilities of care managers, said:

> The duty [of the care manager] should be to the local authority and not the client and I don't understand care managers who say that they should not be asking these financial questions of their clients [and should advise them in their best interests only] – they are working on behalf of the local authority.

This degree of certainty was not evident among practitioners. Care managers were effectively divided; from the questionnaire, 44 per cent said they gave direct advice and information to service users, but 49 per cent reported that this was not their role or appeared unsure about advising service users to access independent advice.

Some interviewees thought that detailed financial information was withheld from them by their department, reflecting a lack of trust. Additionally, a number of care managers thought that they should not give too much information in case they gave the 'wrong advice', including information about protecting assets. Several team managers cautioned about giving the service user too much detailed financial information ahead of the final decision since, as one manager put it:

> We don't want to be both judge and jury. We could give people the wrong advice and channel them into a certain [inappropriate] route.

Revisit training strategies

Managers in all social work and social care agencies are likely to agree that a trained and competent workforce is in the best position to enable the agency to deliver a quality service. However, following the implementation of the NHS and Community Care Act 1990, training in financial assessment in social services departments has not been a high priority for organisations (Bradley et al., 1996; Bradley and Manthorpe, 1997; Manthorpe and Bradley, 2002). Even government-sponsored guidance for practitioners and managers (DoH, 1991) paid little attention to matters of finance. Several years on, this study confirms that care managers continued to receive little training in financial assessment. Whilst almost two-thirds (60 per cent) of care managers had received some training in this area, the average amount was only half a day, even though many had been engaged in this work since the introduction of care management in 1993 and the field is frequently changing.

However, some senior managers held differing views concerning training. They thought that induction training in financial assessment was sufficient and that it was the role of the finance team to help with ongoing instruction. However, we found that, although informal links between the finance section and care managers were generally satisfactory, there was little evidence of formal training or regular updating of practitioners. Managers also require systematic training in order to be able to advise team members as necessary. We noted earlier from interviews with first level managers that many felt they were not sufficiently familiar with the detail of legislation and guidance.

Within a training needs analysis, the importance of regular supervisory systems should not be ignored. In contrast to nursing and medicine, supervision in social work appears well developed and professional, and managerial issues are taken up within this context. While we found in this research that a number of respondents did not bring financial assessment to supervision, nonetheless most had regular supervision which provided their managers with a picture of day-to-day practice and its difficulties. In debriefing sessions with managers to feed back the results of our research, most managers appeared very familiar with the issues raised by frontline staff. Any new configuration of adult services will need to explore and debate the strengths of different models of supervision, particularly if staff other than social workers (for example, nurses) are engaged in financial assessment.

Concluding comments

Throughout the authorities in our study, there was general unease about the charging system. Contradictions and uncertainties abounded concerning policy and practice in this area. Whilst there was evidence of written procedures and guidance, we also found significant inconsistency in the extent to which the guidance was acted on and/or enforced. Ambivalence could be tracked throughout the system and was compounded by the political sensitivities at senior management and elected representative levels. Chairs 'washing their hands' of complicated issues may seem relatively innocuous, but the political message they give and the known local power and influence which they carry, affect the total culture and lack of policy steer in social services departments. Such lessons should inform any proposals to charge for further aspects of health care.

In summary, managers in this area found dealing with financial assessment symptomatic of the pressures they face in modernising social care services. As Martin and Henderson (2001) argue:

> the emphasis is on ensuring that services are responsive to the needs of service users, integrated across traditional professional and organisational boundaries, effective in achieving the outcomes that both individual service users and society as a whole are seeking, and inclusive in identifying and meeting the needs of disadvantaged groups.
>
> (2001: 1)

This is a tall order and skates over the potential conflicts between service users, the 'fluidity' between them and society and the possible different interpretations of what constitutes a disadvantaged group. Managers stand at the centre of such conflicts in respect of financial assessments. However, this research also demonstrates that most frontline practitioners understand their position. While some may view managers with cynicism, most were sympathetic to their position of making hard choices. Managers themselves appeared to accept that making difficult decisions was a choice between options, both of which might have negative consequences.

REFERENCES

Audit Commission (2000) *Charging with Care: How Councils Charge for Home Care*, London, London Audit Commission.

Bradley, G. and Manthorpe, J. (1997) *Dilemmas of Financial Assessment*, Birmingham, Venture Press.

Bradley, G., Manthorpe, J., Stanley, N. and Alaszewski, A. (1996) 'Training for Care Management: Using Research to Identify New Directions', *Social Work Education*, 16, 2, 26–44.

Bradley, G., Penhale, B., Manthorpe, J., Parkin, A., Parry, N. and Gore, J. (2000) *Ethical Dilemmas and Administrative Justice: Perceptions of Social and Legal Professionals Towards Charging for Residential and Nursing Home Care. A Summary of the Finding*, Hull, University of Hull.

Department of Health (1998) *Modernising Social Services*, London, Stationery Office.

Department of Health, Social Services Inspectorate, Scottish Office, Social Work Services Group (1991) *Care Management and Assessment Practitioners' Guide*, London, HMSO.

Manthorpe, J. and Bradley, G. (2002) 'Managing Finances', in Adams, R., Payne, M. and Dominelli, L. (eds), *Critical Practice in Social Work*, Basingstoke, Palgrave.

Martin, V. and Henderson, E. (2001) *Managing in Health and Social Care*, London, The Open University/Routledge.

Means, R. and Smith, R. (1998) *Community Care Policy and Practice*, Basingstoke, Macmillan.

O'Sullivan, T. (1999) *Decision Making in Social Work*, Basingstoke, Macmillan.

Sutherland, S. (1999) *With Respect to Old Age – Royal Commission on Long Term Care*, London, Stationery Office.

PART II

MANAGING TO CARE

Jill Reynolds

INTRODUCTION

All managers need to focus on the primary task of the organisation – 'What are we here to do, and what is my part in it?' (Burton, 1998). For managers involved in care the answer is likely to involve providing some kind of assistance that helps people to maintain or extend their independence. Already we are in a contested and value-laden area. Is it care that people want? Does independence mean not having to rely on others or does it mean autonomy? Where children are concerned, independence may be a rather long-term goal and terms like 'quality' and 'proper development' or 'protection' become part of the task. Again these are words that contain different meanings, the interpretation of which may change the management agenda.

The readings in this part of the book have been chosen for their capacity to shed light on the multi-faceted nature of care. Not all readings focus directly on the manager's role, and you will have to do some of the work yourself in making the connections between leading themes and their implications for managers. The tensions between centrally directed modernising policies and the need for managers and their organisations to be responsive to what the users of their services really want lie at the heart of many of these chapters. Mike Evans describes and reflects on a 'bottom-up' approach to implementing policy guidance. Consultancy work with managers focused on the Best Value requirements that public bodies continuously improve their services in relation to economy, efficiency and effectiveness. The programme used an often neglected resource – the practice wisdom of managers and practitioners. Through the exchange of 'stories' based on day-to-day events, reflection groups looked at how these observations could become a resource for the organisation to learn and develop.

The reading from Pine et al.'s 'Participatory management in a children's agency' also offers a model of consultation that draws on a wide range of experience. The ideas of staff, court officials, foster parents and birth parents contributed to improve the agency's performance in reuniting children placed in foster care with their own families. The benefits of a participatory approach to managing are explored, along with the variables that seem important for work of this kind to be effective. The example is from the USA, and it may raise questions for you of the different contexts of care work in that country as well as some reflection on how far down the road to encouraging worker and user participation UK agencies may be. One interested group that do not appear to have been consulted in this process are the children concerned. The next reading turns to research on children's views: 'Remember my messages.' When one in five children in care do not report anything positive about the experience, and only 57 per cent are able to state with any certainty that they have a care plan, you may like to think about what the messages are for managers. This is a key reading for anyone working in or with residential care for children. Moreover, managers of any service that involves children can learn from this chapter and think about their responsibility to set a tone that enables workers to be responsive to children's wishes and concerns.

David Piachaud calls for a broader vision of public policy for childhood. One in three children in Britain live in poverty and there is a good deal more to be done in tackling this problem. Piachaud points out that the quality of children's lives and their opportunities in later life depend on much more than their material circumstances. Nutrition, health, lack of stimulating childhood experiences, exclusion from normal social activities, while linked to poverty also have wider influences. These include the impact of television and commercial pressures. Again, the direct implications for managers are not spelt out, but participation in work to combat social exclusion is one strand. A broader vision might be a strategy to shift the manifold influences on children's lives towards goals that focus on the quality of those lives.

Ayesha Vernon and Hazel Qureshi explore the meaning of an emphasis on outcomes of services for the people who receive them in the next reading. Government rhetoric obscures the potential for conflicting views on what independence truly means. This article summarises research with disabled service users whose views were collected through in-depth interviews and focus groups in a northern city. If the outcomes for service users are truly to be central, then managers may have to re-examine the core aims of their service. So far, commitment to promoting independence as valued by those interviewed seems limited. The article considers direct payments as a strategy for promoting the independence of disabled people.

The centrality of values in driving the work of the manager is emerging in this set of articles, as is the notion that there is nothing unproblematic about what these values should be. Stephen Pattison takes an ironic look in the next reading at the ethical vacuum in the heart of health service management and the attempts to fill this with professional codes, locally generated philosophies or utilitarian tools such as 'Quality Adjusted Life Years'. He takes as a case study the widespread take-up of appraisal as a symbol of good practice. Pattison suggests that this popular device can become a time-consuming irrelevance, or worse a mechanism of control with enormous potential for inducing guilt and shame in organisational members.

Guneratnam's exploration of dilemmas in dealing with racial harassment among service users is concerned with the values of anti-oppressive practice. She offers a detailed analysis of the way that staff talk about how they manage episodes of racism. How does a nurse respond to a patient or his family who express racist views in the direct hearing of black patients? Is it more important to behave professionally towards the patient or to challenge his racist comments? Her fascinating research study unravels some of the complexity of emotions and power relations within professions and between staff and service users. There are important implications for managers here. In seeking to create a climate that enables staff to deal with racist remarks, managers need to recognise the implicit dilemmas, and avoid simplistic approaches that impose a single 'correct' line.

But does research really help to change practice? Janet Lewis points out in her reading on research findings and practice change that research results do not speak for themselves. She suggests that to be really useful, evidence has to be converted into knowledge. This requires the addition of the experience of practitioners and service users to be added to the researcher's interpretations. If researchers really want to help managers and practitioners to develop and improve what they are doing, they need to start where people are. Work has to be done through personal interaction rather than the written word and organisations need to have a strong focus on the change process itself to enable managers and practitioners to act on relevant knowledge.

The final contribution to this Part is Judi Marshall's classic piece on an ecological understanding of occupational stress. She suggests that workers in public services confront fundamental existential conflicts as essential ingredients of their job. Added to this are other people's projections of stereotypes of occupational groups, and the burden for workers of carrying the society's unresolved anxieties surrounding these issues. There are links here with the approach taken by Obholzer in Part IV of this book. Marshall raises the question of what constitutes effective and healthy coping strategies. Moves to increase contact between caring professionals and the users of their services may be experienced as also increasing the stress load. Questions remain as to how managers who care can support their frontline staff, acknowledge with honesty the inherent stresses in the job and still keep a focus on the needs of service users.

REFERENCE

Burton, J. (1998) *Managing Residential Care*, London, Routledge.

THIRTEEN

THE QUEST FOR QUALITY: REFLECTING ON THE MODERNISING AGENDA

Mike Evans

Source: NISW Briefing Number 30.

Introduction

This chapter outlines the development of a consultancy programme for a group of managers on 'Managing the workforce at a time of upheaval and change: understanding the factors which affect the workforce, and the organisational response to those factors'.

The aim was to develop a set of principles that managers could use to ensure service quality and standards were formed by using a 'bottom-up' approach to implementing policy guidance and regulations. Legislation and government guidance stress the importance of user-centred rather than service-based provision of support and care. This provides a framework for change. Yet, paradoxically, the many resulting directives, and the organisational changes in social services departments, may have really added to the tendency to define practice from the 'top down'.

The Competent Workplace perspective which underpinned the consultancy (see below, p. 110) offers an approach to reaching the aim of user-centred services. It is based firmly on the idea that what is experienced by service users is the *service*. For support and care to be effective, there must accordingly be a bottom-up approach, with maximum utilisation of the talents of the workforce. To aid this cultural shift, managers were brought together in 'reflection groups' to discuss 'events' affecting their workplace.

The competent workplace: key principles

Purpose

To raise performance and morale by moving from:

- control to partnership
- blueprints to a model of reality
- passivity to maximum use of the workforce as a creative resource.

Approach

What the frontline workers do: how this is experienced by the users of the service represents what the service *is* (the actual rather than the ideal). It cannot be assumed.

How do we discover it? By listening to frontline workers and service users.

How can we learn to listen? Through emphasis on partnership with both service users and frontline staff rather than purely relying on prescriptive or procedural control.

Value for money

The workplace is a costly investment. To gain maximum benefit from this, it is important that the workplace stimulates:

- curiosity and questioning about current practices
- a distinct culture of experimentation rather than a personal, pathology, bureaucracy or reactive/crisis-driven culture
- recognition of each individual's contribution, irrespective of status
- recognition and encouragement of creativity (new solutions to old problems).

Aims

1 To minimise worker passivity at all levels: the workplace should have maximum control over its business.
2 To avoid detailed work prescriptions: they become part of the problem rather than the solution.
3 To remember policy intentions only have true meaning when transformed into policy action.
4 To recognise that common purpose and standards are achieved in many different ways by each individual team and facility.
5 To support difference: the job of management is to provide both support and challenge to individuals and teams that is explicit, with realistic goals that are negotiated.

6 To realise development agendas (the learning/development culture) for teams and facilities arising from their work as they experience it.

7 To collaborate with workers on action-based learning as the major focus for development.

8 To build styles of management that utilise the knowledge in the workforce for working on problems (the model of reality) through a partnership model.

9 To manage the workforce at a time of upheaval and change through understanding the factors that affect the workforce, and the organisational response to those factors.

Background

The government White Paper on Modernising Social Services (Department of Health, 1998) requires all sectors to undergo a massive strategic overhaul of the way services are delivered. At the same time, there has been a blizzard of key policy directives and dramatic expectations about 'modernising' social services. 'Cultural change' is invoked, and the importance of organisational learning emphasised. However, the main focus is on the need to ensure the governance of services in a much more prescribed and transparent way. The consultancy set out to examine how best to manage these expectations.

Best Value destination, best practice journey

The focus in local authorities is on the new requirements for 'Best Value' outcomes: that is, pre-determined performance targets and national standards, which can be identified and measured. Best Value requires local authorities and other public bodies to make arrangements to secure continuous improvement in services, in relation to economy, efficiency and effectiveness; to publish annual Best Value performance plans; and effect a process of regular performance reviews designed to raise standards and reduce costs. Running alongside Best Value, joint reviews between the SSI and the Audit Commission challenge the ways in which local authorities deliver services up and down the country.

Meeting these new requirements necessitates a shift in the behaviour of both frontline managers and their organisations if they are to embrace the notion of organisational learning and modernise. To manage the expectations and requirements produced by these perspectives, managers in the consultancy programme developed a culture of 'appreciative inquiry'. Appreciative inquiry is about the 'co-evolutionary' search for the best in people, their organisations, and the relevant world around them. Within this paradigm, managers become 'critical friends' to each other and travelling companions on the journey to best practice, by developing team self-audit tools, listening to feedback from service users, and developing a culture in which conversation forms an aspect of the organisation's learning, linked to its core business of providing a quality service.

The key principles of the Competent Workplace were linked with organisational theories which underpin the concept of a learning organisation and knowledge management.

Garvin (1993: 53–70) sees learning organisations as skilled at five main activities:

- systematic problem solving
- experimentation with new approaches
- learning from past experience
- learning from best practices of others
- transferring knowledge quickly and efficiently throughout the organisation.

Nonaka and Takeuchi (1995) define knowledge management as the way companies generate, communicate and leverage their intellectual assets. New knowledge is not simply a matter of mechanistically 'processing' objective information. Rather, it depends on tapping into the tacit and often highly subjective insights, intuitions and ideals of employees.

Explicit knowledge is formal, systematic knowledge easily transmitted from one person to another in the form of language (verbal, mathematical and numerical). What is transmitted is thought of as a translation of already existing tacit language into a codified form. Immediately, a particular assumption is being made about the nature of language; namely, that it is a formal, objective system of symbols located outside people and employed by them as a tool to translate already existing ideas and concepts into a form that can be readily transmitted to others.

Tacit knowledge is particularly important in this way of thinking. It is personal in the sense of being located in the minds of individuals. It is, therefore, a subject phenomenon of insight, intuition and hunches, below the level of awareness. This makes it hard to formalise and communicate. It is rooted in action and shows itself as skills or knowledge, lying in the beliefs and perspectives ingrained in the way people understand their world and act in it. In other words, tacit knowledge takes the form of mental models that are below the level of awareness (Nonaka and Takeuchi, 1995: 8–11).

Practice wisdom

This notion of knowledge management was promoted by focusing on the 'practice wisdom' found at the frontline among managers and their teams, and encouraging them to develop team self-audits based on their day-to-day experience with service users and the community. Often we discovered that the fruits of that practice wisdom were discarded on the cutting room floor of supervision sessions, because their description did not fit the rigid requirements of the audit pro forma of the organisation.

The government document *A Quality Strategy for Social Care* (Department of Health, 2000) notes the lack of reliable evidence about what works best in social care. Developing an evidence-based culture and discovering 'what works best in social care' requires us to engage with frontline managers on gaining insights from day-to-day practice in a more systematic and meaningful way. Such experience is often described as the 'stories' that practitioners tell each other about what is worrying them, or when they think they have achieved good outcomes for people using services. Yet these 'stories' are a major resource for developing frontline practice and services. It is from this experience that we can learn what works best, where teams need to acquire or seek more knowledge and expertise. Workers often feel that the only time the organisation listens to their experience of day-to-day involvement is when they are required to fill in some monitoring form (whether as 'feeding the beast' of bureaucratic demands or in response to 'when things go wrong').

Although learning at different levels does take place, there appears to be little connection or 'loop back' between day-to-day activities and the strategic plans, the bigger picture of social care within the community and policy directives. Frontline managers' experiences of these gaps, disjunctions and contradictions provides a major resource for improving the climate for change.

The organisational framework

We developed a framework for organisations to use in implementing the modernising agenda.

- Staff are encouraged to be innovative in the way they provide services, within the complexity of the terrain which service users occupy. Organisations are required to become much more resourceful in planning services for individual needs (needs led/Best Value outcomes).
- A means for expressing and actively addressing the varied and complex needs of society is provided (advocacy and empowerment).
- Individuals are motivated to act as citizens in all aspects of society (participation and social inclusion).

- There is the capacity to work within the tight prescriptive framework of government expectations by promoting certainty (expressed through such initiatives as Quality Protects, Best Value, Working Together and the Framework for Assessment).
- Pluralism and diversity in society are promoted by protecting and strengthening cultural, ethnic, religious, linguistic and other identities (enabling diversity and equality).
- Services with greater independence and flexibility are created (responsive learning organisations).
- The concept of appreciative inquiry is raised.

Learning on the run while remaining within the framework

This framework was adapted to the specific context in which the consultancy took place, including consideration of how the stresses and uncertainty experienced by staff should be managed, while at the same time ensuring this did not distract them from focusing on the final destination, providing a quality service. The managers were given opportunity to 'think outside their box', and to reflect on the issues of change and upheaval in a more collaborative, systematic and responsive way. Liberated from traditional ways of line managing, they could try innovative approaches.

In effect, the group became a new 'community of practice', in which a more joined-up learning approach could be developed, linked to knowledge management. This required new skills and a withdrawal from the traditional ways of working that operate in the linear 'command and control' culture. The 'old order' of service-led thinking had not equipped staff for the 'new order' of needs led/Best Value service delivery. The managers were encouraged to examine their own effectiveness and to explore new methods of managing these new challenges, and to share these experiences within the management group. Maintaining a quality service always remained top of the agenda.

Reflection groups, events and stories

We worked collaboratively to discover how practice is supported or undermined by organisational structures, systems, procedures, management style, political activity. The experience of engaging with staff at a number of levels in the organisation was invaluable. Space was allowed for people to 'think out loud' on a range of issues. One of the consistent features was the frankness and openness of staff at all levels in talking about the issues facing services throughout the consultancy period.

The challenge for managers became how to manage the range of tensions within complex situations, and still ensure quality and certainty. The 'reflection groups' provided a platform for everyone in the service to be given time out to reflect on their own needs, the needs of service users and their families. Some even renamed the groups 'safe havens' – this spoke volumes about the levels of anxiety staff felt.

However, the reflection groups were required to provide 'added value', otherwise their effectiveness would be limited. One of the key added value outcomes was the importance of the 'stories' that were beginning to emerge from the 'events' that happened on an almost daily basis. Each event had a knock-on effect as to how policy, procedures and practice should be managed. Stories were given equal space and status in the clinical process of setting objectives, outcomes, benchmarks and performance indicators. The experience of frontline workers thus became information that could be structured as a resource for the organisation. The result was a clearer understanding of the fragility of strategic planning, and that a traditional linear management style was not appropriate for the fast-flowing demands placed upon managers. Dependency on long-term direction or certainty proved to be fatally flawed. At times, we felt that with each week there was a change of direction, outcome or expectation. Reflection groups provided the mechanism to deal with the flaws, redirections and u-turns in policy, and linked support to the workforce with more systematic behaviour.

And the future . . .

We are now at the crossroads in our journey together. New methods of dealing with new expectations about services to the public require managers to rethink the way services are managed, whether these expectations are the result of policy directives, the increasing expectations of service users and their families, or feedback from Joint Reviews. Local authorities must create the culture in which managers can develop the skills essential for meeting new policy challenges. Monitoring 'outcomes' alone is not a satisfactory measure of 'quality', nor its only measure (Balloch, 1998). Listening to the 'stories' based on day-to-day 'events', and capturing these to inform the working of the organisation as a whole, is even more essential. Only thus will the knowledge developed by workers working with service users and their families inform practice and service development.

REFERENCES

Balloch, S. (ed.) (1998) *Outcomes of Social Care: A Question of Quality?* London, National Institute for Social Work.

Department of Health (1998) *Modernising Social Services: Promoting Independence, Improving Protection, Raising Standards*, London, The Stationery Office.

Department of Health (2000) *A Quality Strategy for Social Care*, London, Department of Health.

Garvin, D.A. (1993) 'Building a Learning Organization', in *Harvard Business Review on Knowledge Management*, Boston, Harvard Business School, pp. 47–80.

Nonaka, I. and Takeuchi, H. (1995) *The Knowledge-Creating Company: How Japanese Companies Create the Dynamics of Innovation*, Oxford, Oxford University Press.

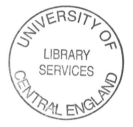

FOURTEEN

PARTICIPATORY MANAGEMENT IN A PUBLIC CHILD WELFARE AGENCY: A KEY TO EFFECTIVE CHANGE

Barbara A. Pine, Robin Warsh and Anthony N. Maluccio

Source: *Administration in Social Work*, 1998, 22, 1.

[. . .] In this article, the authors examine participatory management, using a case example drawn from their experience as consultants to a public child welfare agency. The approach to consultation called for the formation of an interdisciplinary task force comprising agency staff, foster parents, court personnel, and community service providers, with the aim to improve the agency's performance in reunifying children and families separated by foster care placement. A case example is used to illustrate successful planning and implementing of participatory approaches, especially in large bureaucratic organizations.

The "what" and "why" of participatory management

Participatory management is, quite simply, a commitment to carrying out a set of strategies that involve workers in organizational decisions. It is the currently dominating management theme as organizations move from traditional, hierarchical structures toward the empowerment and interdependence of team-oriented approaches (van Vlissingen, 1993; Grosnick, 1993; Burbidge, 1994). In its broadest sense, participation means having a role in solving problems, making decisions about policy and operations, and evaluating the organization (Vandervelde, 1979; Toch and Grant,

1982). Participation is not, as Kanter (1983) notes, a single mechanism or program. Rather, it involves a wide range of activities, such as strategic planning, total quality management, organization development, conflict management and team building and development. [. . .]

A case example of participation: rewards and requisites

In 1993, the authors were invited by administrators in a state child welfare agency to assist them in a participatory management project to evaluate and improve the agency's family reunification services – that is, services aimed at reuniting children placed in out-of-home care. The authors had developed a model for such a project, which calls for the formation of a task force to conduct a self-assessment of the agency's family reunification service delivery system and develop an action plan for change.

The agency was ready to undertake this evaluation for several reasons: staff members had just begun to rethink and strengthen the commitment to family-focused service delivery; there were plans to provide new and more resources for children and families whose case goal was reunification; and the agency's top administrators were looking for a model for planning and carrying out those changes. With the active assistance and support of the agency's Commissioner and Deputy Commissioner, work began with formation of a task force charged with examining the agency's family reunification program and making recommendations for improving it.

The task force was made up of volunteers representing the full range of staff members involved with reunifications, including administrators, supervisors, line staff, trainers, attorneys, staff members with financial responsibilities, foster parents, collateral providers, and birth parents. During five full-day meetings, each held a month apart, this team used a set of guidelines ... to identify the strengths and weaknesses of their service delivery system in relation to family reunification. The guidelines helped the team to evaluate each of twenty-five components of the service delivery system, including those related to the agency, such as roles and responsibilities of social workers and foster parents, cultural competence, and staff development; those connected to direct practice, such as preparing families and children, assessment and goal planning, and visiting; and those associated with inter-organizational relations, such as court and legal systems, schools, and external reviewers.

The guidelines specify the key elements that need to be in place in relation to each of the twenty-five components, if the agency's service delivery system is to be effective in achieving the goals of family reunification. (For example, in relation to the agency's policies and practice around visiting, one key element of a successful program is as follows: "Children are returned home only after they have safely had unsupervised visits in their own home, including overnight visits and visits lasting several days or more.") The assessment process required that the team review each of the key elements, and through discussion and problem-solving, decide where their current system was weak and then generate ideas for improvement. Although task force members, a diverse group by design, had different viewpoints on the problems and issues, these were discussed and through a process of negotiation and renegotiation, a set of recommendations was developed.

Rewards

The project had an immediate, positive impact on the agency. The most tangible result was a set of 65 recommendations for improvement in family reunification policy, program, training, and resources. Every one of the ideas was well-conceived, viable, and could be implemented. The ideas were wide-ranging and included, as just one example, the development of a pamphlet for parents whose children are about to be removed from their care. The pamphlet, already in print, explains parents' rights and provides helpful information for them about how to contact the agency and their child's foster family. It has been enthusiastically received by families and staff members around the state.

Another of the 65 recommendations was that staff members should be involved in grant proposal review, selection, and evaluation of grant proposals from community service providers. This was based on the conviction that only those agencies demonstrating a commitment to reunifying families should receive agency funds. In addition, the task force recommended that a formal mechanism be established through which agency staff members experiencing problems with community providers could be heard during contract negotiations with these providers. These recommendations were made to the state agency's top management, and an Implementation Team was formed to carry them out. In keeping with good participatory management practice, the Team included selected members of the task force in order to help ensure ownership, continuity, and a range of perspectives.

Although beyond the scope of this paper, which reports a set of events from a particular point in time, it is important to note that the agency began immediately to act on a number of the recommendations including a comprehensive redrafting of policies and procedures on family reunification.

Of equal importance were the following additional benefits to the agency in using a participatory management approach:

■ The intense focus on a specific area of child welfare practice gave staff members who participated in the process an increased understanding of family reunification and a renewed belief in the importance of family.

- Staff members received a tremendous morale and creativity boost by reflecting on their work and developing plans for needed change. The energy and enthusiasm throughout the work team sessions was palpable demonstrating that, as Kanter (1983) has noted, "the human energy is there waiting to be plugged in" (p. i).
- Staff members became much more familiar with the services of the community agencies that were represented in the evaluation process.
- The difficulties of creating and maintaining a responsive child welfare system become very apparent to staff members, as did their roles in helping to shape service delivery. The result was a "we're in this together" attitude.
- Empowerment of staff members through participation in the project encouraged them to continue to evaluate the recommended ways of improving the system.
- Participating staff members learned more about each other's job responsibilities and areas of competence and thus were better able to use their colleagues' expertise.

Perhaps the following quotes, the first from a top manager, and the second from a task force member, best capture the spirit of this agency's experience with participatory management:

> Taking this approach is an opportunity to convey our trust in staff. If we trust people enough to decide that a child is safe to return home, we should also trust them to come up with useful policy recommendations.

and

> There seemed to be a special closeness of people gathered for a common purpose – to create a better system to help families. It was refreshing to have my input valued. I believe real good will came from this effort.

Requisites

...Variables to success with participatory management approaches ... include leadership attributes of administrators and team leaders, and planning and structural mechanisms. These variables will be discussed below and illustrated with examples from the case situation described above.

Leadership. No other variable is more critical to the success of efforts to involve staff in organizational decision-making than leadership at the top. Administrators who see themselves as primarily responsible for communicating a vision to others about the organization's future, setting the organization's direction, and finding ways to cope with ever present change are more likely to view participation as critical and to value a team approach. Indeed, the ability to use participatory approaches effectively is now seen as another way of measuring overall management competence (Donnell and Hall, 1980). Equally important is the ability to know when to use a task force approach – for example, when an issue is controversial and consensus is needed, or to ensure that those affected by important decisions are represented when they are made (Kanter, 1983). To use these strategies inappropriately would be inefficient and ineffective.

Another leadership attribute critical to managing change, and thus involving others in planning for it, is a sense of optimism that things can and will be improved, an expectation of a positive outcome (Kouzes, undated). In no other field of social work practice is there a more pervasive need for optimism and focusing on strengths than in child welfare. Related to optimism is a sense of trust among and between staff and managers that problems and challenges will be approached "in a spirit of joint inquiry" (Donnell and Hall, 1980: 64).

Leadership provided by top level administrators in the case example described above was a key to its success. At the time, the agency's top management was shepherding the agency through a period of rapid growth and change, instigated in part by a consent decree in federal court that demanded more responsive policies and programs. In response, the agency developed an overarching child welfare service plan emphasizing family preservation. All of the agency's top management were professionally trained social workers who believed in a family-centered approach. They also recognized the importance of involving staff members, foster parents, and others in shaping and influencing the process to make that philosophy more central to the agency's work, and used their interpersonal skills to publicize enthusiastically the project and recruit volunteers.

The project was not without risks. It represented a major commitment of staff time. Open discussion of problems that prevent or unnecessarily delay families from getting back together requires honesty and courage. There could be blaming among those raising issues; a list of problems with no solutions might result. However, the administrators were confident that members of the task force shared a commitment to improving the agency's services and that the group's leader could constructively manage any conflicts that arose. As one task force member said confidently, "after all, if we keep thinking that we're doing it right, we're never going to improve."

In short, leadership attributes of vision, optimism, shared values, and commitment, valuing a team approach (but knowing when to use it), and trust are critical factors for success in involving others in decision-making and participatory management.

Facilitation skills. Competence in team-building and facilitation are also key attributes. The leader of the task force in the agency we have been describing, a professionally trained social worker and supervisor in her agency, had never before assumed responsibility for leading a project of this kind. With support from the authors, who acted in the role of consultants, she was helped to recognize and draw on her considerable interpersonal skills to organize the work and help the group remain focused. Her low-key style, combined with her enthusiasm for the task, infused each of the five all-day sessions with interest, respect for the views of others, and optimism. Outside of the task force meetings, she generated continuing interest in the project among participants, gently reminding them of tasks that needed to be done in preparation for the next session.

Structures and supports. A number of structural variables can influence success when staff members are involved in teams or task forces to improve programs. The first is related to expectations. Is a team approach to problem-solving widely accepted in the organization? Is participation in such agency-wide activities built into job descriptions (Kanter, 1983)? Are people trained for team and task force roles? Clarification of expectations is essential for participants, their supervisors and their co-workers. How much time will be spent away from the job? Who will cover the participant's workload while she/he is at meetings? What about case crises?

In the agency noted above, a meeting was convened prior to the task force's start that involved all key staff members and administrators affected by the project. At this meeting, the agency's top administrator for the program explained the project, its purpose, why she supported it, what the expected benefits were, and what the project would entail in staff time. She was also able to tie this project into other efforts the agency was undertaking to improve its program. She also made clear that the purpose of the project was to produce a set of recommendations to the agency's top management for improving family reunification services as a whole, thus highlighting that this was to be a systems examination, not a focus solely on practice. Thus, through this meeting she conveyed top management's commitment to, and support of, the project and secured the "buy in" of others. Moreover, throughout the series of task force meetings, administrators and other staff were welcome to, and did, attend and observe or participate in the discussions.

Task force meetings were carefully planned and structured. Participants were given advance assignments to prepare for each session; the system components (of the twenty-five that comprise the assessment tool) that were to be the focus of each all-day meeting were planned at the outset. This enabled the team leader to invite relevant guests to each session (for example, probation officers were invited to participate in the session focused on the agency's relationship with the court system and its influence on family reunification). The sessions were held in an attractive and comfortable location space away from the agency, and lunch and snacks were served.

A second set of structural variables is related to celebration and reward for a job well done. When the set of 55 recommendations was ready, the task force forwarded them to the state agency's Commissioner with a proposal for a full day conference to share findings and plans with other staff throughout the agency. The conference, with keynote addresses by both the Commissioner and the Deputy Commissioner, provided an opportunity to share and celebrate the results of the task force's efforts and begin the process of action planning to make the recommendations a reality.

Rewards took a number of forms. Several task force members gained well-deserved attention through their contributions and received promotions. There were personal rewards as well. As one member said, "I thought I was good at only one thing. Now that I've had the chance to serve in this way, I realize I can expand, and am capable of taking on more responsibility."

Conclusion

Participatory management in the human services is here to stay, as agency administrators and staff members seek to cope with an increasingly complex work environment. As Lee (1994) noted in her discussion of the "feminization of management," "A new model of leadership is in ascendance, one that emphasizes collectivism over individualism, inclusion over exclusion" (p. 26).

Such a new model was exemplified in the work of the multi-level task force in a public child welfare agency that has been described in this article. Through a careful self-study process and intensive examination of the agency's family reunification service delivery system, the task force developed an extensive set of recommendations for strengthening family reunification policies, programs, and practice. The agency was also exposed to a participatory approach for creating change that can be adapted for evaluating other programs and services. Commitment to staff participation is, perhaps, the most important system change an agency can make, for once a collaborative spirit is firmly established and expected, staff members at all levels recognize their part in building a responsive agency.

Implementing these recommendations will not be an easy task, as the agency's internal and external environments are constantly changing, and new challenges arise and must be confronted on a daily basis. Having participated in a joint self-study process, however, agency administrators and staff members are better poised to meet these challenges and contribute to improved services on behalf of vulnerable children and their families.

REFERENCES

Burbidge, J. (1994) Participation: Beyond corporate buzzword. *At work: Stories of tomorrow's workplace*, 3(2), 6–7.

Donnell, S.M. and Hall, J. (1980) Men and women as managers: A significant case of no significant difference. *Organizational dynamics*, Spring, 60–77.

Grosnick, P. (1993) Shifting from functional to empowered teams. *At work: Stories of tomorrow's workplace*, 2(4), 6–8.

Kanter, R.M. (1983) *The change masters.* New York, Simon & Schuster.

Lee, C. (1994) The feminization of management. *Training*, November, 25–31.

Toch, H. and Grant, J.D. (1982) *Reforming human services: Change through participation.* Beverly Hills, CA, Sage Publications.

Vandervelde, M. (1979) The semantics of participation. *Administration in social work*, 3(1), 65–77.

van Vlissingen, R.F. (1993) Beyond democracy, beyond consensus. *At work: Stories of tomorrow's workplace*, 2(3), 11–13

REMEMBER MY MESSAGES: THE EXPERIENCES AND VIEWS OF 2000 CHILDREN IN PUBLIC CARE IN THE UK

Catherine Shaw

Source: The Who Cares? Trust.

Entry into care

Coming into care is clearly a traumatic event for many children. Half the sample described it as being 'scary' or 'confusing'. What can be done to alleviate this? Responses to the survey suggest that information about being in care together with reassurance would help. Thought needs to be devoted as to how, when and by whom such information and reassurance could be delivered.

The research has shown that the first few months in care are also a particularly difficult and unsettling time for a child, associated with negative states of mind and disrupted schooling. Many children would clearly benefit from additional support during this period. Liaison between social services and education professionals is essential. It may be that such support is not always provided nor appropriate services accessed in cases assumed to be short-term placements. Perhaps alternative assumptions should be made, ensuring that young people are enabled to settle as quickly as possible, regardless of the expected duration of their stay in care.

It is clearly worth investing resources into supporting a child's initial placement; after the first six months in care, children who had been *looked after* in a single setting were markedly more positive and settled at school than those who had been moved around.

Formalities

It should surely be a matter of concern that only *57 per cent* of respondents were able to state with any certainty that they had a care plan. One assumes, or would hope, that the true figure is closer to *100 per cent*. If so, why are the children themselves not more aware of their care plans? Have they been sufficiently involved in the planning process?

The research findings suggest that one in three children in public care do not know how to make an official complaint about the way in which they are *looked after*. Why not? Is it simply that they are not being informed? Or are they failing to retain the information, perhaps because the complaints procedure is too complex, or too formal to be readily accessed?

The fact there was greater awareness of complaints procedures than care plans suggests that, for some children at least, being *looked after* is regarded as something imposed upon them from outside. Decisions about their care – to which they can react, for example, by complaining – are imposed from outside, but the impression is given that they are not actively involved or engaged in the process of decision-making and planning itself.

Whilst respondents expressed a number of grievances and gripes about their day-to-day lives in care, when asked specifically what the worst thing was, the message was clear: being separated from their families. The recent legislation recognises the importance of maintaining family links wherever possible. The importance of taking the child's wishes into account in decision-making is also enshrined in the legislation. Why, then, are so many children expressing dissatisfaction with the amount of family contact they have?

Education

...The majority of school-age children felt that being in care had improved their performance at school, and reported attendance rates were surprisingly high. It should be borne in mind, of course, that these are entirely subjective reports, from the child's own perspective, but nevertheless are indications of generally positive feelings about education.

Without detracting from the clearly positive message emanating from the majority of school-age respondents, there should be no room for complacency in the interpretation of these findings. Improved performance is a relative term and may well represent a very minor improvement from a low starting point; low expectations and low attainment are often reported in relation to the education of *looked after* children. Equally, a child's use of the word 'always' when describing school attendance is unlikely to correspond exactly with school attendance statistics, and may be subject to all sorts of qualifications and rationalisations.

The fact that so few children, when looking ahead to their lives in five years time, saw themselves studying is perhaps further evidence of the relativity involved in this area. Whilst respondents may feel that things have improved at school and that they are making better progress in many respects, education does not appear to be regarded as being a realistic option in the long term for *looked after* children.

Homework is important to a child's educational progress and, with the government's recent recommendations of daily minimum amounts of homework for different age groups, is likely to remain high on the agenda in the future. It is a matter of concern therefore that so many respondents who attended school regularly reported never receiving homework. Is this an example of differential treatment or low expectations of children in care by schools? Many of those who do get homework lack the essential support in terms of a quiet place and access to equipment and help when needed. What can carers do to provide a more conducive environment for homework?

Health – physical and mental

There is something of a contradiction apparent in the findings relating to health education. Whilst a vast majority of respondents reported receiving helpful advice and information on a wide range of health issues, many nevertheless admitted to putting their health at risk in various ways. This suggests that, for whatever reason, health education messages are failing to engage many *looked after* children in a way which is perceived as meaningful or relevant to their lives. This may be an issue related to the self-esteem of the individual (which should in any case be addressed); it may also be related to the way in which health education is delivered. To what extent are innovative and imaginative ways of communicating health and safety information to vulnerable children being explored?

The research reveals that the health education needs of younger children were not being met to their satisfaction. Despite the large amounts of health advice apparently available – if not necessarily heeded – to the looked-after population in general, a high proportion of the under-11 age group did not feel sufficiently well-informed about growing up and body changes. Is 'health education' perceived as something required by teenagers only? Are carers fully aware of the needs of younger children, and adequately supported in delivering health and sex education?

Many respondents reported feelings of loneliness or isolation; such negative feelings were compounded by a lack of emotional support in the form of someone special to talk to. Is it possible to ensure that every child in care, or young person leaving care, has easy access to at least one such person? It does not seem to matter who the person is, whether a relative, friend, carer or professional, as long as they are able to 'be there' for the child.

Gender differences in relation to health and emotional issues should not be allowed to pass unquestioned. Why do boys and young men report receiving less health-related advice and support than girls and young women? Are they perceived by carers as having fewer needs or being less at risk? Or are they more reluctant to ask for advice?

Similarly, the fact that girls and young women were considerably more likely to report negative feelings (and less likely to report positive feelings) than boys and young men raises issues pertinent to addressing the emotional needs of both sexes. Girls and young women are expressing negative feelings about their experiences in care; they need to be listened to, supported, and their concerns addressed. Boys and young men, on the other hand, may need drawing out; it should not be assumed that all is well just because they say it is, or that there are no problems, just because none are mentioned.

Types of placement

Some aspects of being *looked after* are experienced in very much the same way across the board (for example 'being looked after' as the best thing about being in care, and separation from one's family as the worst). But, in other respects, the experiences of children in foster care appear to differ fundamentally from those in residential placements.

In some respects, foster placements appear to be more 'successful'; children in foster care feel more positive than in other sorts of placements, their attendance and enjoyment of school are enhanced and they receive more advice on health matters. For the majority of respondents in foster care, this was the case. However, these positive aspects are counterbalanced by a relatively poor level of awareness of the formalities and safeguards provided by the care system. Children in foster care were considerably less likely to be aware of having a care plan or of complaints procedures. Whilst there may be gains from the more personal care and attention provided by a foster placement, when it works, there are potential losses and risks involved in such isolation and ignorance if the placement does not work out.

The converse applies to those in residential care such as children's homes or secure units. In such settings there is a relatively high awareness of being part of a 'system' and the structures and formalities involved, such as care plans, access to files and complaints procedures. Whilst this may invoke feelings of regimentation and impersonality, it does at least provide an environment where children have a greater awareness of their rights and how to exercise them.

However, certain other, more negative, aspects of life in residential care which have been highlighted in previous research, are reinforced by this survey. The higher incidence of risk-taking involving smoking, drinking and abuse of drugs and solvents and poor educational indicators prevail within the residential sector.

It should not, however, be assumed that such contrasting experiences and outcomes are entirely due to the type of care involved. It is important to remember that the individual characteristics of children to a certain extent influence the type of placement provided, and that children in foster care are, on the whole, likely to have fewer problems than those in residential homes or secure units.

Moves and changes

...There is evidence suggesting that numerous moves and changes are associated with a wide range of negative indicators, particularly in relation to a child's education and emotional well-being. More than three-quarters of respondents had experienced at least one move, a substantial minority – including some of the youngest members of the sample – having moved ten or more times. Why are young people in care subject to so much disruption? How could this be avoided? Does enough planning go into selecting an initial placement? Is enough support provided to support and sustain existing placements?

Black children and young people

One of the findings of the survey was that, in some respects, the care experiences of Black children were very similar to those of White children. Where differences do exist, however, their significance should be explored, taking all the findings into account. For example, fewer than half of Black children reported that neither their carers nor other young people at their placement were from the same ethnic background as themselves. In considering this finding, it should be remembered that fewer than 5 *per cent* of Black children reported receiving racist treatment from social workers or carers, but that 19 *per cent* did report receiving such treatment from other young people at a placement.

Leaving care and future prospects

Whilst leaving care was not a subject explicitly addressed in the questionnaire, and care-leavers were not specifically targeted as respondents, nevertheless the findings uncover some relevant issues. A substantial – but unknown – proportion of respondents aged between 16 and 20 can be assumed to have left care already. This age group were particularly likely to report feeling lonely and unsupported. Clearly not enough is being done to support and assist these young people in their transition to independent life.

A broader but related point concerns planning and preparation for the future in general. The fact that a substantial number of respondents did not – or could not – respond to the question about their lives five years into the future should not go unremarked. Are children encouraged to plan beyond the next review meeting? How are aspirations and ambitions encouraged and nurtured?

Universal experiences – bad and good things about care

It was rather disheartening to find that the things that respondents most wanted to change about being in care had not altered at all in the five years since the *Not Just a Name* survey. Specific issues such as bedtimes, pocket money and freedom to go out were widely mentioned, particularly by those in children's homes. Of course, children and teenagers will always want more say in their lives, whether or not they are in care, and it would be ridiculous to suggest that all their demands are met. However, the strength and depth of feeling expressed in this survey suggests that perhaps more could be done in terms of consultation and compromise.

On a more positive note, a substantial number of *looked after* children clearly feel that they are really being cared for within the care system, as expressed in their response 'Having someone who cares' to the question 'What is the best thing about being in care?'.

Do we know enough about young people in care?

Finally, the research process uncovered the difficulties inherent in gathering comparable, consistent, comprehensive and up-to-date information about the looked-after population at a national level. If such data cannot be readily accessed, how can meaningful policy be developed?

The research did not attempt to investigate data-collection procedures and practices at local level, but would suggest that there is much to be gained from local research and consultation exercises. Are local authorities themselves doing enough to monitor the experiences of the young people they look after? Are they aware of particular local issues and needs? Is it assumed, for example, that every young person is aware of their care plan and how to make a complaint? How is information gathered and used? To what extent are young people themselves involved in the process?

Key points [from consumer views on the care system]

■ 'Having someone who cares' was the most frequent response to the question, 'What is the best thing about being in care?'
■ One in five respondents did not report anything positive about being in care.
■ Being separated from their family was the most common response to the question, 'What is the worst thing about being in care?'.
■ 15 per cent of the sample responded 'Nothing' when asked the worst thing about being in care.
■ Large numbers of respondents (particularly those in children's homes) expressed grievances about pocket money, bedtimes and freedom to be out.

SIXTEEN

CHILD POVERTY, OPPORTUNITIES AND QUALITY OF LIFE

David Piachaud

Source: *The Political Quarterly*, 2001, 72, 4.

Britain, as the Commission on Social Justice wrote in 1994, is not a good place in which to be a child. Since 1997 the Labour government has given clear priority to tackling child poverty and has set out the goal of abolishing it in a generation. What is the extent of the problem, and what has been achieved so far? In considering these questions, this article concentrates first on children's material circumstances; then the challenge of making further inroads into child poverty is discussed, looking at wider social influences on childhood, and acknowledging that the quality of children's lives and their opportunities in later life depend on much more than their material circumstances. In the final section it is argued that tackling poverty is not enough. There needs to be a much broader, radical vision of public policy for childhood.

Progress on child poverty

Four million children – one in three – live in poverty in Britain; this is the highest child poverty rate of any major industrialised country apart from the United States. Fifty thousand children aged 8–10 have nothing to eat or drink before going to school in the morning. Many leave school illiterate, innumerate, alienated and a danger to society.

While the experience of childhood is still dismal for millions of British children, this grim picture must be put in perspective. In global terms British children are relatively privileged; very few are seriously malnourished and all go to school. [...]

The government has tackled child poverty in three principal ways: by promoting paid employment through the New Deal and other measures to reduce unemployment; by redistributing money to children with the working families' tax credit, the children's tax credit and increased income support rates; and by tackling long-term causes of poverty such as teenage births and exclusion from school. The estimated impact of these measures is shown in Table 16.1. It will be seen that the measures taken have reduced child poverty by over one million or about one-quarter. This is a remarkable achievement and a good start towards the goal the Prime Minister set in 1999 of ending child poverty in a generation. Yet, despite this progress, child poverty remains much higher than in 1979; and in some respects what has been achieved so far was the easy bit.

In education, basic literacy and numeracy have been given priority, class sizes for under-sevens have been reduced and efforts are being made to reduce truancy and exclusion from school. School test results show these measures are beginning to lead to improved performance.

It is in relation to health that little progress has been made. Providing fresh fruit at some schools is a small gesture towards improving children's diets; obesity is increasing. Alcohol consumption among 11–15-year-olds, lured by the sweetness of alco-pops, more than doubled in the 1990s. Of 13-year-olds, 7 per cent are regular smokers; tobacco advertising and promotion remain unbanned. One-tenth of 11–15-year-olds use other drugs; both hard and soft drugs are increasingly consumed during childhood.

It is abundantly clear that there is a huge disparity in childhood experiences and life-chances. There is much evidence that child poverty is linked to later unemployment, lower earnings, higher mortality and more crime. Employment is closely related to educational level, and those with no qualifications face far worse prospects. Health inequalities remain large: infants born to fathers in unskilled or semi-skilled occupations have an infant mortality rate over 70 per cent higher than those of fathers in professional or managerial positions.

Child poverty and other disadvantages clearly diminish children's

Table 16.1 The impact of five Labour Budgets on child poverty

	All persons	Children		
		All	*One parent*	*Two parents*
Poverty rate,[c] April 1997 policy (%)	19.4	25.9	41.9	21.5
Poverty rate, Labour policy (%)	15.9	18.3	23.7	16.8
Reduction in poverty (%)	3.5	7.6	18.2	4.7
Reduction in poverty (000)	2020	1000	520	480

Source: D. Piachaud and H. Sutherland, 'Child Poverty: Progress and Prospects', *New Economy*, June 2001.
Note: [a] The poverty line is 60% of median equivalised household income before housing costs.

opportunities in life. They also diminish the whole society through the waste of potential, the alienation and disaffection with society that can result and their damaging consequences, and the deprivation of opportunities for succeeding generations.

The future challenge

Much has already been achieved in tackling child poverty: going further remains a formidable challenge.

[. . .]Tackling child poverty and reducing the number of families on very low incomes are important for any government concerned about inequality and social exclusion, and action in this area is something for which the Labour government can take considerable credit. But while it is a necessary condition it is not a sufficient condition for improving children's opportunities and the quality of their lives. Tackling child poverty is not enough.

What is of concern for the quality of children's lives and opportunities is not low family incomes in themselves, but their consequences – for nutrition, stress, lack of stimulating childhood experiences, exclusion from normal social activities. All these are linked to child poverty. It is irrelevant to argue, as some do, that there are many poor children whose upbringing and quality of life are much better than that of some 'poor little rich kids'; in general, poverty does diminish choice and opportunities. But more money is not of itself enough to enhance the quality of children's lives.

Will a reduction in child poverty improve the nutrition and health of children? Simply because worse health is associated with poverty, it does not follow that less poverty will result in better health. Certainly increased income improves spending power. But the nutrition of many children is poor for a combination of reasons. First, in many areas the foods on offer are limited: many peripheral housing estates have only a corner shop with little or no fresh food and high prices. Many of the poorest families lack the mobility to reach the supermarkets which offer more choice and lower prices. Second, families are bombarded with disinformation promoting processed junk foods, crisps and soft drinks – Coca-Cola, for example, spent billions sponsoring the football World Cup to link their product with health and fitness. Third, many parents know next to nothing about nutrition, having learned nothing from their own parents or their schools. Prosperity and falling child poverty have certainly resulted in improved nutrition for many, perhaps most, children; but for a growing number of children the result has been obesity and damaged health in childhood and later life.

The same story could be told about alcohol, tobacco and other drugs. Higher incomes do not necessarily result in improved quality of life for children. [. . .]

One of the key influences on children's material and cultural environments is television. The complex relationship between the media, the quality of children's lives and child poverty is one that cannot be ignored. Virtually all households with children now have television (and most also have videos). In 1997 three-fifths of children aged 9–11 had a television in their bedroom, as did nearly half of 6–8-year-olds: three times the proportions in France, Germany and the Netherlands. The average time spent watching television by children aged 6–17 in the UK in 1997 was 2 hours 30 minutes per day, with another half-hour spent watching videos (Livingstone and Bovill, 1999). Over a year this amounts to over 1,000 hours in front of a TV screen. This may be compared with less than 100 hours, on average, spent reading non-school books, and about 750 hours per year spent in school classes.

[...] Commercial pressures only add to the difficulties of families living in or close to poverty – and hardly assist those on higher incomes. The needs of children – beyond basic food, clothing and heating – are socially defined. Middleton *et al.*'s study of family budgeting found intense pressure on children to have and do things if they are not to be socially and educationally excluded (Middleton *et al.*, 1994). They showed the strength of peer group pressures among children not only to wear the right *things* but also to wear the right designer *brands*; the case is cited of a 13-year-old girl who got beaten up just because her trainers had the 'wrong' label. This pressure is transmitted to parents, often by 'pester power'. The concern of parents, particularly poor parents, to maintain their children's social standing may make such pressures irresistible. Thus, if socially defined needs increase, unless resources increase too then the result is more poverty. Government attempts to tackle child poverty may be doomed to failure if new 'needs' are created by commercialisation faster than any rise in family incomes. Limiting the pressures that over-extend needs may be essential if child poverty is to be effectively tackled; without doing so incomes may never be adequate, except for those engaged in the exploitation of children.

Is it possible to limit the commercialisation of childhood? Certainly it is not easy. [...] Unlimited commercial pressures on children are incompatible with goals such as improving educational opportunities for all, overcoming child poverty and giving freedom to children to develop without exploitation – goals on which the future of society depends.

A broader strategy for improved quality of children's lives

[...] That the influences on children's lives and opportunities are complex is, as illustrated here, not exactly rocket science. Reducing child poverty requires not only adequate incomes but also a limit to commercial pressures, educated and informed consumers, and access to high-quality and reasonably priced food and other goods. Improving education requires not only good schools with highly motivated teachers, but also supportive media and active parental involvement and encouragement. Improving health requires not only a good health service but also – and probably much more importantly – a good diet, less smoking and drinking, and more exercise. In each case the government is actively and genuinely concerned with the 'not only' part, but is virtually ignoring the 'but also'.

The lack of breadth of vision suggest the government's efforts will have only a marginal impact on the quality of children's lives. The opportunities of children are affected by:

a) the families into which they are born and raised;
b) the environment in which they live – physical, social and cultural; and
c) government provision for education, childcare, health and measures to tackle child poverty.

All these interact. The government's Sure Start programme is seeking to influence a), and crime and neighbourhood renewal measures are focused on b). But the largest part of government efforts to improve children's opportunities is directed at c). Let us take a look at each element in turn.

a) In the past the family has been considered a private sphere, and children the chattels of their parents. The only substantial intervention has been to protect children from dangerously violent parents – with limited success. Virtually nothing has been done to improve poor parenting. While parenting is lauded as being of crucial importance to society, parenting skills have to be learned almost entirely by observation or by trial and error. Citizenship may have crept on to the school curriculum, but more basic skills for life have not. It is small wonder that many children of poor parents who may be financially rich or poor) become in their turn poor parents.

b) The physical environment is in many respects worse than in the past, with neighbourhoods seen as less safe, with less opportunity for play and exploration, and more time spent indoors. The social environment for many children is also deteriorating, with neighbours afraid to exercise the guidance and social contact that can help to socialise children for fear of accusations of interference or worse. The idea that children are the concern of everyone seems to be waning. The cultural environment in many ways contributes to a curtailment of childhood and to the treatment of children as commodities and consumers, as discussed above.

c) The Labour government has made much progress in terms of service provision and redistribution, although, again as discussed above, much more remains to be done. But ensuring opportunity for all cannot be achieved with these measures alone. The influence of family and environment – physical, social and cultural – on opportunities is so important that if opportunities are to become more equal, then family and environment must become of more public concern. The boundary between the private and public must be reassessed.

At this point a baying chorus of privileged neo-liberals – including some in the present government – decry any intervention in the private sphere as the 'nanny state' or 'social engineering'. Parents must be free to assault their children violently, to neglect them and to ruin their lives and their opportunities, because families are a private matter. This is dangerous nonsense. If children have rights, then these must be protected. Such protection must extend far beyond the protection of children whose safety is at risk. Damilola Taylor was not 'at risk': yet he lived in a social, physical and cultural environment that resulted in his violent death aged ten.

There are few parents who do not see some aspects of their environment as threatening to their children – whether the danger be from motorists and transport ministers – who choose speed over child safety, from hostile and discriminatory neighbours who threaten the peace of mind, even the survival, of minority children, or from the corrupting influences of media that wish to turn small children into profitable consumers who pester their parents and think the right logo will give meaning to their lives. Yet these threats are treated by many as inevitable and immutable, and the assumption is widespread that it is for the children's parents to protect them or warn them of the dangers – although we know full well that many parents will not or cannot do so. It is as though collective action has been forgotten because it is only children who are being victimised.

It is surely time to think about what we want childhood to be and what we want as a society for children and for their futures. It is sad but true that far more coherent thought, discussion and legislation has been concerned with the rights of women, of disabled people, and of ethnic minorities than with the rights of children. Unknown to most, the UK government was a signatory to the UN Convention on the Rights of a Child. Even though it lacks the force of law, this document sets out rights most people think desirable, for example, rights to education, health, protection from violence and abuse, a standard of living adequate for physical, mental, spiritual, moral and social development, and to freedom from economic exploitation. If the government thinks these are rights children should enjoy, then it should start thinking much more broadly than it has so far about how it can make them a reality; if it does not think they are appropriate, it should say so.

What seems lacking within government is a serious strategy to shift the manifold influences on children's lives towards goals that focus on the quality of children's lives – goals of achieving childhoods that are, as far as possible, happy, healthy and fulfilled and that nurture young people who are civilised and educated. Socialisation of children into humane, respectful and tolerant human beings is incompatible with increasing privatisation of children's lives. Education to develop children's full potential is incompatible with increasing exploitation of children as consumers and commodities.

The experience of childhood has been much improved in recent years in some respects, but not in all. Much remains to be challenged and changed if there are to be genuine opportunities for all. Children's opportunities depend ultimately on the society in which they are born and raised. As Robert Kennedy wrote:

> Too much and too long, we seem to have surrendered community excellence and community values in the mere accumulation of material things. Our gross national product ... counts air pollution and ciga-rette advertising, and ambulances to clear our highways of carnage ... Yet the gross national product does not allow for the health of our children, the quality of their education, or the joy of their play. It does not include the beauty of our poetry ... It measures neither our wit nor our courage; neither our wisdom nor our learning; neither our compassion nor our devotion to our country; it measures everything, in short, except that which makes life worthwhile.

REFERENCES

Livingstone, S. and Bovill, M. (1999) *Young People New Media*, Report of the Research Project 'Children, Young People and the Changing Media Environment'.

Middleton, S., Ashworth, K. and Walker, R. (1994) *Family Fortunes*. London, Child Poverty Action Group.

SEVENTEEN

COMMUNITY CARE AND INDEPENDENCE: SELF-SUFFICIENCY OR EMPOWERMENT?

Ayesha Vernon and Hazel Qureshi

Source: *Critical Social Policy*, 20, 2.

In the UK there is currently a new focus on the basic purpose and object-ives of services, not on organizational structure or the efficiency of the systems alone, but on the outcome of services for people who receive them. The Labour government has defined the promotion of independence as a priority for health and social services, but this outcome can be interpreted in a variety of ways which may not be compatible. As part of a pro-gramme of research into identifying ways of measuring the outcomes of community care, views about outcomes have been gathered from a number of stakeholders – disabled and older service users, family members and social service staff. [. . .]

The programme as a whole included group or individual discussion with 127 service users, 39 of them adults below pension age. The detailed analysis given in this article [is] from two discussion groups and five indi-vidual interviews involving adults below pension age with physical impair-ments.

[. . .]

Outcomes and the meaning of independence

Users identified a number of outcomes, some of which were currently being achieved, and some of which they felt would, if achieved, enhance their quality of life. These included a number of linked outcomes related to the business of daily living such as personal cleanliness, a clean home to one's own standard, ability to move about freely at home and freedom to move about outside so as to maintain social contact and interesting activities. These were continuously underpinned by issues of choice, independence and control over one's life. . . .

Personal cleanliness and comfort

Feeling clean and at ease with oneself was crucial when defining one's quality of life:

> Quality of life is knowing that you're comfortable with yourself and that can be from getting dressed in the morning, washed, feeling that you're clean, you can then face your day comfortably.

[. . .] Quality standards relating to inputs, such as an all-over wash once a week, do not guarantee the required outcome from a user perspective.

> I need washing from top to bottom because I can't wash myself and I can't get behind to wash myself . . . I'm a big lady and I smell . . .

A substantial majority of participants felt that *a clean home to a self-defined standard* was very important:

> The quality of life is knowing that the house is as (you) would like to keep it. There's nothing more frustrating than looking at something. I had a mirror installed in my bathroom and the dust from the wall fell below the sink level near the wall. Every time I went to the toilet I saw this dust, I couldn't reach it and it went on for three months before I realized I could get home help and finally I got this damn wall cleaned. It's keeping your house the way you want to and being comfortable in your own home.

Despite such feelings, a majority felt that cleaning was afforded a low priority by service providers. Consequently, some were forced to rely on family members who were themselves frail or unwell to help clean the house.

Being able to move about freely at home

Accommodation which is unsuitable for a person's physical needs can undermine their quality of life in several different ways. For example, a participant who had arthritis reported how she often slept downstairs apart from her husband due to the difficulty with negotiating stairs. Inaccessible accommodation can also compromise personal hygiene and dignity [. . .]

Freedom of movement outside the home

Being able to go where you want and when you want was identified as one of the most critical factors in determining one's quality of life. One person reported that she had become virtually housebound since becoming impaired as she could not use public transport:

> Accessible buses would be a big help; since the injury to my back I've become a hermit. I stay at home all the time.

Others felt that although there were alternative means of wheelchair accessible transport available if required, having to book a week or more in advance undermined their quality of life:

> You can't be spontaneous and say I'd like to go to such a place today.

Being able to go where and when they wanted was also linked to being able to pursue some form of hobby or *leisure activity*. This was felt to be particularly important for those disabled people who live alone and are unemployed:

> To be able to follow some interests . . . so you don't just exist. You have actually got an interest in life whether it be tapestry or painting or whatever.

Similarly, *social contact and company* are valued because they prevent isolation and break the monotony of being confined in the home with nothing to do. [. . .]

Disagreements about priority outcomes

The definition of outcomes regarded by service providers as reasonable to expect seemed to some users to be pitched rather low. Whereas personal assistance within the home was readily accepted as a need (even if the user valued social contact more highly), support for integrated living was often viewed as a 'want', and thus defined by service providers as illegitimate, as the following comment from a homecare user demonstrates:

> There seems to be a split between needs and wants, days out are a kind of a want and you can really do without them. . . . I just feel that it's not unreasonable to have the occasional social event. . . . I don't think it's unreasonable to expect that, because it's something that non-disabled people wouldn't think unreasonable for themselves to be doing. . . .

[. . .]

Control over services

Thus, for these individuals, independent living is about access to and control of a range of community-based services which enable them to identify and pursue their own lifestyle. The opportunity to employ people of their own choice to provide the assistance needed gave those using the local personal assistance scheme more control over their lives:

> I have two personal assistants working for me and basically they can do anything that I need doing. . . . The advantage of that is that you pick somebody . . . I know who's coming, . . . it's a matter of choice and flexibility because, . . . if I needed extra hours, I could ask one of my PAs to spend a whole day with me if that's what I wanted from that particular day so it gives you more of a choice.

[. . .]

Clearly, choice, flexibility and control over when and how support is provided is at the heart of maintaining quality of life, and, as summed up by one user in our study, an integral part of what is meant by independence:

> I think the whole thing we're talking about is maintaining independence, being able to live your life the way you choose to live it.

Choice about sources of assistance was part of independence, for example people might prefer to receive services rather than be dependent on family or friends. Where services were inadequate to achieve desired outcomes, then people remained dependent on informal help [. . .]

Attitudes towards self-sufficiency and autonomy

Staff did argue that there were individuals who, in their view, preferred to remain dependent, and to have tasks performed for them which they could have undertaken themselves. However, these instances were regarded by staff as exceptional. The general view from our discussions with disabled people was that they do not want to be passive recipients of services. Some wanted help if tasks took too long, and/or required too much effort. Others, however, preferred to do tasks themselves, whatever it took, and enjoyed the sense of achievement, self-worth and independence this provided. [. . .]

Having roles 'taken over' and being given no opportunity for participation, and no say in how things were done, could be a painful experience, particularly when the obligations of parenthood were involved:

> You should get involved in whatever they're doing, like if it was caring for your children, you should be involved like sitting and talking while your kids are in the bath. I always got ushered out the bathroom so I never felt part of caring for them . . . I felt like I was in the way.

[. . .]

Another user pointed to the variability of her needs for assistance, and the importance of help being available when she needed it:

> I have a lot of carers coming in to see to me. I have one about five to eight in the morning and she . . . helps do things, you know, she gets me my slippers on, because I can't get them on . . . and then I get washed and if I need help to dry and put my clothes on. Sometimes I'm worse than others with the arthritis and if I'm stuck, well she'll help me.

The key factor in this is choice and control: being able to choose the occasion and degree of assistance required to enable the person to reach the outcomes they define as important in the way they prefer. [. . .]

Disabled people's views on quality

Definitions of quality from the perspective of those on the receiving end of services may be considerably different from those of professionals and service agencies. The earlier discussion of outcomes has a number of implications for definitions of quality from a user perspective. Service users are more interested in what services can do for them, in the effect on their lives. They also emphasize that the way in which services are delivered – the extent to which the behaviour of workers is or is not empowering – is a crucial and necessary component of quality (Beresford, 1997). The definition of quality in service provision is value-led as Priestly (1995: 7) points out:

> Definitions of quality (used to judge both disabled people's quality of life and the quality of the services available to them) are derived from and determined by a variety of dominant and oppressive social values about the role of disabled people in society . . . in this way the social construction of quality is inextricably bound up with the social construction of disablement.

[. . .]

Participants were asked what made a good quality service and what a poor one. Poor quality services failed to deliver the outcomes identified, thereby undermining independence. An ideal service was identified as one in which people had a say in how things were done, and, if desired, had assistance to perform tasks themselves.

Having a say – control over services and meeting user-defined standards

Control over the people who might provide a service and over the timing of tasks were both important, because they affected the likelihood of satisfactory interactions with staff and the degree to which people could achieve their own goals, for example, could meet the standards of parenting which they found acceptable:

> When I came out of hospital . . . the home help didn't come till half past eight (or) nine o'clock. But my children get up at half past six. . . . By which point [my youngest son] has gone a full night with a nappy on. It's just a general restriction all the time because you have to stick to set hours . . . it's just the lack of control that's the main problem.

The users have no part in the recruitment process for these people working for the agency. It's the lack of control. . . .
[. . .]

Competence

Competence was usually defined in terms of ability to achieve user-defined standards, being well-informed about the user's individual needs and ensuring that these were met. There was evidence of variable standards of home care, with some services being of an unacceptably low quality, for example, where cups were inadequately rinsed after being cleaned with disinfectant. There were particular concerns over the standards of domestic cleaning and cover at weekends and evenings.

Waiting times

Delays in obtaining needed assistance were criticized. Participants felt that the delay between initial request and assessment was too long, and were particularly concerned about the time they had to wait between assessment and the provision of equipment or adaptations. Such delays undermined their independence and sense of control over their lives [. . .]

Information to support choice

Lack of information on what services are available is often cited as a barrier by disabled people to their achieving a range of opportunities and services (Evans, 1998). [. . .] As the old adage says, knowledge is power. Without adequate knowledge of services, individuals are powerless and dependent on the judgement of professionals. Not surprisingly, then, there is an overwhelming consensus among all user groups of the value and necessity for clear and accessible information so that they can make informed choices about what services will best meet their needs:

> I think it's nice actually to know what they are specifically. Now I can assess better in my mind whether I actually want to use it or not, if I know what the thing out there is.

Most felt that they had no way of accessing such information. Therefore, it was greatly appreciated when on a rare occasion a social worker had listed all the options available:

> She said 'Now let me tell you what we can provide you if you need it'.

And she spelled out everything that I could, all the services I could get ... who to call and what to ask for. . . .

[. . .]

Value for money

The introduction of charges had undoubtedly concentrated people's minds on the question of value for money, and perhaps had the positive consequence that it led to less tolerance of unsatisfactory services. Value for money was inextricably linked with competence, achievement of desired outcomes and the degree of control users had over services. People felt that if they were paying for a service, it should be of an acceptable standard; they resented paying for a substandard service:

> Well I actually had to end my private agency service for the same reason, being on income support. £4 plus out of your money each week was a lot of money to pay for somebody who did something so unprofessionally.

Value for money was essentially defined in terms of achieving user-defined standards:

> Half the time you find somebody to do your ironing and my friend she'd have to come round and do it again ... I got to the stage of thinking 'I am paying for this service'. I felt awful phoning up and saying 'This person cannot iron' or 'This person cannot do this'.

Being asked to pay for a service even when it was not delivered was also an issue:

> Twice they didn't turn up when they were supposed to and they didn't let me know either. So I was left without being washed and I still had to pay the full money and I was narked over that.

Participants were concerned that the introduction of charging for services might prevent people from taking up services they needed, and staff, in their discussion groups, reported instances where they felt that people had refused services which they needed because of unwillingness to pay charges.

Staff attitudes

People's perceptions of the quality of service they were receiving were, to a large extent, shaped by the attitude of the workers who provided the service: [...]

> My family aide worker, she ... dealt totally with my children on a one to one. ... And by the time she came to leave, my children were heart-broken ... because she ... wasn't a family aide worker by the end of it, she was a friend. I mean I'd have trouble like I say with the home help shopping, she'd throw me in back of her car and whip me up shopping. And we didn't tell anyone we were doing it.

[...]

In contrast were examples where staff focused too heavily on the impairment rather than the individual:

> Sometimes they can be really negative about you, rather than having a positive approach. They don't see you as a person, they just see you as a disabled person not being able to do things ... it used to undermine my confidence and I had very low self-esteem.

Undoubtedly, therefore, the single most important factor identified by service users in determining a good quality service was the attitude of those providing the service. [...]

Respect, dignity, being treated equally, trust and reliability were all identified as critical factors in how service users felt about the service they received. At their best, relationships with staff maximized choice and control, reinforced self-esteem and dignity, and made users feel genuinely valued and cared for; at their worst, they could enforce dependency and passivity, erode self-esteem and be intrusive.

Conclusion

[...]

The outcomes outlined in this article can be a basis for defining the objectives of social services for disabled people and can provide a basis for understanding quality. A quality service from a user perspective is one which delivers the outcomes users are seeking, both in terms of specific aspects of quality of life (such as personal cleanliness, ability to move around freely both in the home and outside, parenting one's own children and accessing meaningful activity and social participation) and also in terms of the important aspects of process (enabling people to have control over their lives, being treated as valued human beings with legitimate needs, being able to choose when to have, and not to have, assistance in relation to their personal goals and preferred ways of living). These outcomes can apply without difficulty to interagency activity: indeed inputs across several agencies may be essential to achieve them. The accounts of workers who did provide information for choice, and who did respond to a disabled mother's own perceptions of her needs, illustrate that the desired quality can be delivered through conventional services, as well as direct payments, but other accounts suggest that the commitment to promoting independence in the sense of autonomy remains limited.

[. . .]

REFERENCES

Beresford, P. (1997) 'Identity, Structures, Service and User Involvement', *Research Policy and Planning* 15(2): 5–9.

Evans, C. (1998) 'User Empowerment and Direct Payments', in S. Balloch (ed.) *Outcomes of Social Care: A Question of Quality.* Social Services Policy Forum Paper, No. 6.

Priestley, M. (1995) 'Dropping "E's": The Missing Link in Quality Assurance for Disabled People', *Critical Social Policy* 44/45: 7–21.

EIGHTEEN

VIRTUES AND VALUES

Stephen Pattison

Source: 'Virtues and values', *The Faith of the Managers*, London, Cassell, 1997.

[. . .] The rhetoric of ethics and values, expressed in the high tones of moral vision, runs deep in some parts of management theory (see Beauchamp and Bowie, 1993; Solomon, 1993). It is difficult, however, to evaluate how far moral vision affects practice. Within the British public sector, finding ways of articulating and interpreting ethical and value issues for managers and groups has been problematic. The importance of recognizing and dealing with these issues in management has been equalled by a corresponding ignorance of how to do it.

I . . . look at concern for ethics and values within public service management as a way of highlighting some of the problems that arise when organizations and their managers aspire to be ethical and moral.

Explicit concern about ethics in the public sector

Explicit concern about ethics and values has only recently become an important feature of organizational management in the public sector. A number of factors have contributed to this change.

First, the whole management function has become more important and significant. It has been revised and upgraded to become more 'professional'. There are now, for example, attempts to specify common standards and skills for managers. It is usual for professions to have a code of ethics to which members are required to adhere. This helps regulate standards, as well as enhancing clear professional identity.

At a more practical level, significant decision-making and responsibility have been devolved downwards to smaller independent purchaser and provider units. In the absence of precise central guidance, many managers perceive a fairly urgent need for greater guidance and for more skills of value judgement, for example in trying to determine how resources should be deployed on behalf of a local community. In the past, it was mostly professionals who were perceived as needing to make overtly ethical decisions; now this responsibility is shared by managers.

Ethical and value issues become both more apparent and more contested when radical change takes place. Custom, tradition and 'common sense' can no longer serve as a complete guide to behaviour. Public service organizations have undoubtedly experienced radical change over the last few years. Many of the changes which have taken place have been driven by a powerful moral vision of free-market values. This has served to make ethical concerns more visible.

There is now an ethical and value 'market-place', as much as in any other kind of market-place, in the public sector. Lack of specific guidelines coupled with organizational change and fragmentation in public services controlled by local contract rather than direct central management means that the details of responsibility and judgement are not filled out. Individual managers at the local level therefore have a clear responsibility to formulate and choose their own values and ways of realizing them.

Public bodies have become much more politicized and overtly value driven. Politics, however, which from Plato onwards has been the art of debating social values and determining the public good, has been edged out of the public domain with the exclusion of elected, representative politicians from responsible bodies. This has left an ethical vacuum which contributes to the present need to develop managerial ethical codes, competence and awareness as a partial substitute. As in the world of business, from which managerialism has taken much, the place of politics is taken by ethics. At the same time, the consensus on the Welfare State and the meaning of the public-service ethic has disappeared (see Klein, 1989). We are in a period of exploration and change.

Ethical issues and dilemmas

That managers in the public sector face important ethical issues and dilemmas is not in doubt. Here is a list of issues that might face any manager in health care:

- How are the competing interests of the individual patients and patients as a group to be reconciled?
- How are competing principles of individuality, privacy, preservation from harm, informed consent and professionalism to be harmonized?
- How should scarce resources be allocated between different needy and deserving groups?
- What weight is to be given to patients' preferences/beliefs?

■ Does respect for the autonomy of individual patients override the health of the nation, for example in immunization and screening campaigns?

■ Which professionals should have the dominant voice in making decisions about individual patients or indeed about the allocation of resources?

■ What is the role of managers in inter-professional disputes?

■ To what extent should managers act as champions of those like elderly and mentally ill people whose rights may be threatened?

■ When is it right to intervene in someone's life for their own benefit but against their will?

■ What significance and resources should be given to health promotion and illness prevention for the sake of generations yet to come when present needs of sick people are still unmet?

■ What responsibility does the manager have to the general public as opposed to the health care services?

■ How much should a manager tell members of the public about health service plans – what obligation does she have to inform and consult with the public about proposals which may affect their future?

■ What personal ethical and religious beliefs and practices should be tolerated and encouraged by the manager within her organization?

■ How should a manager behave ethically towards her employers and her employees?

■ How should ethics impinge upon contracting with its competitive and therefore secretive implications?

■ What is the relationship between the law and ethical principles, for example that of confidentiality? (adapted from Wall, 1989)

These issues have been supplemented and sharpened by various difficulties and problems that have arisen recently. For example, there are concerns about probity in corporate governance, corruption and failure of judgement in public bodies, and the increasing need to make conscious, controversial decisions about the use of ever-scarcer resources. In these circumstances, it is not surprising if public-service managers feel a bit at sea, rather confused and isolated, terribly responsible for many things at different levels and needing to get it right first time, without really knowing what 'right' means any more.

Strategies for filling the ethical vacuum

In the absence of any clear, easily accessible guidance from ethical tradition and of authoritative consensus on methods to be used or values to be adopted, various strategies have been employed to fill the ethical vacuum between legal requirements and individual conscience in public-service management. Central government has tried to provide guidelines for corporate governance to enhance its reliability and credibility (Department of Health, 1994). Professional bodies like the Institute of Health Services Management have issued statements of values which provide some guidance for managers, but only at a high level of generality (Institute of Health Services Management, 1994). There is some impetus towards providing detailed codes of practice for managers that are modelled on the professional codes of, for example, doctors or nurses. Here there is the danger either of vagueness or over-specificity for managers who may have to deal with very different issues in different contexts in different ways. To help overcome these problems, some people suggest that the main thing is for organizations at a local level to develop their own philosophies and codes, formulated as a kind of ethical 'Ten Commandments' which can be hung upon the wall of every office and against which behaviour may be measured.

Some managers repose much of their hope for responsible, ethical decision-making and behaviour in consulting with the public by various means, for example using referenda or reference panels on priorities and resources. [. . .] In practice, such populist methods often yield results that would be professionally unacceptable, giving, for example, low priority to mental health needs or the needs of the elderly. Another method that may be used to supplement management decision-making is the employment of utilitarian techniques like 'QALYs' (Quality Adjusted Life Years). [. . .]

All the above techniques and initiatives contain elements of arbitrariness and subjectivity. At best, codes, QALYs and the rest are simply guides and aids to judgement. They cannot remove the responsibility for judgement, decision and action from individuals and groups of human beings. Managers play a crucial role in ensuring that appropriate decisions are made in ethical ways. To do this they need the confidence and skills of appropriate ethical judgement and discernment. If these skills and this confidence are not easily to be found (and presently they are not) a real vacuum of moral responsibility can emerge.

[. . .]

The inevitability of values and ethics

While attempts to help managers manage more ethically in both private and non-profit organizations are still in their infancy, this does not mean that organizations lack ethos, norms and practices, some of which are explicit, others implicit and unacknowledged. Organizational members 'swim' in a sea of values, adding their own value preferences together with the ethical decisions and performances to this sea. It is not a matter of choosing whether or not to have ethics and values in management. Rather, it is a question of which values should be selected and affirmed and whether to be unconscious and uncritical or conscious and critical of them.

I [now] examine one of the ways in which ethos and values are incul-

cated in the individual by the process of Individual Performance Review
(IPR). [. . .]

Governing the soul: appraisal and Individual Performance Review

Appraisal, or IPR, is, in some ways, the most personally immediate sign
and sacrament of the modern managed organization. In most organizations, some kind of appraisal or performance review is now mandatory
for employees. It has been one of the elements of private-sector management practice that the British government has been most keen to promote
right across the public sector. Many charities and non-profit organizations
have also introduced it voluntarily in the name of good management practice.

The nature of appraisal

Systems of appraisal, and the uses to which it is put, vary between and
even within organizations. Three elements are typical of all appraisal
schemes. First, it is usually individual performance that is the subject of
appraisal: individuals are usually appraised by a single other individual
who often has direct managerial oversight of their work. Second,
appraisal requires assessment of past performance against previously
agreed goals or targets. Third, goals and targets are set for future
performance.

Appraisals may take place annually, or more or less often. Appraisal
can be linked to the judgement of whether an individual should receive
additional reward . . . or to the planning of career development and dis-
cerning training needs. Some appraisal systems use a standard form or
format for all employees of a particular kind. Others work with a 'blank
sheet' upon which the appraisee assesses him or herself . . . Like many
types of management technology, appraisal is usually aimed at ensuring
that employees understand and assimilate the objectives and goals of the
organization and their function within it so that they can bend their efforts
to the corporate purpose. Being linked to the overall future-oriented
vision, aims and objectives of the organization, the setting of performance
goals and targets inevitably contains an imperative to personal change.
Although some goals and targets will be about maintenance, that is carrying on doing what needs to be done, the implicit thrust of much appraisal
is towards change and development.

The advantages of appraisal

In a history spanning more than 40 years, appraisal has become steadily
more universal throughout organizations and a staple element of personnel

management. It has many enthusiasts and defenders. It has been character-ized as 'a key management system by which the effectiveness of individual managers is assessed and developed' (Flanagan and Spurgeon, 1996: 67). Its advocates argue that it has many benefits. It gives managers a chance to assess the human resources at their disposal and objectively to review the work and skills of their subordinates so that they fit in with overall organi-zational needs and objectives. It permits a systematic and objective view of an individual's total performance. Career counselling and career develop-ment can be planned using appraisal. It can also be used for planning succession to different posts, assessing suitability for promotion, for identifying problems and poor performance, and for improving perform-ance. [. . .]

From the appraisee's perspective, appraisal may allow for the recogni-tion of past achievement, a sense of being supported, open communication with superiors, and knowledge of how their role and efforts contribute to the overall organizational task. Regular appraisal permits weaknesses and training needs to be identified and remedied, as well as giving a sense of progress and movement within an occupational role. [. . .]

Problems with appraisal

From this kind of description, it might be concluded that appraisal is a kind of universal panacea for the management of people, the holy grail of personnel work. However, even protagonists of appraisal point out some important limitations of this activity.

For appraisal to be effective, a large number of conditions must be met. The objectives of any appraisal scheme must be very clear. If too many objectives have to be met, for example reviewing past performance, deciding on performance-related pay, identifying development needs and opportunities, then a scheme may well fail to meet them. Similarly, some purposes and objectives may conflict; for example, it is unlikely that someone is going to be honest about their failures and performance defects if the appraisal is to be used to determine pay or promotion prospects. Organizational objectives and definitions of effectiveness must be clear if appraisal is to be used to set individual targets. If appraisal is to work well, it should be introduced with the active consent of the workforce. Further-more, it must be an integrated part of a whole philosophy and style of management, not an afterthought, or a 'bolt-on'. This is particularly important if the needs and opportunities identified in appraisal are to be followed through. If there is no action as a result of appraisal, for example if time and money for training are not forthcoming, then people may become cynical and detached about it. Successful appraisal schemes should be flexible and develop over time with the changing needs of the organi-zation. The people who act as appraisers have to be skilled. They and their appraisees will require time to prepare for appraisal. It needs to be understood that honesty in appraisal sessions will not be punished and a non-judgemental attitude needs to be cultivated.

Beyond these ideal conditions, which are often not met in appraisal, there are a number of specific criticisms that protagonists make of appraisal systems. Some kinds of appraisal tend to focus on the traits and personality of the individual being appraised rather than upon actual behaviour and observable performance. The creation of goals and targets that extend only, say, over a twelve-month period can create a short-term view of the individual's role and function. Frequently, appraisal does not acknowledge or deal effectively with the fact that individual performance is often dependent upon, and embedded within, group activity. Then again, appraisal can be too static and infrequent; objectives may be set but not revised over time as situations change...

Appraisal easily becomes an end in itself, detached from other aspects of organizational life such as planning, pay and training. This makes it essentially a time-consuming irrelevance. It can also become too complex and too general, failing to provide swift, accurate and specific feedback to appraisees. If insufficient time is given to the development and implementation of appraisal schemes they often fail. If they are too rigorous and judgemental, appraisees may not be honest. They may then try to select low and loose aims and targets that they can easily fulfil. This can actually lead to diminished rather than improved performance. [...]

The critique of appraisal outlined above has been mostly constructed from sources that enthusiastically commend this activity as a key management tool. It shows that there are so many imponderables and things that can go wrong with appraisal, both in theory and practice, that it must be seen as a highly problematic activity. Most people working in managed organizations will recognize the difficulties and practical problems that arise in its implementation (hasty implementation, lack of employee participation and consent, failure to be non-judgemental and to follow through on needs identified etc.). Notwithstanding the fact that some people actually value appraisal and may feel that they get a great deal from it, the ubiquity and popularity of appraisal schemes which are time- and money-consuming would seem to require an explanation that goes beyond vigorous assertion of their self-evident value.

Appraisal as a mechanism of social control

At least one important, if often implicit, function of appraisal is to contribute to organizational discipline and social control of the individual employee. [...]

To produce employees who have internalized organizational norms and values, even to the level of conforming their emotional responses to that which is organizationally acceptable, requires concerted effort and considerable technology. The one-to-one, confessional aspect of appraisal is one important way in which people learn to internalize, or at least be constantly aware of the fact that their performance and behaviour is constantly being monitored. Performance and values may not be much altered by appraisal in concrete terms. However, the very process of having to account for one's work and activity reinforces the important value that individuals are personally responsible and must account to those who are 'above' them.

[...]

If appraisal systems are organizational 'cultural artefacts' that send out 'clear cultural messages', at least one important cultural message that most appraisal schemes send out is that people's lives and behaviours are constantly subjected to critical gaze from above. Even if individuals find ways and means to hide or partially hide from the all-seeing, appraising eye (which they do), the right to appraise undergirds the right to manage. It is an outward, powerful and visible manifestation of the ethos of top-down control that has enormous potential to produce guilt and shame in organizational members. This occurs almost independently of any particular values and behaviours that might be commended in any specific organizational appraisal process. As such, it can be a powerful symbol or sacrament of the absolute need for employee loyalty and obedience.

Paradoxically, the existence of highly visible external methods of surveillance like appraisal testifies to the continuing recalcitrance and ungovernable aspects of the humans who comprise the workforce, just as the existence of the confessional witnesses to the ineradicability of sin. [...]

REFERENCES

Tom Beauchamp and Norman Bowie (eds) (1993) *Ethical Theory and Business*. Englewood Cliffs, NJ, Prentice Hall, 4th edn.

Department of Health (1994) *Report of Corporate Governance Task Force*. London, Department of Health.

Hugh Flanagan and Peter Spurgeon (1996) *Public Sector Managerial Effectiveness*. Buckingham, Open University Press.

Institute of Health Services Management (1994) *Statement of Primary Values*. London, Institute of Health Services Management.

Rudolph Klein (1989) *The Politics of the NHS*. London, Longman, 2nd edn.

Robert Solomon (1993) *Ethics and Excellence*. New York, Oxford University Press.

Andrew Wall (1989) *Ethics and the Health Services Manager*. London, The King's Fund.

NINETEEN

'WE MUSTN'T JUDGE PEOPLE ... BUT': STAFF DILEMMAS IN DEALING WITH RACIAL HARASSMENT AMONGST HOSPICE SERVICE USERS

Yasmin Gunaratnam

Source: *Sociology of Health and Illness*, 2001, 23, 1.

[...] In this chapter, I will use the concept of 'dilemma' (Billig *et al.*, 1988) to examine and theorise aspects of anti-discriminatory practice in a hospice setting. [...] I argue that ... specific inter-relations between philosophies of hospice care and anti-discriminatory discourses play a significant role in constructing the nature of staff dilemma in their responses to incidents of racial harassment. I begin this analysis by first describing how dilemmas have been conceptualised by Michael Billig and his colleagues (1988), and then move on to explore representations of the anti-discriminatory dilemmas talked about by hospice staff.

Dilemmas

Billig *et al.* (1988) have used a rhetorical approach to argue that dilemmas are a ubiquitous part of everyday life in which both ideology (values and beliefs) and common-sense ('lived ideology') contain inherently contradictory themes. This social–psychological framework draws attention to the links between the structural–political foundations of ideology and individual representations and negotiations of meaning in everyday life. As such, ideology is not seen as dictating unproblematically the way in which individuals should think, feel or act. Rather, ideology and common sense are seen to consist of contrary themes that produce valuable dilemmas and 'puzzles'. [. . .]

Dilemmas for anti-discriminatory practice

Within St Elsewhere, a key site of tension in inter-cultural relations could be heard in re-occurring accounts of the racialising of public space within staff interviews. Staff often talked about finding themselves involved in the management of spatial boundaries between service users from different ethnic groups. Accounts included difficulties in managing 'noisy' mourning rituals in shared hospice bays (Gunaratnam, 1997), and the management of racism directed at staff and service users. Participants in all of the groups talked about racism from white service users as presenting significant and common dilemmas for practice. The following case discussed in a group with white British nurses, relates to a story in which a white Englishman was placed in a shared bay with three black men:

ROZ: It was the patient's wife who made racist comments and the patient never said 'yea' or 'nay'. And they were both white and then he, he was admitted into a bay that had three, um, three black men. Two from Jamaica and one from Ghana and, um she made loud racist comments that she thought it was disgusting that her husband should be in a bay with three black men on their own

KATE: (gasps).

INTERVIEWER: Did they, did these men understand and hear the –

ROZ: Oh yeah. Yes. One of them was, they were all, one was in his 50s and the two other were late 60s and were both very sort of gentle, god-fearing type men and, I think chose to let it wash over them. But the chap who was in his 50s was rightly angry about it and he's in fact one of the patients that I've learnt most from about dealing with that kind of situation when people are making racist comments. Because I felt incredibly embarrassed about it. I felt, really, really dreadful about it and this woman was making loud comments about 'How these dark people come in all loud during the day and night and they're noisy and they bring in smelly food' . . . (. . .). And he was angry that she was such a dreadful woman. He was angry at her and at her attitude. Um, and I, and amongst the staff as well, was always saying that we, that we welcomed all people regardless of colour that everybody was equal in our eyes and that her comments were not welcome. That they were racist. . .

INTERVIEWER: Was it one, was it one, one staff member who took responsibility for that or did it –?

ROZ: We had to respond to it as she said it, so that if she said something in our hearing, or directly to us. I mean I just couldn't believe how blatant she was, um, that we had to counter it at that point –

INTERVIEWER: And was that a decision taken at a team level or–?

ROZ: Yeah.

INTERVIEWER: Right

ROZ: And then, I, I didn't want my other patients to be exposed to this woman any longer, so we had a big debate about whether this white bloke should be moved into a, a side room and I felt that I didn't want my other patients to be exposed to his wife but I also felt that was giving his wife exactly what she wanted. So in the end I [. . .], I went and spoke with the, the chap who was in his 50s and just used him. It was happening over a weekend of course, so you don't have, I mean Social Work or Chaplaincy to talk to and try and mull over these issues.

GILL: That's right. Yeah.

ROZ: So I went and spoke to him, because he was, he was all sort of dynamic, business person, you know, really set up. He's coped with racism in this country and has, you know, has succeeded financially. So I actually went and picked his brains about it and he said 'No'. He felt that that man should stay there and that they would cope with it and the other three blokes were really supportive. And I think I learnt a lot about that and it also made me feel less frightened of actually discussing racism with, with people who aren't white because, I think I've always been embarrassed to sort of discuss it before, because I felt so shameful, so responsible for it.

Representations about the management of this incident of racial harassment, are framed in triumphalist terms, in which collaboration across a multiplicity of power relations (staff/service user, white/black, female/male) are represented as challenging racism, whilst also empowering the speaker. These representations are used in ways that enable Roz to talk about her own emotions and to speculate about the emotions of the black service users (particularly the younger man). Interestingly, although Roz aligns herself repeatedly with the black service users, and in opposition to the racist wife, her language in relation to emotions constructs boundaries of a racialised difference, in which her prevailing feelings of embarrassment and shame as a white woman are talked about in contrast to the apparent passivity of the older, 'god-fearing' men, and in her view, the justifiable anger of the younger black man. In this way, Roz's narrative also produces racialised and age-based differences within her normative evaluations of emotional responses to racial harassment.

Most markedly, despite the organisational and professional context within which the incidents had taken place, Roz talks about her emotional responses to the incidents in personalised terms. She draws upon anti-discriminatory discourses in describing her attempts to manage the wife's racist remarks. She does not initially, however, make reference to organisational responsibilities or boundaries; instead, appropriate responses to her dilemma of how spatially to contain the racism are said to have been negotiated and discussed with colleagues and with the younger, black service user. It is only as the discussion develops (in response to my following up of an earlier point), that another key source of dilemma is identified and explored: how and when is it appropriate to challenge racism by service users?

Challenging racism

INTERVIEWER: Gill, you were just talking about it earlier, when you were saying that, you know . . . people might make comments, but you make a decision at one point whether you're going to sort of counter that or not. So how do you make those kinds of decisions?

GILL: Well speaking personally, I always counter it but (sighs) –

INTERVIEWER: As, as soon as it happens, or – ?

GILL: Um, yeah, yeah. I mean it depends . . . on the comment, I suppose. But I, I would pick up on it and say, you know, I mean, it tends to be 'Darkies', as you (to Roz) said actually. A, a lot of my patients will refer to black people as 'Darkies', you know in a derogatory fashion. Um, . . . sometimes, you know they'll say it in a sentence and you think, 'did they just say what I thought they said?' And you know, so I wouldn't respond until I was completely sure maybe, or, or maybe I'd get on to, sometimes you can work, you know the conversation around to, you know – I don't know, just discussing, um, not you know, I wouldn't necessarily bring up black people, you know as a subject, but sometimes you can get around to it again and I, I would bring it up then.

INTERVIEWER: What kind of thing do you say?

GILL: Um (. . .), what kind of thing do I say? Um (. . .), I probably say, 'well, who do you mean? You know Darkies?' You know, if they're saying something like that, um, I say 'Well why are you calling, you know, people that?' you know and say to them that, that's not acceptable, 'They're human, just like you and I . . . What's the colour of a skin?' you know, but, I, I wouldn't be as cross as I would be socially if somebody had said that to me –

ROZ: Yeah (laughs).

GILL: I would, you know 'cause, I really, really let rip if someone was racist in front of me socially –

INTERVIEWER: So what's the difference?

KATE: We're professional.

GILL: Professional. That, that is the difference and, and I, to a degree, I am always worried that I'll upset my patient as well. I mean, my patient is my priority.

KATE: They can be very rude to us, but we can't actually.

GILL: Yeah. I do accept a lot of rudeness. I do accept a lot of rudeness to myself, but I, to another patient I wouldn't, you know, I mean, if they were, were very, you know, if I could hear a comment being said about another patient, it doesn't matter if it's a racial comment or whatever, I would always counteract back, you know, whether, or investigate what they, you know, if they're talking about, you know, but there is a professional limit, you know –

ROZ: Yeah, it's like we're, I, it's a really hard balance. I don't know if we ever get taught it –

GILL: Yeah. Yeah.

ROZ: It's like we're not here to judge. And there are some things that are blatantly outrageous and that affect other patients and therefore we have to counter it –

GILL: Yeah.

ROZ: But, there's other things, that, like if somebody makes a sexist comment or something like that (. . .). There, there are some that you just have to think 'Right, that's how they are', and there's others that really affect –

KATE: I suppose it's what –

INTERVIEWER: No, no, go on.

ROZ: I was saying, I suppose it's what you feel the sort of boundary within your institution is. But that's really hard. Like we have to be all-embracing. We mustn't judge people. We have people here who sort of, whose um, er, lust (laughs), I don't like or, I don't know (laughs). You know, there's things about them that I think 'ugh'. But yet I have to care for them and give exactly the same care and I think, I think the sort of, the (. . .) (sighs), no matter how racist somebody is there's, there's some point along the scale at which it's not, it's not acceptable and that you say something. But I couldn't tell you exactly where that is –

KATE: No.

ROZ: You'd have to give me hundreds of examples and –

GILL: Yeah, it's different –

ROZ: Yep, 'challenge that' and 'no that one would have to be put on hold'
. . . .

In exploring issues of anti-discriminatory practice within the discussion, it appears that for the nurses there are several facets to the dilemmas that they talk about. Throughout the discussion they talk about their responses to racial harassment and racism within the hospice as reflecting personal, professional and organisationally influenced choices. Such choices are portrayed as a part of broader, tried and tested strategies in which incidents are first 'investigated', contextualised, confirmed and challenged subsequently within universalistic discourses of 'sameness'. Significantly, appraisals of racist incidents and the choices that the nurses talk about in addressing them are far from consistent or straightforward, but are contoured by ambiguities and contradictions.

For example, a significant theme in the discussion arose when Gill introduced differences between her professional and social selves as also contouring the nature and forcefulness of her responses to racism. This narrative theme began by Gill suggesting that her professional role often acted to constrain her challenging of racist incidents. Here, discourses involving a primary concern for the wellbeing of the 'patient', together with more explicit gendered, professional themes of emotional control and distancing were used to justify imposed limitations upon her accounts of the challenging of racism. This scenario, however, is simultaneously undermined, and the dynamics affecting her reported responses are more qualified in her following more ambivalent statement that she would always interrupt and challenge racism towards other service users – within her professional 'limits'. [. . .]

Despite the 'messiness' of Gill's narrative, the dilemmas and themes within her account appear to be recognised, and are picked up and addressed by both Roz and Kate. The starting point in unravelling the dynamics of such professional responses for Kate, is that within their professional roles, nurses *have* to accept levels of 'rudeness' from service users. From Roz, there is the suggestion that such levels are negotiated intuitively within the *felt* boundaries of the organisation. Here she uses Kate's more general description of 'rudeness', to introduce issues of sexual harassment from service users. Within this context, dilemmas involving anti-discriminatory discourses of inclusion and non-judgemental care are positioned differentially onto gendered and racialised power relations and their relation to constructions of professionalism.

Through her example of sexual harassment, Roz suggests that despite her personal revulsion for such incidents, she is compelled by her professional role to inhibit how these feelings may affect her care. She further indicates that she is more tolerant of sexist behaviour from service users, drawing upon essentialist options to suggest that sometimes the extent of such behaviours are so deep-seated, that individuals are unchangeable, 'that's *the way they are*'. However, when she moves her focus onto incidents of racial harassment, no allowances appear to be made for the extent and nature of racism expressed by service users. Issues concerning the impartial delivery and quality of care are also left behind in favour of dilemmas concerning the calibration of 'acceptable' and 'unacceptable' levels of racism and the corresponding appropriateness of professional responses.

For Roz, Kate, and Gill a central part of the dilemmas they talk about involves the 'technical' difficulties of identifying absolute criteria against which judgements can be made about the challenging of racist incidents. The combined message is that: 'it depends'. Whether or not racism and racial harassment are challenged cannot be taught, but come down to intuitive matters of individual judgement (and by implication, dilemma) that have to be developed according to the dynamics of each case. Dilemmas are thus framed as a necessary and productive, although frequently hidden, part of anti-discriminatory practice, if only in relation to racism. In fact, a specific silence within the discussion relates to the differential investments that the nurses talk about in interventions around incidents of sexual and racial harassment, that construct a double-standard for levels of professional tolerance and practice.

[. . .]

Conflicting roles and expectations

[. . .] At the time of the fieldwork . . . St Elsewhere did not have a formal organisational policy for dealing with racial harassment. Within the context of this procedural gap, however, organisational initiatives on equalities issues were talked about as creating an ambivalent organisational atmosphere. The normative commitment to equal opportunities evident in this atmosphere was sometimes talked about as making it particularly difficult for staff to explore, and address openly, dilemmas of anti-discriminatory practice. As one member of staff put it:

> I feel that the climate now, with equal opportunities and everything, that it is unacceptable at a professional level to be racist. So it is really difficult to be able to ask for help, it would be a bit like identifying yourself as having racist tendencies . . . I think all the drive against racism in organisations has sometimes also been counterproductive and has pushed it underground. Racist people are more circumspect now, but for people who may be just naive, it is more difficult to ask for help. To come forward is a way of making yourself vulnerable and it's not easy to express and explore things. It feels very frightening and daunting . . .

By talking about the emotional impact of equal opportunity policies within the hospice, this part of the narrative also refers to processes of interaction and contradiction between the seemingly rationalistic frameworks of formal organisational initiatives and the emotional dynamics that surround them. Expressing ambivalence, ignorance or uncertainty about race equality issues within such a context is talked about as stigmatising, leaving no room for the tolerance of 'naiveté', or an exploration of matters where racism is implicated. There is a paradox here. The speaker uses her narrative to draw attention to the restrictive effects of the drive against racism. But her account can also be seen as providing evidence for the relative 'success' of equal opportunity initiatives in drawing upon and manipulating wider social norms to shape an organisational climate within St Elsewhere, where the overt expression of racism at a professional level is unacceptable.

The tensions in this instance are also positioned at the level of formal organisational policies and discourses that have to combine and use appropriate levels of challenge and support, structure and ambiguity, and rationalism and emotion to enable positive organisational changes. In order to be successful, for example, equality initiatives have to be seen to generate and police rationalistic, public, codes of discipline. These codes must challenge and deter discriminatory practices, whilst also enabling open questioning, communication, and a clear understanding of the organisation's goals in situations of difficulty and uncertainty. However, while certain aspects of such policies can provide guidance for work-place behaviours, they can only ever provide a framework for the development of meanings, attitudes or values that are honed in the detail of everyday practice.

It is here that the ideological nature of dilemmas has specific relevance and can be used to gain insights into more fundamental relations between the agency of individual practitioners and the structural limits within which they operate. . . . There were professional variations in the nature of talk about anti-discriminatory dilemmas within the hospice. Within these variations – that were related to the occupational structures, history and the organisational context of different professional groups – some individuals were better located to be able to address and challenge the ethnocentrism of particular hospice philosophies and models of care. Thus, although structural power relations and the ideologies that accompany them can be constraining, they are also vulnerable to the actions of individuals. Such actions and negotiations, however, also take place within structural limits (Connell, 1995), and it is in this vital area that further research and analysis is necessary if we are to gain a more multi-dimensional understanding of the nature of racialised power relations within health care organisations.

Conclusion

[. . .] Recognition of dilemmas can . . . be of practical value to service providers. For instance, because dilemmas are by their very nature unresolvable, it is inappropriate to impose and also to expect staff to follow a single, 'correct' line of action in relation to anti-discriminatory practice. The formal recognition of staff dilemmas can thus facilitate a move away from 'political correctness' to what Cohen has referred to as a 'relative autonomy' rule which recognises that a variety of different modes of intervention are required to address different sites and forms of racism: 'within the comforts of immutable definitions and impermeable boundaries, or the moral certitudes that go with them' (1992: 97).

Attention to dilemmas of anti-discriminatory practice can thus present positive opportunities for the development of policy and the emotional 'climate' surrounding equal opportunities within organisations, which may in turn help to transcend rigid and moralistic notions of 'correctness'. This does not necessarily mean that staff decision-making and practice should become unaccountable, or that feelings of 'getting it right' and 'getting it wrong' will disappear (Gunaratnam, 1997). Rather, it could mean that processes of searching for appropriate forms of professional practice, the discourses that different groups of professionals can draw upon, and the emotions that go with this, can be explored more openly as a valuable part of professional and service development.

REFERENCES

Billig, M., Condor, S., Edwards, D., Gane, M., Middleton, D. and Radley, A. (1988) *Ideological Dilemmas: a Social Psychology of Every Day Thinking.* London, Sage Publications.

Cohen, P. (1992) 'It's racism what dunnit': hidden narratives in theories of racism. In Donald, J. and Rattansi, A. (eds) *'Race', Culture and Difference.* London, Sage Publications.

Gunaratnam, Y. (1997) Culture is not enough: a critique of multi-culturalism in palliative care. In Field, D., Hockey, J. and Small, N. (eds) *Death, Gender and Ethnicity.* London, Routledge.

TWENTY

THE CONTRIBUTION OF RESEARCH FINDINGS TO PRACTICE CHANGE

Janet Lewis

Reading based on J. Lewis (2002) 'The Contribution of Research Findings to Practice Change', *MCC: Building Knowledge for Integrated Care*, 10, 1, 9–12

Introduction

There is now a great deal of talk about 'evidence-based practice' but few attempts to understand the relationship between evidence and practice, or to query what constitutes 'evidence'. In many ways evidence-based practice is a fashionable myth – and sometimes a con. This is not because evidence is unimportant, it is that it can be very difficult to decide what the 'evidence' is; and evidence can only ever be a small part of the package of what constitutes practice. Factors other than evidence are very important to practice development – the financial resources available; the skill of the people delivering the service; the extent to which there is organisational stability or upheaval; and what the core objectives of the organisation are. This means that practice can almost never be *based* on evidence – it can certainly be informed by evidence, and I think this is what we should be aiming for.

It can be a con because people will say 'we should do this because the evidence says so' when what they mean is that they think it should be done – and they have found a bit of evidence that they think confirms their view. This approach is particularly prevalent when, as now, policy and practice are expected to be evidence-based. This does create particular dilemmas for policymakers. After all, if you are in the business of policy change you are committed to particular perspectives. But really to assess the evidence, particularly when it is saying something counter to what you want to hear, requires you to be rather dispassionate. The two do not go easily together. Often, too, evidence is a threat – it can cast doubt on cherished assumptions and widespread practices. In these circumstances, it is often suppressed.

These problems around the concept of evidence-based practice do not mean that evidence is unimportant. Simply that there is a need to be aware that the evidence alone may be insufficient to bring about changes in practice. There is also a question of what constitutes 'evidence'. While it sounds easy, 'evidence' is not a straightforward idea. This chapter will elaborate on some aspects of this and then go on to examine the relationship between evidence and practice.

The lack of transferability of 'evidence-based practice' to social care

The idea of evidence-based practice started in medicine in relation to drug-testing and similar interventions. 'Evidence' was considered to be provided by the results of studies based on randomised controlled trials (RCTs). One difficulty in transferring this model of evidence to social care is that, by its very nature, it is very difficult to set up RCTs in relation to social care provision. Because of the pressure to move to an evidence-based approach, the neatly narrow definition based on RCTs has now expanded to cover all kinds of research – and, one sometimes thinks – all sorts of random good ideas as well.

The context for research in social care is that much of practice is based on individual professional judgement made within complicated contexts. The form of support and services offered in response to social care needs is much more varied than a more straightforward decision as to whether to prescribe one drug from a number that have been shown to be effective for a particular condition. The range of possible causes of people's social distress or difficulties means that the decision about the help to be provided is going to be taken in the light of a variety of factors. These involve very different situations to study in comparison with the circumstances in which a controlled drug trial is carried out. It is, however, possible to evaluate the impacts of the judgements that are made and draw some conclusions about 'what works' in social care. But the results of evaluations of social care are usually much less precise than whether using a particular form of treatment is successful.

There are, therefore, difficulties in producing the kind of results, within social care, that pass the threshold of what is considered 'evidence' in the medical field. This may be the reason for a further difficulty which is that the evidence of what works in practice has not been collected as routinely as it might be. Research on social care, as in many areas of social policy, is often more concerned with identifying problems and the ways in which particular policies are *not* working, rather than providing examples of what has worked successfully in particular settings. But this is changing, and a number of funding bodies, both within and outside government, are supporting substantial bodies of research concerned with assessing 'what works' (see, for instance, the Department of Health's policy research programme, or the Home Office (1998) and McGuire's (1995) work on reducing offending behaviour).

The relationship between research results and evidence

What constitutes robust 'evidence' in the social care field depends substantially on people's views about the findings from research. There is a naïve assumption, held it seems by many politicians, that research results speak for themselves – that once the findings of a piece of work are available it is clear what action should follow. This is not the case in reality. Anyone who has done any research knows that writing it up and making sense of it are in many ways the most difficult parts. Facts uncovered by research do not speak for themselves. They need to be interpreted and put in context. The way in which a researcher identifies the key points to pursue in the analysis and the conclusions that they draw are the thing that differentiates research findings from *evidence*. One device for looking at the relationship between various factors is to turn them into equations. In this case what is being proposed is that:

Evidence = Research 'findings' + interpretation of the findings

One of the reasons for articulating it in this way is to emphasise the complexity of what constitutes what we call 'evidence'. Producing good research findings is difficult enough in itself; their interpretation is also a complex task. Different people could well draw out completely different interpretations from the same research findings.

Evidence defined in this way is also limited because it is relying on the interpretation of findings from one perspective – that of the researcher(s). To make *evidence* really useful it has to be converted into *knowledge*. This requires the researcher's interpretation to be augmented by the experience of practitioners and of service users. This too can be summarised in an equation:

Knowledge = Evidence + practice wisdom + user experience

The elements of practice wisdom and user experience are added because, even if the research findings provide a basis for strong evidence, there are other kinds of information and experience that are important in understanding what action to take. The contribution of the experienced practitioner is often overlooked by researchers. Experience can provide an understanding about things like the causal relationships between circumstances and outcomes, the effects of changes over time, and the impact of changing structures and organisations which cannot easily emerge from research. The experience of the service user is crucially important to developing an understanding of what aspects of services make a difference to their lives and to the processes that make for good provision. If ways can be found of building 'practice wisdom' and user experience into the processes of change, it might be possible to talk about developing 'knowledge-based practice' rather than 'evidence-based practice' – which would be a good thing.

The co-production of knowledge

Peter Beresford has written and spoken extensively about involving service users in research (Beresford and Evans, 1999; Beresford, 2001a). He has raised in particular the question of who can legitimately interpret the experience of service users, and makes the point that some service users feel that only they can appropriately analyse and interpret their experience. No doubt some practitioners feel the same – that it is only by becoming a researcher/practitioner that practice experience and perspectives can be properly understood and interpreted. I take a different view, in that I consider that good researchers can be sensitive analysts of all kinds of experience.

But it is clear that practitioners and service users are two important groups to involve in the research process. A number of researchers are already working in a collaborative way, by involving service users and practitioners in the development of the research idea and sometimes as members of the research team. For example, the research projects funded within the Joseph Rowntree Foundation's programmes of research on social care and disability and those funded by the National Lottery Charities Board (now Community Fund) put the involvement of service users as a key requirement before a proposal can be considered. There are therefore a growing number of examples of research projects that have been 'participatory' in the way they have involved service users. But the involvement of individuals in a particular project does not necessarily mean that the results of the project constitute *knowledge* rather than *evidence*.

In a recent article Beresford (2001b) has suggested that the development of the knowledge base needs to be seen as *co-production* between researchers and services users as equals. This seems an excellent way of seeing this relationship and an important principle that we should be pursuing. But the co-production should also include practitioners and service providers. Knowledge could then be genuinely co-produced by involving the various elements identified in the equations.

But there are some real disincentives for a co-production to happen, even where everyone is keen on it. There are few incentives for researchers to spend time discussing their research findings with practitioners and service users before they write their final reports and there are no incentives at all for them to stay with the issues and convert their 'evidence' into knowledge. The imperatives of the world of the short-term contract, and the pressure on university staff through the Research Assessment Exercise to publish in academic journals, do not encourage co-production. Equally there are many practitioners struggling to keep the ship afloat who have little time to contribute to wider discussions about the interpretation or use of particular research findings in their daily practice. Many service users, too, know what their experience is and want to get on with living their lives.

It is therefore likely that only small groups of practitioners and service users will wish to engage in the process of converting evidence to knowledge across a number of research projects. This is a different level of engagement from involvement in a particular piece of work. It would be good to create a forum or equivalent through which such testing could happen. The new Social Care Institute of Excellence (SCIE) could have a role here. Many responsibilities, and hopes and expectations (probably too many), have been put on SCIE and it would be unreasonable to expect it to be able to fulfil them all. But setting up a *practice and user panel* to help to create knowledge from evidence would be beneficial. The panel might also test research findings against experience and make recommendations about their general appropriateness for practice, rather in the way that the Consumers' Association tests other kinds of products.

The relationship between knowledge and practice

As mentioned earlier, having 'knowledge' is not enough to make change happen. I have argued elsewhere (Lewis, 2001) that a number of factors needed to be in place for knowledge-based change to happen, including: practitioners taking ownership of the problem, wanting to change, having the knowledge and having the resources. These factors are likely to be important. But implicit in these ideas was a linear relationship between the various factors. Despite knowing – from experience and observation – that one thing does not lead to another, this continues to be the assumption. This is a trap into which I, and many people keen to promote the dissemination of research findings, continue to fall. We seem to assume a chain of action from research findings, through evidence and knowledge, to individuals immediately changing what they are doing. This, of course, is not how it is. But what is the appropriate perspective to have on the relationship between knowledge and practice?

Rather than seeing this relationship as a linear one, my view now is that there are two chains of activities, which run in parallel. There is a *knowledge chain*, which is what I have described above. This is the process of moving from *research findings*, through interpretation of these to *evidence* and, through contextualising this evidence and adding the perspectives of practitioners and service users, to *knowledge*. The knowledge which comes from a piece of research needs to come together with knowledge from other areas to form a *knowledge pool*. ('Knowledge pools' are now a fashionable idea with a number of organisations, including the Government's Centre for Management and Policy Studies in the Cabinet Office, who are developing them for different purposes.) This pool should be much more than the sum of its parts as it would allow the knowledge gained from small studies to be put together and for results to be aggregated across a range of perspectives. The other chain relates to the world of *practice delivery* when it is concerned with making changes.

As suggested earlier, the impetus for *practice change* does not normally come from research findings or from reading. Most practitioners see research findings as irrelevant to their day-to-day work. They are also too busy to go searching for new ideas. But most staff are able to identify a number of ways in which things could be done better and are keen to improve what is going on. If the space is created for staff to identify what they want to do differently, they will often start to ask how this can be done and what would be a better way of doing it. At this stage, knowledge from research can provide useful evidence – and meet a need.

The *practice–delivery chain* that is proposed therefore starts with the practitioners – with their problems, issues, concerns, etc. If ways are found to work with groups of staff in an organisation to address the issues, there is likely to come a point when it is appropriate to feed in *knowledge* from the existing pool that will contribute to decisions about, for example, what changes to make. This is the point at which the two chains connect (see Figure 20.1).

It is important to point out that, although the connection, when it is made, may well be through the conventional mechanisms for conveying information – the written word – stimulating the desire to have this information is likely to involve some more personal interaction.

The key points to draw from the relationship are that:

1   if researchers want to help service providers and practitioners develop and improve what they are doing, based on research, it is necessary to start where practitioners are, rather than with the findings or knowledge derived from research, whether past or recent.
2   if you want to start 'where people are' the initial work has to be through personal interaction, not via the written word.

The implications

A number of implications flow from the identification of two chains of

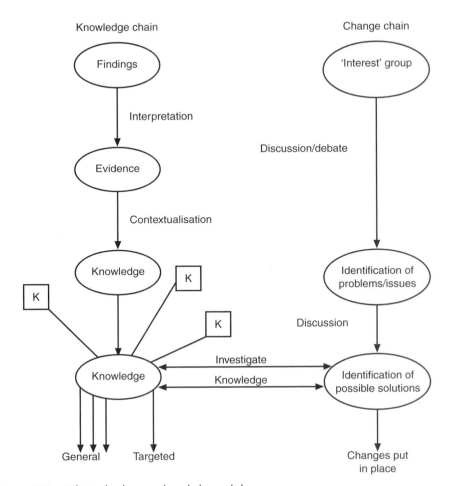

Figure 20.1   Relationship between knowledge and change.

activity, running in parallel. If we are committed to change based on knowledge, as opposed to guess, prejudice, whim or fashion, we have to continue to expand the knowledge pool. Where possible, the contents of the pool should be co-produced by researchers, practitioners and service users. The knowledge pool of co-produced knowledge should grow.

We also have to continue to disseminate the findings from research, and the contents of the knowledge pool, in accessible formats so that people know what is in the pool. They may need assistance to find the information they want. Making Research Count and Research into Practice[1] are

1 Information can be found at www.rip.org.uk for Research into Practice and at www.uea.ac.uk/swk/research/mrc/welcome.htm for Making Research Count.

organisations that can play a key role in making links between practitioners and the knowledge pool. SCIE will have a role here too, although it is too early to know exactly what it will be.

However, if we are serious about the introduction of *knowledge-based change* there needs to be a stronger focus on the change process itself. Organisations can be managed in ways that encourage appropriate change and the use of relevant knowledge. Gerald Smale's book on mapping change and innovation (1996) provides a useful framework for thinking about the processes involved in practice development. He showed that change is possible but there are no quick fixes. Just focusing on information and 'evidence' is not enough. More resources probably need to go into practice-focused development work.

REFERENCES

Beresford, P. (2001a) 'Social Work and Social Care: the Struggle for Knowledge', *Educational Action Research*, 9, 3, 343–53.

Beresford, P. (2001b) 'Evidence-based Care: Opening Up the Discussion', *Managing Community Care*, 9, 6, 3–6.

Beresford, P. (2002) 'User Involvement in Research and Evaluation: Liberation or Regulation?', *Social Policy and Society*, 1, 2, 93–103.

Beresford, P. and Evans, C. (1999) 'Research and Empowerment', *British Journal of Social Work*, 29, 671–7.

Department of Health, Policy Research Programme – text index, http://www.doh.gov.uk/research/rd2/prindex.htm (accessed 11 March 2002).

Home Office (1998) *Report of the What Works Project: Strategies for Effective Offender Supervision*, London, HMSO

Lewis, J. (2001) 'What Works in Community Care?', *Managing Community Care*, 9, 1, 3–6.

McGuire, J. (ed.) (1995) *What Works: Reducing Offending. Guidelines from Research and Practice*, Chichester, Wiley.

Smale, G. (1996) *Mapping Change and Innovation*, London, HMSO.

TWENTY-ONE

TOWARDS ECOLOGICAL UNDERSTANDING OF OCCUPATIONAL STRESS

Judi Marshall

Source: *International Review of Applied Psychology*, 1986.

Introduction

I am using this article as an opportunity to draw together three themes in my current speculations about the nature of stress, and about our abilities to understand and map it appropriately. My initial interest was the potential value of focusing on particular occupational groups separately, to achieve complex understandings of the environmental and personal pressures which contribute to individual experiences of stress. I have called the resulting patterns, which amount to equations of risk, 'stress profiles'. I soon learnt that these profiles need to include not only the nature of, and fit between, job or organizational factors and individual characteristics, but also an appreciation of these within their wider context. Most research models take into account the mutual interaction between individual, role and organization. By drawing on notions of self-perpetuating ecological systems, particularly elucidated by Bateson (1973), I shall be taking a still more comprehensive approach to stress. This appreciates that the individual, their job and organization are embedded in a social system (see Figure 21.1).

From this perspective, stress is an aspect of the system as a whole (I shall sometimes refer to stress as being 'in a system', a notion to which I return towards the end of the paper) and cannot meaningfully be attributed to any particular part, such as an individual worker, alone. In this article I shall concentrate on how system characteristics contribute to indi-

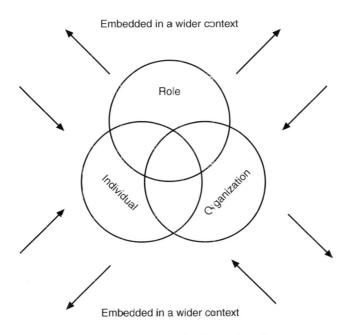

Figure 21.1   Towards an ecological understanding of stress.

viduals' experience of stress. I shall leave consideration of how individuals, and occupational groups, complement contextual forces and perpetuate the total system to a later occasion.

An ecological profile takes the shape of an interconnected pattern of significant elements. This pattern should be meaningful in relation to the phenomenon I am studying. The critical predicament is where I draw the boundaries around and within it. Even if I take certain elements – potential stressors, for example – as my foci, this selection must be derived from, and in harmony with, a more broadly-based (and potentially dynamic) appreciation of the whole area of *relevance*. In relation to stress, an occupational group's social status, functions in society and methods of occupational socialization are some of the more obviously relevant aspects.

My belief in the importance of 'ecological understanding' makes me suspicious of studies which take a handful of factors to sum up a particular area of someone's life. I want to know whether, and how, these isolated concepts make sense in a broader picture. Ecological understanding is not therefore proposed as a replacement for more focused approaches to research, but rather as an invaluable complement to them, and a significant perspective in its own right.

In the tentative theoretical perspective I am adopting, what I mean by 'stress' becomes contentious. My initial focus was on the ill-effects (physical, cognitive, emotional and behavioural) experienced by the job-holding individual, and these remain my dominant concern. Moving towards the proposed ecological approach I suggest that other people's anxiety and tension, and general social denial of stressful issues contribute to, and are in turn reinforced by, the focal individual's experience. In the following pages, therefore, I use the one label 'stress' in relation to these individual, interpersonal and societal aspects of disturbance. This usage reflects a real complexity in the area. An ecological appreciation requires suspending bounded notions of cause and effect, and moving towards a more systemic way of thinking. In this article I experiment with this approach but do not achieve it wholeheartedly. Nonetheless, in these first theoretical steps, I am wary of labelling as 'stress' only one dimension of the interconnecting field which requires understanding. [. . .]

As my first steps towards elucidating the ecological approach to stress, I shall focus on three processes through which contextual forces contribute to stress for workers in public service roles.

1   The implications for the worker concerned of confronting fundamental existential conflicts as essential ingredients of their job.
2   Other people's projections of relevant stereotypes onto the occupational groups.
3   Their place as 'carriers' of society's unresolved anxiety surrounding these issues.

I shall use the role of nurse to illustrate these processes in practice . . . with occasional examples from . . . other . . . professions.

Conflicts inherent in the job

A core dilemma for nurses is their relationship to death through their care for the sick and dying. At a personal level this raises anxiety about their own forthcoming death. This anxiety is most likely to surface in their direct contact with patients. Studies show that an individual factor which makes nurses vulnerable to stress is becoming too attached to a particular patient. They are most likely to identify with someone similar to themselves or to someone they love. Many of the coping strategies nurses use reduce the opportunities for emotional involvement of this sort. They may, for example, de-personalize patients, refer to them by their illness rather than by name, or keep busy with their tasks and avoid spending too long in conversation. Even the significance of deaths can be reduced by routinizing procedures for dealing with corpses, and by 'counting deaths' (remembering how many deaths they have been involved with) so that each is only one more in a tally of professional experience. This is not simply a personal matter for the nurse – the context tells us more. Because we deal so poorly with death and its anticipation culturally, their anxiety is heightened and prevented from socially acceptable expression. Confronting death becomes more stressful and coping more difficult because of these contextual features.

Being responsible for patients' lives and potential deaths is a related, equally significant potential cause of stress for the nurse. The profession maximizes clarity about responsibility, enshrining this in clear hierarchic structures and working procedures (Menzies, 1970). This helps to alleviate stress by reducing the weight of responsibility on individuals. Amongst social workers, case meetings serve similar functions by diffusing responsibility for difficult decisions amongst a team of professionals. These 'solutions' may, however, become 'problems' at another level, as individuals experience frustration and lack of autonomy. All four public service occupations experienced some pressure from their openness to public opinion about the quality of their work performance. Most commentators suggest that demands for social accountability are strengthening, and will contribute increasingly to pressure in the future.

Receiving others' projected needs

Playing such significant social roles, nurses (and police, social workers and teachers) are the recipients of other people's stereotypes, conflicts and anxieties. They become symbols rather than individuals. Their functions conjure up archetypes – idealized roles with powerful social, cultural and historical significance; our heroes and heroines and villains. Often these idealizations themselves enshrine ambivalence. 'Mother', for example, represents both unconditional, nurturing love and the potential to smother and destroy.

Nurses are particularly aware of and constrained by others' expectations that they are caring, devoted, Florence Nightingale types, contributing to patients' cure. In crises they are expected to act professionally, with detached concern, and not to express, or even to have, their own emotions. This image is the crystallization of our hopes and fears when faced with illness. For the nurse, it has several implications for potential stress. It fosters their best image of themselves, but conflicts markedly with their daily experience of their work – the often unpleasant practicalities of dealing with blood, excrement and illness, for example. It heightens their own sense of inadequacy when patients become more ill or die. And it constrains them from revealing (or fully experiencing?) their emotions and publicly discussing the less-glamorous aspects of their experiences. Their role thus becomes one of managing other people's anxieties at the expense of coping with their own. We learn again from taking an ecological approach that immediate personal pressure is accentuated by societal connotations.

Some of the stress experienced by members of the police service can be similarly interpreted as the projection of societal needs and conflicts on to this professional group. Interested researchers have long tried to identify characteristics of a 'police personality', consistently citing suspiciousness, conformity, rigidity and cynicism as possibilities. Evidence of variations, between cultures and geographic regions, has, however, confounded these attempts to generalize. Instead, Vastola (1978) suggests that police characteristics mirror the nature of their local or national community:

> Simply put, the police personality is merely a reflection of the dominant cultural personality of citizens with whom police primarily interact.

Professional groups as carriers of societal anxiety

We can, then, see these occupational groups as 'carriers' of the anxiety attached to significant social issues. They seem essentially to be receivers, sensitive and responsive to their environment, largely unable to protect themselves from these sources of pressure. There are, however, also forces which foster their separation and isolation. These can be interpreted as protective social mechanisms: an essential conflict is enshrined in a particular group, which is then isolated to contain the attendant anxiety and stress. This is also beneficial for members of the occupational group who make their own contribution to maintaining the boundaries. One means by which separation is achieved is through professionalization. Professional standards, often reinforced by legislation, provide rules for handling the paradox. Fundamental issues about socialization versus independence and authority versus self-direction, for example, are concealed by having schools, stipulating attendance requirements and using examinations to evaluate 'learning'. For the individual teacher (or other professional meeting similar circumstances) this will mean less flexibility in interpreting his/her role. Apparent deviance can be heavily sanctioned because of the need to keep professional behaviour within bounds. Teachers are not, for example, expected to expose pupils to moral beliefs currently judged 'unorthodox', or to be openly deviant in their own lifestyles.

Another means of achieving similar effects is through social isolation. This also has marked, if possibly protective, benefits for the occupational group concerned. Living with the conflicts between image and actuality defined above, they often favour mixing with 'like' individuals who understand their experiences, and share similar perspectives of 'reality'. Society can foster such polarization by failing to acknowledge this 'reality', or denying it legitimate means of expression. The various profiles in Cooper and Marshall (1980) suggested that the public service occupations featured here do tend to close in upon themselves. Poor relations with the general public and, for the police and nurses, 'unsocial' working hours, join the search for shared meanings already mentioned as motivations. There are benefits and costs to individuals of restricting their social contacts to work colleagues. The resulting cohesive social groups can provide much needed emotional and professional support, and thus act as buffers against stress. Alternatively, those who do not 'fit in' successfully will feel particularly isolated. This is given in nursing as one reason for leaving the profession. Mixing together socially strengthens occupational norms and image, provides more opportunities for normative socialization towards shared values, and can eventually reinforce initial barriers of misunderstanding, and polarize potential conflicts, with other social groups.

Barriers may also exist around these professions within the work environment. The detailed profiles suggest good relations with colleagues and immediate superiors, but relatively poor communications with more distant administrators and/or senior management. For nurses this difference is because they do not feel administrators appreciate the 'true' nature of their work.

In this section I have explored several strands in possible ecological stress models for four public service occupations. Further development must await more first-hand material, another opportunity, and the refinement of my conceptual model. I shall now turn to my third and final speculative theme.

Drawing implications from ecological stress profiles

A full ecological stress profile for an occupational group would provide a complex, dynamic, interconnected understanding of relevant factors. In this final section, I shall use the tentative material developed above to illustrate two possible uses of such models. The first draws on their illumination of coping behaviour, the second on their value in helping us manage potential change.

A key question once we take this approach to stress is what constitutes adaptive coping. The very nature of the pressure identified means that there are no simple answers. An ecological understanding of stress has (at least) two levels of relevance: the micro level of individuals performing their particular job, and the macro level of societal issues. Unless the total system changes, adaptive coping at one level typically increases experienced stress at the other. Measures taken recently by the police service in the London area of Notting Hill illustrate this paradox. Notting Hill has an annual West Indian carnival, during which there have sometimes been street riots directed at the police. To minimize tension in the area, the police have adopted a 'low key' policing policy, keeping interventions in the local community to a minimum. This has alleviated stress at the macro, societal, level. At the micro, individual, level tension has, however, increased in several respects. Police officers are experiencing frustration because they cannot take action in cases of day-to-day crime (which they see as a core purpose of their job), as this would be provocative. Some officers have been attacked on the streets. Local residents are complaining because petty crime is on the increase.

For the four public service occupations featured here, the balance seems to be towards societal rather than individual benefits in coping. This follows from their social roles. The institutionalization of these occupations is an indication of society's unresolved stress. If we as individuals were more competent at dealing with the existential issues in which they specialize we would need them less. Nurses, police, social workers and teachers are society's formalized coping mechanism, and their needs as individuals are therefore by definition subservient to general social needs.

The self-sustaining nature of this disturbed pattern of unresolved pressure, projection and avoidance-based coping, is the basis for my suggestion that stress is 'in the system' and cannot meaningfully be attributed to any one part of it alone. Stress is a system characteristic, even though it is primarily expressed through individual experience. Hence there is a certain inevitability in jobholders' exposure to potential stress. The individual nurse can take some action to minimize pressure, perhaps by privately holding beliefs (that death is inevitable and acceptable, say) which conflict with social norms. But she or he cannot leave or fundamentally reshape the system if they continue to accept their core task as sensitivity and service to public needs. Within the total system, then, any path for coping is conflict-ridden and limited because it is barred by the social definitions and imperatives which give the occupation its base of meaning. As a result, all of the four occupational roles discussed here incorporate, probably in varying degrees, emotional repression and denial as essential elements. This adaptation, however, makes it still more difficult for individuals to manage the core paradox of their work successfully and maximize coping at the micro level. Whilst a high risk of stress is an ever-present aspect of these roles, experienced stress is usually managed to tolerable levels by individual defence mechanisms and institutional coping strategies. Members are likely to experience most stress when their occupation's core conflict is accentuated. For the police, dealing with street riots is probably a critical incident. It brings to the fore their power for aggression and oppression, which is generally submerged by the peace-keeping image. Running a seminar recently for educationalists, I learnt that being on the receiving end of relatively student-centred teaching brought critical issues about their own roles to the surface. Our refusal (as staff) to give them 'right answers' provoked a rebellion, followed by reflection on their own assumptions about knowledge and learning.

In the sense that conflict is buried in each role all the time, these jobs can be seen as intrinsically about stress management. Usually their holders keep stress to manageable proportions. An individual's ability to maintain this balance will depend, in part, on character structure and life style. I have left these aspects out of my model so far, and am unable to do them justice here, but their significance must not be underestimated. Occupational choice is highly related to personality and personal values. I suspect that many of those who go into nursing, the police, teaching and social work do so because they have developed soundly-grounded coping skills for the conflicts the roles incorporate. Others, who more often receive attention in the available research literature, choose their jobs because their own anxiety is particularly great, and they need to achieve a sense of mastery. The stress implications of how individuals sustain the system of which they are a part, in their occupational choice and interpretation of their role over time, requires further development.

The second use to which I wish to put the ecological approach to stress is that of a framework for exploring possibilities for change – which is often the course advocated as a result of stress research. For this we need to understand how the significant elements fit together, and hold themselves, and each other, in place. These forces typically promote stability in the overall system, and will be mobilized by any attempt to change any part's functioning. Often they are the processes which manage uncertainty and anxiety to tolerable levels. They may appear maladaptive or trivial to the uninformed observer, but have their own force of necessity. Ecological stress maps help us understand the wider context in which elements we wish to change are embedded. Unless these are taken into appropriate account, powerful forces for stability can overwhelm, or completely subvert, changes which seem sensible from a rational, cognitive perspective.

There are many examples of organizational change attempts which result instead in 'more-of-the-same' with new surface appearances, because the organization's ability and needs to stay the same were underestimated. The same things can happen to an individual's good intentions. A common example is stressed executives who decide to make changes to their life style to avoid coronary heart disease. They take up exercise (or some other preference), with the same competitive attitude with which they pursue work. The new activity soon becomes an additional pressure rather than a balancing force, because their underlying philosophy remains unchanged.

It is interesting to consider suggested changes to the work practices of nurses and the police from this perspective. A recent trend in nursing has been towards more sustained contact between a particular nurse and patient, for the latter's benefit. Given the above stress profile we can now predict that such arrangements are likely significantly to increase stress for the nurse. If no other factors in the pattern are modified, to help balance additional pressures, they can be expected to accentuate previous strategies – such as de-personalization of patients – as means of coping. Similarly, community policing has been suggested to improve relations between police and the public. In city areas in which police are abused or attacked on sight, more factors must be addressed to prevent such initiatives breeding more rather than less suspicion and polarization.

Reflection

What type of ecological awareness is appropriate to understanding a particular occupational group's experience of stress will depend on the core definitions of its role. In this paper I have concentrated on professions with similar, unusually critical, relations with society. The appropriate context is usually identified via one key factor which has the potential to explain others. In a study currently being undertaken by one of my research students at Bath (Marcia Evans), 'change' soon took on this key integrating role for technical and sales staff in the computer industry. Changes in technology are what the industry is all about, but when it impacts organization procedures and structures, computer people become less clearly enthusiastic. Annual reorganizations, and the difficulties of planning satisfactory career routes when new jobs are continually being created and old ones abolished, are two very significant sources of stress.

There can be no neat ending to a speculative paper such as this. I have explored some of the possibilities for understanding stress ecologically for four occupational groups. My conclusion is that this is a promising approach, with room for further development.

REFERENCES

Bateson, G. (1973) *Steps Towards an Ecology of Mind*. London, Paladin.

Cooper, C.L. and Marshall, J. (1980) *White Collar and Professional Stress*. Chichester, John Wiley.

Menzies, I.E.P. (1970) *The Functioning of Social Systems as a Defence Against Anxiety*. London, Tavistock Institute.

Vastola, A. (1978) 'The Police Personality: An Alternative Explanatory Model.' *Police Chief*, 45(4): 50–2.

PART III

MANAGING IN CHANGING CONTEXTS

Julie Charlesworth

Introduction

The readings in this Part explore the impact of organisational, institutional and policy changes on discourses of management and the role of practitioners, managers and service users. Change is often feared and, as this collection illustrates, it can have both negative and positive consequences. However, there is nothing new about having to cope with change, and the collection of readings begins with John Adams, who sets debates on change within their historical context, detailing how changes in workhouse and poor law policy affected staff. By doing so, he illustrates how the pressures of changing legal and policy frameworks have resonance for different managers and professionals across the decades. Adams shows how the transition from workhouse to residential home was problematic for wardens, with traditional attitudes towards care hard to shift and widespread resistance to change thereby creating conflicts within homes. Policy emphasis was largely on buildings and environments, but with belated attention to staffing and training. As Adams demonstrates, incremental changes to policy on workhouses eventually helped bring the welfare and quality of life of residents to the fore.

Moving into more recent times, several of the readings explore the impact of changing structures on practitioners, professionals and notions of professionalism. John Clarke continues the historical focus by exploring discourses of managerialism under the New Right in the 1980s and 1990s. His critique shows how management assumed a greater importance in welfare with the government's mantra of more and better management to counteract the perceived failures of bureaucrats and professionals. As an integral part of this new discourse, change was supposed to be welcomed and embraced. Clarke asks whether it is possible to overcome the perverse effects of fragmentation without reverting to centralisation.

Peggy Foster and Paul Wilding also examine the problems faced by care professionals over the past few decades, with challenges to their expertise and the government's search for greater accountability from the professions. They focus in particular on social work and its increasing 'proceduralisation', bureaucratisation and changes in patterns of training towards a competency-based approach. They argue that such change has had both negative and positive effects. On the negative side there is exclusion of professionals from policy making, the imposition of external methods of scrutiny and appraisal and an expectation that professionals would shift loyalty to their institution rather than their professional body code of ethics. On the positive side, service users' views are more actively sought. However, they outline concerns that the overall effects of change could lead to demoralisation within professions and affect relationships with clients.

Gordon Causer and Mark Exworthy's discussion continues the themes of managerial–professional conflict, arguing that the relationship between professionals and managerial professionals is more complex than purely explaining it through a dichotomy of roles. They develop a typology capable of exploring the ways in which professional and managerial activities relate to one another, thereby allowing for the reality that individuals interpret their role in different ways. Martin Kitchener, Ian Kirkpatrick and Richard Whipp explore the impact of what they term 'new public management' on professional supervision work through a study of the management of children's homes. They assessed the extent of change in social services departments, particularly in supervisory structures, styles and practices. Their evidence suggests that shifts towards a more bureaucratic model of control are more contested than one might have expected and that radical change in supervisory systems is extremely problematic.

An extensive literature exists on the virtues of partnership and collaboration in both public and private sector organisations and the need to work on an interprofessional and interagency basis has become increasingly important in health and social care. The reading from Bob Hudson, Brian Hardy, Melanie Henwood and Gerald Wistow reviews the wide-ranging debates and theories seeking to explain why organisations collaborate and, in doing so, develops a framework for understanding rationales for partnership, issues of legitimacy, collaborative capacity and purpose, power and trust, and sustaining interagency relationships. Sally Hornby and Jo Atkins also look at collaboration but shift the debate towards the role of practitioners (here called 'faceworkers') in collaboration between service users and their helpers (or carers). The organisational context and structures of power can be experienced as constraints by these frontline workers as they develop helping relationships. Hornby and Atkins explore the impact of psychological defences used by members of the multidisciplinary team (see also Obholzer in Part IV). They call for the expertise of faceworkers, users and carers to be incorporated into decision making and planning at all levels of the organisation.

Vivien Martin examines the practicalities of what it means to be a manager in the twenty-first century and the tensions and ambiguities between the theory and practice of management. She discusses how the style and practice of a manager can impact on service delivery and how it is important for managers to reflect on their practice, in order to develop management conducive with improving the quality of both care and working life. In a similar vein to other readings in this book, she also offers insight into how managers experience stress arising from conflicts in their different roles and objectives.

Jan Horwath and Tony Morrison look at attempts to introduce change through a wide-ranging programme of new guidance in children's services, focusing particularly on the *Framework for Assessment of Children in Need and their Families*. The authors examine the challenges posed by new guidance and how organisations bring different agendas to strategic plans for themselves and partner agencies. They look at the suitability of models of change in providing a structure for planning, implementing and reviewing change and also highlight the importance of reconciling different organisations' understandings and interpretations of new guidance and utilising an interagency approach. The models discussed provide guidance on the process of change management, together with a means of assessing readiness to implement change.

The final reading in this Part on managing in changing contexts illustrates the usefulness of a systems approach in social work management. Andy Bilson and Sue Ross present a case study based on their in-depth work with social care practitioners and managers, and explore issues of how information is used in organisations. For example, they illustrate its linkages to power and politics within organisations.

These readings illustrate clearly that, although the reasons for change may vary over the years, there is much to be learned from different circumstances and time periods about understanding processes of change and managing their effects.

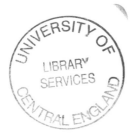

TWENTY-TWO

THE LAST YEARS OF THE WORKHOUSE, 1930–1965

John Adams

Source: *Oral History, Health and Welfare*, Borrat, J., Perks, R., Thompson, P. and Walmsley, J. (eds), London, Routledge, 2000

The recent celebrations marking 50 years of the National Health Service revealed much about British attitudes to health and social welfare, as the spotlight remained almost totally focused on the advances in acute medical care taking place in prestigious hospitals. The fact that 1948 also saw the abolition of the Poor Law and sweeping changes in the system of care for many vulnerable groups in society passed almost unnoticed. [...] For several decades the former workhouse buildings were both an essential resource for the new NHS and a constant reminder of the past that had been renounced. As the tide of opinion turned against institutional care and in favour of care in the community, the former workhouses and asylums provided easy targets for reformers. Now that this transition looks much more problematic than once it did, there is a fresh incentive to re-examine policy in terms of the continuities between the old and the new.

In this chapter, based on interviews with the staff who administered the workhouses, an attempt is made to begin this process of re-assessment starting from the passing of the Local Government Act, 1929. [...] It could be argued that as so many former workhouse buildings still survive, and often continue to provide care services for very similar groups such as older people and people admitted for reasons of mental illness or distress as they have always done, the workhouse is still with us, run by masters under the new guise of 'patient services managers'.

This chapter is based on material derived from tape-recorded interviews and informal discussions carried out over the past 12 years with 10 leading members of the former Association of Health and Residential Care Officers. [...]

The workhouse master in context

The workhouse has proved to be one of the most enduring features of both the English townscape and rural landscape, despite the ambivalence or even open hostility with which it has been regarded throughout its existence. Many of the remaining buildings date at least in part from the years immediately following the passing of the Poor Law Amendment Act of 1834 which required groups of parishes, known as Unions, to underwrite the heavy cost of construction. [...]

Those framing the legislation, however, believed that they had created a system which, unlike the prison, provided an ever-present incentive for the inmate to leave. This was the principle of 'less eligibility' which meant that the discipline, labour and restrictions imposed by the workhouse regime should encourage those who could support themselves by their own efforts outside to do so. For those who were genuinely unable to cope outside the institution, the aim was to provide all the necessities of life in a way that made the workhouse 'a place of comparative comfort' (Crowther, 1983: 41). This may have been the intention of the central authorities, but the fragmentation of a system administered by locally elected Boards of Guardians allowed a number of scandals of neglect and abuse to occur in the early years. [...] The subsequent Parliamentary Committee of Inquiry, and the campaign for action led by *The Times*, resulted in major organisational changes and also focused attention on the key posts of master and matron. The rapid development of a new national network of institutions which required a wide range of skills and personal qualities to be deployed in often difficult circumstances meant that guardians had no existing occupational group with its own standards and traditions on which they could draw. As a result, appointments were made on the basis of experience which appeared to be relevant to the new occupation. [...]

It is inevitably the worst cases of cruelty and neglect by workhouse masters that drew most attention at the time and provide such compelling material for the modern historian, but it is necessary to balance these accounts with those of efficient and humane masters who gave good service to both guardians and paupers. [...]

In the same way that the scandalous behaviour of some of the early workhouse masters of the 1840s and 1850s has come to be seen as typical for all subsequent holders of the post, so the changing nature of the workhouse itself has often not been fully appreciated. There is a tendency for local histories to dwell in detail on the regime in the middle years of the nineteenth century and then move abruptly to the 'coming of the welfare state' in 1948 as if nothing of significance had occurred in the interim....

By 1914, the 'mixed' workhouse ... still existed in many places, but some unions had built separate infirmaries for the sick or specialised institutions for the aged and 'cottage homes' for children (Crowther, 1978). Even where separate accommodation had not been developed, the character of the workhouse had changed. It had ceased to be the main focus of society's efforts to grapple with unemployment, with all the social tensions and disciplinary problems which that brought, and had become instead a refuge or hospice for those who were unable to cope alone in the society which lay outside its wall. Now more than ever the master of a workhouse needed to have managerial abilities which were coupled with the insight and imagination to ameliorate the worst aspects of institutional routines in order to improve the quality of life for the long-stay inmates. Given the importance of the role which workhouse masters played for more than a century in administering and delivering services at a local level for most of the vulnerable groups within society, it is surprising how little attention they have received from historians. [. . .]

Having previously reviewed some of the literature on workhouse masters, hospital stewards, superintendents of public assistance institutions and the wardens of local authority residential homes, I was expecting to meet men who were, to use some of Peter Townsend's adjectives, 'blunt', 'hearty' or 'extraordinarily rough-hewn and Micawberish' (Townsend, 1962: 86). To my great surprise, I found myself interviewing articulate professional men who could have been retired hospital consultants, architects or solicitors. [. . .]

The dominant impression was of two distinct cultures of care co-existing in the 1930s: one characterised by traditional workhouse discipline; the other provided role models for a more compassionate and caring interpretation of the role of master and this was to influence these new recruits:

> I suppose there were always bad masters and bad matrons – I've come across a few of them – but generally the masters and matrons were very humane people; tolerant of all the things that happened. And in many ways they were looked upon as the 'head of the family'.
>
> (Mr Lewis)

It could be argued that from the decision to interview former office-holders in an occupational association, the views expressed would inevitably be those of an elite group rather than typical of officers as a whole. Yet the recognition that such an elite actually existed helps to correct the general view of Poor Law Officers as an undifferentiated occupational group characterised by low expectations and lower achievements (see Crowther, 1983). In my view, it was the consistent failure of both government and campaigners to recognise the positive contributions that this elite group could make to the evolution of policy which led directly to some of the fundamental problems which still afflict residential care. In particular the refusal to recognise and support the officers' attempts to achieve professional status based upon a specific educational programme undermined the status of residential care officers and set the scene for several decades of neglect of their educational and training needs. [. . .]

Professional qualifications in the workhouse

The characteristics which distinguish a profession from other occupations have been widely debated by sociologists, but there is no doubt that Poor Law Officers regarded the possession of a specialist body of knowledge confirmed by the gaining of a certificate or diploma as its hallmark. [. . .] Once the decision had been taken to develop courses, the question of their content had to be addressed. For the master of a mixed institution such as a workhouse, it proved to be impossible to identify a specialist area of knowledge that was appropriate so a generalist collection of subjects had to suffice. Lionel Lewis described his studies in 1932:

> [. . .] You did books and accounts, mercantile law, English, buildings and construction. I had to know how to do a specification for building . . . this ward needs redecorating, it's so-and-so and so-and-so, prepare a specification for any building work and any painting work to be done. I took my exam in 1936 – we held the highest certificate that you could get at that particular time, so in effect you had qualified yourself to run a hospital or an institution.

[. . .] In practice, as officers keen to move in a 'professional' direction were only too well aware, the members of a public assistance committee were as likely to be swayed by their own judgements of character as they were by the possession of a certificate when they came to appoint a master:

> I remember somebody saying that someone had got the job [of master]. They asked him, what are the qualities of a master? He said, I think he should be a jack-of-all-trades, a good husband and a good father – and he got the job!
>
> (Mr Frank Hinchliffe, born 1917)

By the end of the 1930s the distinction between the roles of superintendent of a 'mixed' public assistance institution and that of steward in a local authority infirmary was becoming more marked and in 1943 stewards established their own section of the National Association of Administrators of Local Government Establishments. [. . .]

The creation of the National Health Service meant that administrators from the voluntary and municipal sectors had to compete for the new posts, with the former having the prestige of their former jobs to assist them, but at least the new career structure with its recognised professional qualifications was now in place. One of my interviewees succeeded in obtaining the most desirable post – Group Secretary – in the new structure, and became, as he described it, 'lord of all I surveyed' (Mr Dawber). Three of the others were successful in becoming a hospital secretary, the next rung down in the hierarchy but with the opportunity for close contact with patient care. For the rest, either by choice or because their institution did not have enough beds to qualify them as hospital officers, the future lay in residential care for older people after 1948.

The early years of the new service

In addition to the formal qualifications described above, progression in a career in the public assistance institution required ascent up each rung of the ladder with every promotion usually involving a move to another part of the country. . . . It was possible to gain the top post of master while a single man, but it was more usual to apply for the joint appointment of master and matron as a married couple (Adams, 1992). While the main change that hospital administrators had to face after 1948 was a new system of accounts, those running the former workhouses which had now become residential homes found that they were faced with a completely new philosophy of care but few of the resources to put it into practice. [. . .]

The fact that the new local authority residential homes for older people began their existence in many areas in the former workhouse buildings is well known, but what is less widely appreciated is that the tone of life was often set not by new residents moving in from the community but by a hard core of former workhouse inmates. Control over the more challenging elements in this population had been maintained by a system of punishments administered by the master, but under the new system control had to be maintained with no sanctions to fall back on:

> [Prior to 1948] you could stop their privileges – stop them from going out, stop their tobacco, stop the sweets, or whatever it was, so you had certain punishments you could inflict. Because immediately the '48 Acts came in, you had nothing – nothing at all. So that everything was completely taken out of your hands and very often that was one of our complaints. That the 'residents', as we used to call them then,

could do exactly what they wanted. I mean they could throw hot cups of tea at attendants – which they did quite often – and hit them with sticks, and there was nothing you could do about it.

(Mr Lewis)

Having set up a new system of residential care which aimed to sweep away the old Poor Law attitudes, practices and training schemes, successive governments failed to put new arrangements in place. As a result, the new wardens were left to struggle on as best they could. [. . .]

By the 1960s there was an increasing realisation that residential care services were in crisis and that the new world envisaged in 1948 had largely failed to materialise. The scene was set by the publication of Townsend's major survey of residential homes for older people, published in 1962. He was able to show that many vast former workhouse buildings were still in use despite the ambitious plans to replace them with small, purpose-built homes. . . . This concern culminated in the setting up of a committee of inquiry into the staffing of all types of residential homes by the National Council of Social Service, under the chairmanship of Lady Williams (Williams, 1967). The Williams Committee concluded that the staff shortages which characterised residential care were attributable to the lack of status in the eyes of the general public who fail to appreciate that 'this is a profession that requires specific training'. [. . .]

The Williams Committee was able to diagnose the national lack of training and relate that to high levels of staff turnover and resultant poor care, but the oral evidence collected in this project is able to show something of the potential that they were arguing could be released from well-educated staff with professional aspirations. Although it is an aspect of the history of care which has received very little attention from historians, the former workhouse officers from this elite sample were often fully involved in contemporary efforts to improve care.

[. . .]

Conclusion

If history is the story of winners and losers then there has been no doubt as to which category is appropriate for the former workhouse masters. As the representatives of a system that was criticised from all sides and finally swept away in 1948, they have been consigned in the popular imagination to a place in the Victorian chamber of horrors. . . . The central fallacy, however, lies not in mistaking the exceptionally brutal for the average but in imagining that a service as large and complex as the Poor Law and Public Assistance could be replaced overnight with a new and different creation. In practice, the same staff had generally to care for the same residents in the same buildings as before the changeover. This inability to recognise essential continuities in the new system led to a total failure to support progressive and innovative approaches to care demonstrated by the professional organisation representing masters and the collapse of educational initiatives. The Association of Hospital and Welfare Administrators, as the organisation was named at this period, recognised that the qualifications which it had struggled so hard to establish would become obsolete in 1948, so it proposed that they should be replaced by new qualifications ... to give professional status to the non-medical lay administrator. This proposal came to nothing and as the government itself had no proposals to put in their place, the result was the almost total lack of appropriate training opportunities for residential staff noted by Lady Williams in her Report nearly 20 years later (Williams, 1967).

While the Association's lobbying efforts were undoubtedly hampered by its links with a discredited Victorian past, it finally put itself beyond the pale with its campaign launched in 1944 as 'One Code for all the Social Services and one only', ... (Morgan, 1944). This was directly opposed to the philosophy of the new services which lay in a divide between 'health needs' which were to be met by the NHS and 'social needs' which were to be the responsibility of the National Assistance Board and local social services departments. To supporters of the new plans, this campaign appeared to be an attempt to mould the new arrangements on the all-embracing lines of the Poor Law and so was easily dismissed as reflecting the self-interest of a group of reactionary staff (see Roberts, 1970). It highlighted the difficulty, and ultimately the absurdity, of making a distinction between the health and social needs of frail older people (see Brumpton, 1948; Moss, 1948; Townsend, 1962: 35). . . . By failing to support the professionalising aspirations of an elite grouping of former masters, the reforming post-war government sowed the seeds of continuing structural problems in the health and social services.

REFERENCES

Adams, J. (1992/3) 'Master and matron: work and marriage in the public assistance institution', *Royal College of Nursing History of Nursing Society Journal*, 4(3): 125–30.

Brumpton, C.S. (1948) *Memorandum on the Possible Effects of Legislation in Connection with the National Assistance Bill and the Repeal of the Poor Law Acts, upon the Administration of Local Authority Welfare Establishments*. Blackburn, NAALGE.

Crowther, M.A. (1978) 'The later years of the workhouse 1890–1929', in P. Thane (ed.), *The Origins of British Social Policy*. London, Croom Helm, 36–55.

Crowther, M.A. (1983) *The Workhouse System 1834–1929: the history of an English social institution*. London, Methuen.

Lewis, Mr Lionel (born 1914).

Morgan, W.E. (1944) *The Future Institutional Service*. Blackburn, NAALGE.

Moss J. (1948) *Hadden's Health and Welfare Services Handbook*. London, Hadden, Best & Co.

Roberts, N. (1970) *Our Future Selves*. London, George Allen & Unwin.

Townsend, P. (1962) *The Last Refuge: a survey of residential institutions and homes for the aged in England and Wales*. London, Routledge & Kegan Paul.

Williams, G. (1967) *Caring for People: staffing residential homes*. London, George Allen & Unwin.

TWENTY-THREE

DOING THE RIGHT THING? MANAGERIALISM AND SOCIAL WELFARE

John Clarke

Source: *The Sociology of the Caring Professions*, Abbott, P. and Meerabeau, L. (eds), second edition, UCL Press, 1998.

This chapter summarizes recent work about the relationship between managerialism and the restructuring of social welfare.

It is clear that managerialism has formed part of a sustained attempt to reform the old institutional arrangements of the welfare state in Britain. [...] In particular, it promised to discipline those embodiments of 'producer power', the welfare professionals. I do not want to get bogged down in a discussion of whether such occupational and organizational formations are or are not 'real' professions, or even whether they are semi-, pseudo- or quasi-professions. ... [T]here are reasons to take seriously the public representation of such formations as professions. For the moment, however, I think it is more useful to consider the characteristic forms of organizational co-ordination in the practice of state welfare work.

Colleagues and I have found it useful to treat professionalism and bureaucracy as the characteristic modes of organizational co-ordination that dominated the institutional arrangements of the old welfare state (Clarke and Newman, 1997; see also Cousins, 1987). By 'modes of co-ordination', I intend to refer to the complex set of rules, roles and regulatory principles around which the social practices of organizations are structured. These modes generate typical patterns of internal and external social relationships and, in particular, privilege certain types of knowledge. We have used this idea of modes of co-ordination partly because it undercuts the naturalizing effect of the word 'managing', in which the commonsense meaning of 'running things' is elided with the more specific prescriptions of a managerialist mode of co-ordination (this is taken up later). By starting from these ideas of bureaucratic and professional modes of co-ordination, it is possible to develop a view of welfare agencies as organizational regimes in which different modes of co-ordination co-existed – in the characteristic form of 'bureau-professional regimes'. The reason for this rather circuitous approach to treating social welfare organizations as combining professionalism and bureaucracy is that much discussion of welfare restructuring has proceeded as if the old welfare state was either dominated by professionals or was entirely bureaucratic. The effect of emphasizing either one of these is to miss the internal complexity of the organizational forms, labour processes and significant intra-organizational struggles that characterized the bureau-professional regimes of state welfare (Clarke, 1994; Cochrane, 1993).

There are two further uses of this conceptual framework that are significant for what follows. The ideas of modes of co-ordination and organizational regimes provide a way of thinking about differences of organizational form within the welfare state – for example, the different sorts of organizational structures, cultures and processes that characterized the range between the NHS, on the one hand, and (what used to be) the Department of Health and Social Security on the other. In this range the co-existence of professional and bureaucratic modes resulted in very different forms and distributions of power and privileged different sorts of organizationally-valued knowledge. The second value of the framework is that it allows some degree of analytical grip on the (uneven) combinations between these regimes and a third mode of co-ordination – that of political representation. The effects – and discomforts – of this articulation have tended to be most visible at the level of the local state – around education, social services and housing, for example (Cochrane, 1993). [. . .]

Naturalizing managerialism

In part, the new role for management derived from the New Right's ideological insistence on the innate superiority of the market over the state as a means of allocating resources. In this view, 'managers' inhabited the world of market action, and were thus the natural bearers of its entrepreneurialism, its dynamism and the full gamut of 'good business practices' from which organizations in the public sector needed to learn. To some extent, this imagery of management was concerned with rather old-fashioned virtues of organizational co-ordination – the 'hard-headed' control of costs in the pursuit of greater efficiency, not least through intensified labour productivity. But it also drew on the more dynamic celebration of the manager-as-hero being articulated in the new managerialism – particularly in those new conceptions of the manager as leader and corporate culture shaper, inspiring the unending pursuit of quality and excellence (Clarke and Newman, 1993; Pollitt, 1993; Flynn, 1994). Both, however, centred on one essential precondition for 'transforming' the dull professional bureaucracies into modern organizations – the establishment or enhancement of 'the right to manage'.

The legitimation of managerialism as a new mode of co-ordination for social welfare organizations involved a double discursive tactic. On the one hand, public sector organizations were subjected to a *logic of universalism*. This defined all organizations as essentially the same. It suggested that all organizations face similar tasks; all need to be co-ordinated to pursue their goals efficiently; managers have the capacity to create efficiency; therefore, all organizations need to be managed. On the other hand, public sector organizations were also subjected to a *logic of isomorphism*. This implied that successful organizational performance is to be found in the private sector, and since public sector organizations deviate from the 'norm' of the private sector, so public sector organizations must become more 'businesslike'. Managers provide 'good business practices', so public sector organizations need to be managed. In the process, the demand that public services need 'more and better management' was legitimized.

These legitimizations of the 'natural' desirability of management as the obvious way of running organizations (reflected in the increasing use of the phrase 'well-managed' to describe successful organizations) were supported by a further discursive tactic. This involved the articulation of the differences between management and the other pre-existing forms of co-ordination in the welfare state, juxtaposing the virtues of managers with the failings of bureaucrats, professionals and politicians. So, where bureaucrats were rule bound, inward-looking and inert, managers were innovative, externally-oriented and dynamic. Where professionals were paternalistic, self-regulating, building a mystique to protect their power, managers were customer-centred, created transparent organizations and were tested in the 'real world' of the marketplace. Finally, where politicians were dogmatic, interfering and changeable, managers were realists, capable of taking a strategic view and – if given the 'freedom to manage' – able to 'do the right thing'.

It is difficult to find any reform of social welfare in the 1990s which did not draw on and contribute to this installation of a managerial mode of co-ordination – from the creation of agencies (Benefits, Child Support, etc.) to the reorganization of health and social care. I have tried to summarize the main dimensions of the ideological and organizational salience of managerialism and managerialization.

Managerialism is:

■ *an ideology* centred on expanding the right to manage in the pursuit of greater efficiency in the achievement of organizational and social objectives;

■ *a calculative framework* which orders knowledge about organizational goals and the means of their achievement, typically around an internal calculus of efficiency (inputs–outputs) and an external calculus of competitive positioning within a field of market relations;

■ *a series of overlapping discourses* which articulate different – even divergent – conceptions of how to manage and what is to be managed (Total Quality Management; Excellence; Human Resource Management; Business Process Re-engineering and so on).

Managerialization is:

■ a process of *establishing managerial discretion/authority* over corporate resources (material, human, symbolic) and decision-making about them;

■ a process of *establishing calculative frameworks* that define the terms and conditions of decision-making, and are embedded in patterns of internal and external processes;

■ a process of *creating forms of managing and types of managers*. It might be suggested that there are three forms of 'managing' visible in the restructuring of social welfare: managers; hybrids; and a 'dispersed managerial consciousness'.

[. . .]

'Perverse effects': managerialism and social welfare

This section traces some of the consequences of managerialism for the provision of welfare services. . . . The four shifts are encapsulated in the ideas of 'core business', 'ownership', 'audit' and 'corporate culture'.

The idea of an organization's *core business* is a corollary of processes of service fragmentation (between providers) and forms of quasi-market competitiveness. It represents the managerial attempt to define the focus of attention of the organization – either externally-oriented in terms of competitive positioning, or as the internal management of 'waste and inefficiency'. Such specifications order the priorities of different potential calls on organizational resources and are formulated within a range of possibilities that are constructed by external or statutory requirements and internal organizational politics. Perhaps more important, the specification of core business legitimizes withdrawal from previously undertaken activities that become redefined as 'inessential'. [. . .]

The effects of defining core business overlap with the issue of *ownership*. The creation of ownership – of missions, targets, and responsibilities – has been one of the most sought-after effects of the managerial revolution. Its aim is to construct commitment and motivation among staff in the pursuit of corporate objectives (Clarke and Newman, 1993). Nevertheless, there is a conception of ownership which highlights a darker side of such initiatives: this is the view of ownership as 'proprietorialism' or 'possessive individualism'. . . . It is, therefore, not surprising to find the new field of welfare provision being characterized by ownership conflicts: over who owns customers (their needs and the resources that might accompany them); who owns service responsibilities and the resource implications that they bring; and who owns those practices that take place in the interstices between organizations or departments. [. . .]

What Michael Power (1993) has referred to as the *audit explosion* indicates the growth in both internal and external evaluations of performance and compliance. In part, such processes may reflect the increasing impossibility of 'trust' between citizens and service providers, between government and its agencies, or between purchasers and providers (Walsh, 1995). But they are also strategic responses from the centre aimed both at extending the disciplines available to regulate the periphery, and overcoming the dislocating relationships of an increasingly fragmented or, perhaps more accurately, dispersed state (Clarke, 1996). Nevertheless, they also have perverse effects on welfare services. They transfer scarce organizational resources from what Power calls 'Level 1' to 'Level 2' activities: from service production or delivery to information and monitoring systems (with an emphasis on guaranteeing procedural correctness). [. . .] Organizations, units and individuals are likely to find themselves pursuing objectives and targets in which they may have little confidence (waiting list reductions or telephone answering rates) and which may even draw attention and resources away from activities perceived as more significant to the service in question.

[. . .]

The enthusiasm for creating new *corporate cultures* poses rather different problems (Newman, 1996). At a mundane level, this enthusiasm seems to have inversely proportionate effects on staff motivation and morale, producing credibility gaps and collective cynicism. More significantly, the attempt to elaborate corporate cultures reflects the processes of fragmentation and dispersal and the impact of competitive field of relationships, so that individual fortunes (what used to be called careers) are seen as increasingly tied to the success – or at least survival – of the particular organization rather than a professional field. One counter-tendency to this is to be found in the combination of competition and the growing possibilities of local wage bargaining which has the potential for creating 'transfer markets' for high performers. A second counter-tendency is to be found in the search for increased managerial authority over labour – in particular over its disposability – since affective attachment or loyalty to corporate cultures may be undermined by the lack of evidence of corporate loyalty to employees. . . .

Despite such problems, it is clear that public sector managements have discovered the attractions of corporate cultures and their enthusiasm (or missionary zeal) has once more put professionalism in social welfare at the centre of tensions. [. . .]

Doing the right thing? The politics of managerialism

The title of this chapter derives from the frequently quoted assertion that the difference between administrators and managers is that where 'administrators do things right, managers do the right thing'. But it also raises the question of whether, in the context of welfare restructuring, managerialism has been doing the Right's thing. Managerialism has been both the beneficiary of and the conduit for Conservative policies for social welfare and the wider reconstruction of the relationship between state and society. The New Right's obsession with dismantling the institutionalized forms of social democracy led to a view of managerialism as a lever to break open the power bloc that the old welfare state represented. As I have suggested earlier, 'management' performed a double role as the organizational proxy of the market (embodying 'good business practices') and as a means of disrupting and disciplining the old forms of organizational co-ordination – bureaucratic, professional and political.

The conditions for managerialism playing this role can be traced back to the mid-1970s in the points of overlap between the emergent agendas of both the New Right and the new managerialism. As we have argued elsewhere (Clarke and Newman, 1993, 1997), there were a number of affinities between these projects. They shared: a hostility to bureaucratic organization; a commitment to entrepreneurial dynamism and competition; a drive towards deregulation; and, above all, a demand for the 'freedoms' necessary to give managers 'the right to manage'. Such affinities created the grounds for an alliance between the political and the organizational forces for change. But I am not convinced that it is satisfactory to treat managerialism simply as the organizational 'proxy' of the New Right. This does not mean that managements have not pursued elements of the Conservative reforms with great enthusiasm, since they clearly have. But thinking of the relationship between managerialism and the New Right as an alliance (rather than a hierarchical structure of strategists and implementers or leaders and subalterns) opens up issues both about the limits of the alliance and the prospects of managerialism after the New Right.

There are a number of potential sites of antagonism or tension within this alliance that have been particularly visible in recent years. The first concerns the allocation of responsibility. Several authors have seen the managerialization of social welfare as a way of moving (or attempting to move) hard choices out of the political arena into the realm of managerial responsibility (see, for example, Salter, 1993). This dispersal of decision-making (through agencies and quangos, and into multiple or fragmented sites) has applied most to the problems of budgetary management and service priorities. But it has not always been successful, since questions of services and priorities have tended to resurface at the political level despite government attempts to gloss them as 'operational' or 'managerial' matters. Indeed, some of the issues have returned to the political realm precisely because those in managerial roles have refused 'responsibility' (in community care and the Gloucestershire test case; in the 1995 conflicts over school budget setting, and so on).

There are also problems about how managements choose to exercise their new-found freedoms to manage, since the pursuit of local objectives may not deliver the nationally-desired aims. Consequently, political intervention has been required in what had been identified as the realms of the market or NHS management as the 'wrong results' appear (for example, in the 1993 'over-achievement' on contracts, leading to ward closures). In a rather more dramatic way, the 'Romeo and Juliet' saga in Hackney highlighted the potential for local management to produce unintended consequences. 'Local' management contains the permanent possibility of new alliances or of managements being themselves co-opted to local values, objectives or missions. As the organizational hinge between government policy and 'local' users – staff and other 'stakeholders' – managements find themselves trying to reconcile potentially conflicting interests. Although, as Taylor-Gooby and Lawson put it, the twin strategy of centralization and decentralization aims to ensure that 'power over the essentials is retained centrally while the management of inessentials is decentralized' (1993: 133), it is harder to guarantee that the choice of what to decentralize can anticipate what will be 'essential' in practice.

Finally, there are continuing problems about the 'freedom' of managers to manage. For the New Right, this has primarily been interpreted as needing the combination of deregulation and the removal or reduction of trades union 'interference'. But there has been a tension between the political concerns of policy-making and the wish of managements to be able to behave like 'real managers'. So, the decision to retain a role for Regional Health Authorities provoked dismay among Trust managers who saw it as an unwanted inhibition of their autonomy (see also Harrison et al., 1992: 122–8). Similarly, many 'business units' in local authorities and other public sector institutions complain of being artificially confined by wider corporate agendas, policies and costs which stop them from getting out there and 'doing the right thing'. At a number of different levels, the dispersal of the state and decision-making has established instabilities at the intersection between centrifugal and centripetal forces – or between pressures towards further fragmentation and stronger integration.

I raise these issues because they serve as reminders that managerialism was not simply or solely a proxy for New Right policies. It is also a social and organizational force with its own trajectory that was not wholly circumscribed by Conservative programmes. Recognizing that difference also requires us to consider the longer-term salience of managerialism for the future of social welfare.... We could view managerialism as 'apolitical' and subscribe to the claim that it is merely the technical means of implementing whatever objectives the 'national board of directors' decides upon. There are clearly attractions to this view, not least the implication that social policy becomes a matter of deciding on new 'targets' and embedding them in the nexus of corporate missions, strategic plans and indicators for performance audit.

And yet, I confess I cannot quite bring myself to believe in this vision of managerialism's technocratic innocence. In the end, I return to the view that all modes of organizational co-ordination are implicated in the construction of particular regimes of power. While the managerialist mission may be to 'empower everyone', I lack a sense of trust (in my multiple identities as a social scientist, a service user, a manager and one who is managed). As a result, I am left with a series of as yet unanswered questions. Is it possible to discipline managerialism as a form of social and organizational power – and how might this be accomplished? Put another way, the problem with the claim to 'do the right thing' is that it is self-referential. By what means can the rest of us judge whether it is 'right', or exercise control over the managerial autonomy legitimated by the claim? Is it possible to overcome the perverse effects of dispersal and fragmentation without reverting to centralization? Is it possible to restore some collective conception of the public, the public good and public service which does not reproduce the post-war mythology of the one-dimensional nation, which at the same time escapes treating diversity as the individual differences of autonomous customers? Is it possible to develop a conception of management as stewardship, responsible for the preservation and enhancement of the public realm, rather than management as entrepreneurialism, chasing the next big transformation?

REFERENCES

Clarke, J. (1994) 'Towards a post-Fordist welfare state?', *Local Government Studies* (Winter).

Clarke, J. (1996) 'The problem of the state after the welfare state', in May, M., Brunsdon, E. and Craig, G. (eds) *Social Policy Review* 8, London, Social Policy Association.

Clarke, J. and Newman, J. (1993) 'The right to manage: a second managerial revolution?', *Cultural Studies* 7(3): 427–41.

Clarke, J. and Newman, J. (1997) *The Managerial State: Power, Politics and Ideology in the Remaking of Social Welfare*, London, Sage.

Cochrane, A. (1993) *Whatever Happened to Local Government?*, Buckingham, Open University Press.

Cousins, C. (1987) *Controlling Social Welfare*, Brighton, Wheatsheaf Books.

Flynn, N. (1994) 'Control, commitment and contracts', in Clarke, J., Cochrane, A. and McLaughlin, E. (eds) *Managing Social Policy*, London, Sage.

Harrison, S., Hunter, D., Marnoch, G. and Pollitt, C. (1992) *Just Managing: Power and Culture in the National Health Service*, Basingstoke, Macmillan.

Newman, J. (1996) *Shaping Organisational Cultures*, London, Pitman.

Pollitt, C. (1993) *Managerialism and the Public Services* (2nd edn), Oxford, Basil Blackwell.

Power, M. (1999) *The Audit Explosion*, London, Demos.

Salter, B. (1993) 'The politics of purchasing in the National Health Service', *Policy and Politics*, 21: 171–81.

Taylor-Gooby, P. and Lawson, R. (1993) 'Where do we go from here? The new order in welfare', in Taylor-Gooby, P. and Lawson, R. (eds) *Markets and Managers*, Buckingham, Open University Press.

TWENTY-FOUR

WHITHER WELFARE PROFESSIONALISM?

Peggy Foster and Paul Wilding

Source: *Social Policy and Administration*, 2000, 34, 2.

[. . .]

From golden age to disillusionment

Looking back with all the advantage of theoretical and empirical insight we can now see that the 1950s and 1960s were a golden age for welfare professionalism. These were decades in which policy makers trusted welfare professionals to shape and run the social services without 'outside' interference from elected politicians, public officials or consumers. As Rudolf Klein has pointed out, in the 1950s the medical profession not only determined which issues were or were not put on the health policy agenda, it also 'to a large extent succeeded in defining certain areas as out of bounds to non-professionals' (Klein, 1989: 57). [. . .] In 1969 the Children and Young Persons Act made 'need' the criterion for public intervention. Need is a matter of professional judgement. Social workers therefore became key decision makers in relation to children and young people. In these years, doctors, teachers and social workers were granted a major role in policy making, power to define needs and problems, power in resource allocation, power over people, and substantial control over their area of work (Wilding, 1982).

In the 1970s and 1980s, however, a critique of the position, roles and functions of welfare professions developed. The historically taken-for-granted assumptions about the professions fitted less easily with a more plural, less deferential, more educated and more critical society. Academic critiques of welfare professionalism were fuelled by a succession of child abuse tragedies, hospital scandals, educational disasters and planning debacles.

Academic analysis moved from seeking to understand the characteristics which supposedly distinguished professions from mere occupations, to analysing how professions had gained and exercised power over their area of work (Johnson, 1972). Professional power was in turn linked to professionals' relationship to the state – redefined as capitalist and patriarchal. Professionalization was conceptualized not simply as an aspect of a benign and inevitable process but as an occupational strategy aimed at monopolizing practice and increasing financial rewards – a collective mobility project.

Radicals argued that professional power was a cloak for class power legitimated by dubious claims of expertise, political neutrality and an ethic of service (e.g. Doyal, 1979). The radical left characterized professionals as agents of the capitalist state employed to maintain a particular social and economic order and to blame the victim rather than change the system. Feminists meanwhile accused the professions of being bastions of male privilege and patriarchal control. The medical profession, for example, was accused of attempting to control female patients in the interests of patriarchy (Dale and Foster, 1986).

The charge from the New Right was that professionally dominated services like the NHS were always unresponsive to patients because there were no built-in incentives to put clients' needs first. They were monopolies lacking the essential stimulus of competition. They were also wasteful of resources because professionals, like bureaucrats, were self-interested budget maximizers rather than altruistic servants of their clients and the common good. [. . .] Whereas professionalism had been the dominant ideology of service provision until the mid-1970s, the 1980s and 1990s saw what Inglis described as 'the moral ascendancy of managerialism' (quoted in Troman, 1996: 475).

The New Right critique was reinforced by the emergent consumer movement which argued the right of consumers to a voice in the planning and running of services. What the consumer movement asserted was the value of a different kind of expertise – experiential knowledge – as opposed to the theoretical and distance-learned knowledge of professionals.

From the late 1960s there was a succession of tragedies and scandals in health, education and social services in which professionals were deeply and damagingly implicated. There were the scandals in mental handicap hospitals (Martin, 1984). There was the long succession of child abuse tragedies starting with Maria Colwell in 1973 (DHSS, 1974). In education there was the William Tyndale inquiry (Auld, 1976). Inquiries found serious failures of basic professional competence and care for very vulnerable people. The standing – moral and expert – of the professions suffered serious damage. Colleague and peer-group maintenance of standards was more and more seen as not working. Sharp questions were asked about the way professional power threatened or abused the rights of users – people with mental illness committed to mental hospitals, children who were made the subject of care orders. There was an issue of rights, due process and grievance procedures (e.g. Wilding, 1982: 103–8).

Industrial disputes also damaged the altruistic service image of the professions. There were the social workers' strike, the long-running teachers' dispute in the mid-1980s, and the doctors' threat of industrial action over new contracts. Hatcher, for example, sees the 1985–6 teacher dispute as ending the model of what he calls 'incorporated professionalism' where the state could be relied on to 'incorporate' professional definitions and ideas in all policy proposals (Hatcher, 1994: 55).

A new line of criticism also developed in terms of ideas of professional accountability and the rights of service users. Professionals in many areas, it seemed, were not really accountable to anyone. As criticism developed of professionally dominated services, so professions were exposed to new lines of attack. 'To the teachers I would say,' said James Callaghan in the famous Ruskin speech in 1976, 'that you must satisfy the parents and industry that what you are doing meets the requirements and needs of their children' (quoted in Harrison and Pollitt, 1994: 8). This speech initiated a search for a more accountable education system via new forms of political and managerial intervention. Accountability to themselves, to a professional ethic or to their professional peers was criticized as little more than a figleaf on a naked unaccountable, unmanaged, unresponsible independence.

Finally there was a wide-ranging critique of the nature and validity of the expertise on which the whole edifice of professionalism rested – the ability of doctors to improve health (e.g. Illich, 1975), the ability of social workers to grind young delinquents into responsible citizens (e.g. Brewer and Lait, 1980), the capacity of teachers to inculcate basic literacy and numeracy and socially acceptable standards of behaviour. In essence it was a challenge to the professions' cultural authority. The declining faith in professional expertise led to what Freidson calls a loss of 'ideological monopoly' which had allowed a profession to dominate policy and lay perceptions of problems and supposed solutions (Freidson, 1994: 31).

The attack on the welfare professions

When the New Right came to power in 1979 the writing was – in retrospect – on the wall for the traditional world of welfare professionalism. . . . They saw the professions as a powerful vested interest, effectively accountable to no one – politicians, managers or consumers. They were inefficient, the inevitable result of their insulation from the bracing competitive stimulus of market forces. They were ineffective in achieving society's aims for particular services. Their claims for expertise were scarcely supported by experience and their claim to an ethic of service which legitimized their lack of normal accountability was dismissed as the most specious of special pleading. 'Professions' were seen as very much secondary to management as an instrument of effective social policy.

The Thatcher aim was to bring welfare professionals firmly under political and managerial control, to enhance consumer power to induce greater professional responsiveness, to improve efficiency and effectiveness by various strategies. [...]

Social work

What happened to social work in the 1980s and 1990s can be explored under two main headings: increasing 'proceduralization' (Banks, 1998: 213) and 'bureaucratization' (Howe, 1992), and the move from a professional-style education towards competency-based training. Both these developments contributed to an erosion of professional autonomy and influence.

Social work was a residuary legatee of the liberal hour of the 1960s. The creation of social services departments in 1971 was a milestone in its development. In the next five years the number of social workers doubled. But in 1974 the Report of the Inquiry into the death of Maria Colwell was published (DHSS, 1974), and this – with the wisdom of hindsight – was a milestone of a rather different kind marking the beginning of the ebb tide of social work's march towards professional status.

The critique of social work which developed in the 1980s had five central strands. There was strong criticism of social workers' competence with much reference to the damning findings about social workers' failure in child abuse cases. There was an attack on the supposed fragility of social work's knowledge base. There was criticism from the government and its supporters of the basic ideology of social work with its emphasis on understanding rather than blaming, on treating rather than punishing. Social workers were charged, too, with fostering irresponsibility – for freeing people from a sense of responsibility for their own actions, for encouraging them to look to the state for help rather than relying on their own resources or their families. Finally, their supposed service ethic was questioned following strike action in the mid-1980s. Social work intervention and social workers' judgements were therefore problematized. Social workers did not intervene when they should have done, for example in the Beckford case (London Borough of Brent, 1985); they intervened when they should not have done, which was the charge in Cleveland (Secretary of State for Social Services, 1988). Individual judgement therefore had to be reduced and controlled by the institutionalization of good practice through the promulgation of guidelines. Guidelines, and the audit which they allowed, replaced trust – historically a central element in professional relationships with both managers and clients. [. . .] As the Department of Health put in *Protecting Children*:

'It is now generally accepted that this formal procedural framework is essential to the effective management of child protection' (quoted in Howe 1992: 501). All this meant a redefinition of the role of the social worker in relation to child abuse cases. In Howe's view the social worker's role became that of 'investigator, reporter and gatherer of evidence'. The result was that 'the social worker loses much of her professional freedom' (1992: 502).

[. . .] The child abuse tragedies, the subsequent inquiries, and the government response to them led to a much more restricted kind of social work – bureaucratized, proceduralized, guideline practice. As Banks puts it: 'Proceduralization can be viewed as a way of circumscribing professional autonomy' (Banks, 1998: 214). The space for autonomous, individualized professional judgements which social workers had gained in the 1950s and 1960s and which reached its apotheosis, perhaps, in the 1969 Children and Young Persons Act was sharply narrowed.

The second major area of change relevant to an analysis of what happened to social work in relation to its professional status was changes in patterns of training. In the 1980s and 1990s there was much debate about the nature and content of social work training – partly fuelled by the supposed failure of social workers in relation to child abuse tragedies and partly driven by the Conservative government's concerns about the ideological content of social work courses. The result was a strong movement towards a competency-based approach stressing specific competencies rather than a liberal professional education. In Dominelli's view: 'This is leading to the demise of the autonomous, reflective practitioner' (1996: 153), 'the Taylorization of professional tasks' and 'the proletarianization of professional work' (ibid.: 163).

The stress on competency-based training has a number of implications. It increases government and employer control over training inputs and outcomes because competencies can be prescribed very specifically and tested for their achievement. It gives managers clear yardsticks for supervising and controlling social workers. It 'bleaches out' (Dominelli, 1996: 172) the political nature of social work. It divorces social work from a focus on the whole person by its focus on specific competencies, skills and tasks. Professional work is essentially about focusing on the whole person – it is human-centred rather than task- and competency-centred.

What were the outcomes for professionals?

[. . .] First, the professions have been far less centrally involved in the policy-making process. Politicians from both the left and the right now appear to feel confident to implement major changes to welfare policies without gaining the agreement of those welfare professionals responsible for implementing such changes. [. . .]

Second, a whole range of external forms of scrutiny and appraisal have been imposed on welfare professionals during the 1980s and 1990s, although there are one or two aspects of professional practice which are still only to be judged by those with equal professional qualifications. For front-line professionals, however, increased scrutiny and inspection of their day-to-day work is an infringement of their previous professional autonomy, whether it comes in the guise of peer audit, appraisal by a more senior professional colleague, or inspection from an outsider who may or may not have professional qualifications. Some of the most controversial and feared Ofsted inspectors, for example, have been professionally qualified ex-teachers.

Third, the creation of internal markets within the NHS and the state school system and the privatization of much residential care within the personal social services has broken up very-large-scale state monopolistic suppliers and thus weakened in various ways the power of service providers who can no longer assume that most welfare clients have only two options – to take the service on offer or go without. In order to promote competition within the state sector more and more league tables are being published to encourage both consumer choice and competition between welfare providers to push their particular institution to the top of the league tables. [. . .]

Fourth, management as an activity within welfare services has increased dramatically during the 1980s and 1990s, both quantitatively in terms of the extra numbers of staff designated as managers and qualitatively as those who previously played a back-up role increasingly exert far greater control over these 'front line activities'. Again, some of these managers such as the non-teaching heads of large comprehensive schools and medically qualified chief executives of hospital trusts could still be deemed to be welfare professionals but their priorities tend to be the interests of the organization they run rather than the interests of either their front-line professional colleagues or the individual clients of their organizations. [. . .]

Fifth, a major theme of social policy making in the 1980s was a new emphasis on the rights of welfare clients or 'consumers' as the New Right preferred to call them. The days when parents of primary school pupils could be told not to cross a white line drawn in the school playground or parents of hospitalized children could be restricted to set visiting hours have now gone for good. Welfare clients are not only encouraged to play a more participatory role in their individual interactions with welfare professionals but they are also, at least in principle, now given more rights to choose between competing welfare services. [. . .]

Evaluation

The changes we analyse above have been dramatic and radical. Clearly, any assessment of their significance and of what has been gained and lost is heavily influenced by value judgements and at this early stage can only be very provisional but some of the issues are plain.

Emerging criticism of the position of the welfare professions in the 1970s focused on four main issues: the absence of effective political control, the general lack of accountability, the absence of a genuine 'voice' for users, and professional dominance in key areas of policy making. In all these areas there have been striking changes.

1 Professional dominance has given way to a more managed, more democratic professionalism. Reconciling the two inevitably conflicting sources of authority – professional and managerial – needs a lot more work and experience but the pendulum has swung strongly in favour of a more managed and more accountable professionalism and towards a more bounded autonomy. We see that as an advance.
2 We see the expansion of audit, appraisal and inspection as a step forward to a more accountable professionalism. Clearly, it is important to know what professionals do and how effectively and efficiently they do it. Major discrepancies in, for example, the success/survival rates from similar medical interventions on similar types of patients are simply unacceptable.
3 Service users have emerged from a state of virtual social exclusion to a place at least on the edge of the stage. They have gained a 'voice', embryonic rights to a certain specified standard of service and more accessible and easier-to-use complaints systems.
4 Professionals are no longer seen as the arbiters of public policy in their areas of expertise. Their exclusion from the discussions which preceded the educational reforms of 1988 and the health service reforms of 1990 was a watershed in the extension of political power over professional work.

[...] Freidson aptly captures the potential downside of the changes of recent years:

> If they [professionals] are to be mere passive employees without a strong organized voice in the allocation of the resources which are essential for doing good work, they will find it difficult to remain committed to doing good work. If they are to play the role of merely providing whatever is demanded by consumers and authorized by those who pay for it, they will find it difficult to preserve a sense of the value of their schooled judgement. If they are to be merely loyal servants of

the interests of their employers or their own 'business', they will have difficulty sustaining any independent commitment to serving the good of both individual clients and the public. And if they are to be required to work within ultimately mechanical, albeit permissive, standards established and enforced by professionals who act as their administrative and cognitive superiors, they will have to forsake the communal and collegiate principle that is distinctive of the professional mode of organizing work.

(Freidson, 1994: 215)

Four clear and specific issues can be drawn out of Freidson's passionate cry of concern.

1   A reduction of the autonomy of individual welfare professionals as a result of closer management control of resources may be desirable on a number of grounds – and may also be inevitable. But it may significantly affect the ability of professionals to do high-quality work in particular situations, as Freidson suggests, and it may also – more generally – affect morale, motivation and commitment.

2   Professional independence is an important countervailing power to the ever-increasing power of the modern state, under which welfare professionals might eventually become simply servants of state purposes. Professional independence is not the product simply of professional imperialism but of the uncertainty, complexity, and ultimately individual nature of much professional work. Good professional work in medicine, teaching, or social work requires the space for individual judgement. [...]

3   Promotion of consumer power without careful assessment of the consequences entails losses as well as gains. One such cost is the development of more adversarial relations between professionals and service users – witness the huge increase in complaints and legal actions against doctors in recent years. Clearly in the past complaining was too difficult and costly for many of those with grievances. But the new consumerism has been both a spur to a more responsive professionalism and to a new and more adversarial rather than a more constructive partnership relationship between professionals and service users. [...]

4   The attempt to cut the professions down to size has employed certain obvious instruments: political control, management control, law and regulation, inspection and audit. What it has neglected either to cherish or to build on is the potentially positive elements in traditional professionalism: the service ethic, the principle of colleague control, and the commitment to high-quality work. There has been no attempt to build on these aspects of traditional professionalism and breathe new life into them.

Conclusion

Politicians, managers and users may now be attacking traditional welfare professionals' autonomy so hard that some of the most beneficial aspects of professional service are in danger of being lost. The new relationship between politicians, professionals, managers and service has yet to settle down into a partnership based on mutual respect and trust. Until and unless this new partnership is achieved, real gains in terms of the quality of welfare service provided may be much smaller than those promised by the radical reformers of traditional welfare professionalism.

REFERENCES

Auld, R. (1976) *William Tyndale Junior and Infants Schools Public Enquiry: A Report to the Inner London Education Authority*, London, ILEA.

Banks, S. (1998) Professional ethics in social work: what future?, *British Journal of Social Work*, 28: 213–31.

Brewer, C. and Lait, J. (1980) *Can Social Work Survive?*, London, Temple Smith.

Dale, J. and Foster, P. (1986) *Feminists and State Welfare*, London, Routledge.

DHSS (1974) *Report of the Inquiry into the Care and Supervision Provided in Relation to Maria Colwell*, London, HMSO.

Dominelli, L. (1996) Deprofessionalizing social work: anti-oppressive practice, competencies and postmodernism, *British Journal of Social Work*, 26: 153–75.

Doyal, L. (1979) *The Political Economy of Health*, London, Pluto Press.

Freidson, E. (1994) *Professionalism Reborn*, Cambridge, Polity Press.

Harrison, S. and Pollitt, C. (1994) *Controlling Health Professionals*, Buckingham, Open University Press.

Hatcher, R. (1994) Market relationships and the management of teachers, *British Journal of the Sociology of Education*, 15, 1: 41–61.

Howe, D. (1992) Child abuse and the bureaucratization of social work, *Sociological Review*, 40, 3: 491–508.

Illich, I. (1975) *Medical Nemesis*, London, Boyars.

Johnson, T. (1972) *Professions and Power*, London, Macmillan.

Klein, R. (1989) *The Politics of The National Health Service*, 2nd edn, London, Longman.

London Borough of Brent (1985) *A Child in Trust: the Report of the Panel of Enquiry into the Circumstances Surrounding the Death of Jasmine Beckford*, London, Brent.

Martin, J.P. (1984) *Hospitals in Trouble*, Oxford, Blackwell.

Secretary of State for Social Services (1988) *Report of the Inquiry into Child Abuse in Cleveland*, London, HMSO.

Troman, G. (1996) The rise of the new professionals? The restructuring of primary teachers' work and professionalism, *British Journal of the Sociology of Education*, 17, 4: 473–87.

Wilding, P. (1982) *Professional Power and Social Welfare*, London, Routledge.

TWENTY-FIVE

PROFESSIONALS AS MANAGERS ACROSS THE PUBLIC SECTOR

Gordon Causer and Mark Exworthy

Source: *Professionals and the New Managerialism in the Public Sector*, Exworthy, M. and Halford, S. (eds), Open University Press, 1999.

The professional as manager

The thesis that professionals and managers stand in a necessarily antagonistic relationship has ... been a recurrent one in the sociological literature. However, this argument has not been without its critics (see for example Child, 1982). As Freidson has emphasized, a key problem with the thesis of managerial–professional conflict is the fact that professional employees are commonly managed by those drawn from within the profession itself, a pattern which has been long established both within the public sector and elsewhere. Consequently, even though managerial controls may entail a loss of autonomy on the part of the individual professional, the fact that managers are either practising professionals or of professional origin may be argued to represent a continuation of the principle of professional control (Freidson, 1994: 139). Freidson's argument emphasizes that professions are themselves internally stratified, with a division between the rank-and-file practitioner and the supervisory or managerial professional (the 'administrative elite') (p. 142).

Even this, however, is arguably an oversimplification, implying as it does a simple dichotomy between practising professionals on the one hand and supervisory and managerial professionals on the other. In many settings a hard-and-fast distinction along these lines may be difficult to make for at least three reasons. First, the group of managerial professionals may itself be internally stratified, with variations in the relative closeness of different positions to day-to-day practice. Second, a number of areas are characterized by the existence of 'hybrid' roles in which the exercise of formalized managerial responsibilities is carried on alongside continuing engagement in professional practice. Third, the role of the rank-and-file practitioner may itself entail activities of a managerial kind, even where the position occupied is not formally designated as a managerial one. This is most obviously the case where the professional employee has responsibility for supervising the work of non-professionals, or of professionals of lesser experience, but it also extends to responsibilities in such areas as the formulation and management of budgets and handling external relations with customers and clients on behalf of the organization (Causer and Jones, 1996a, b).

As this suggests, a mapping of the relationship between professional and managerial roles and functions is not one which may be adequately attained through the use of a simple dichotomy. Rather, it is necessary to develop a more complex typology which reflects the varying ways in which professional and managerial activities may be related to one another. This typology reflects a continuum of roles rather than discrete categories because different individuals in the same formal position may 'interpret' and 'enact' their roles in different ways. We would suggest that in organizations employing significant numbers of professional employees we can identify three broad roles, each of which may itself be differentiated into two types.

First, there is the role of the *practising (or rank-and-file) professional* – those whose primary function is to engage in the day-to-day exercise of professional activities. Practising professionals may themselves, however, be divided into those whose work involves no supervisory or resource allocation activities (the *pure practitioner*) and those for whom the exercise of such responsibilities is an integral part of their activities, even though they are not formally designated as managers (the *quasi-managerial practitioner*).

Second, there are those drawn from the ranks of practising professionals whose primary responsibility is the management of the day-to-day work of other professionals and of the resources utilized in that work – who we may describe as the *managing professional*. However, this group too may display internal differentiation, according to whether or not the managing professional continues, alongside their managerial activity, to maintain some direct engagement in professional practice. The category of 'managing professionals' may therefore be divided into two groups – the *practising managing professional* and the *non-practising managing professional*.

Finally there are those who have an overall managerial responsibility for the activities of professional employees, but are not themselves concerned with the direct management of day-to-day practice. This group, whom we will designate as *general managers*, may, but need not, be drawn from among those with a background in the practice of the profession itself. We can accordingly differentiate within this group between the *professionally grounded general manager* on the one hand, and the *non-professional general manager* on the other.

Of the six groups identified here, five are characterized by their past or present engagement in professional practice, thus emphasizing the complexity of the processes by which professional groups within organizations may be internally stratified. On the one hand, managing professionals (whether continuing to practise or not) and professionally grounded general managers are likely to retain a measure of identification with the professional group, and may well ground their claim to authority in part on this identification. On the other hand, even among practising professionals there will be those whose roles are not those of the pure practitioner, but rather entail undertaking activities of at least a quasi-managerial nature.

The existence of these patterns of internal stratification has significant implications for the nature of professions. To a greater or lesser degree, professional groups have been held together by the notion (or fiction) of equality of competence (Freidson, 1994: 142). The undertaking of managerial activities by professionals at various levels of the organization reflects an erosion of this notion, as a key function of these groups may be to monitor (overtly or discreetly) the practice of other professionals, and to institute corrective action where it is deemed necessary. Thus in so far as there *is* a tension between managerial imperatives and professional autonomy, this will commonly be expressed not through the imposition of these imperatives by managers on professionals, but rather through the work of those professionals who engage in managerial or quasi-managerial activities.

A further implication of this internal stratification concerns the nature of professional careers. Where advancement within the profession entails movement into positions which involve control over the work of others, or decisions on the allocation of resources, such movement will be dependent not simply – or even primarily – on the display of professional competence, but also on the possession of . . . 'managerial assets' (Exworthy and Halford, 1999: 134). A distinction may be drawn between the older professions, such as medicine and the law (in which the possession of such assets has traditionally been of restricted significance), and the newer professions embedded in both public and private bureaucracies (where their importance for both professional roles and professional advancement has always been greater). However, it may be argued that recent developments have had the effect of promoting a greater degree of internal stratification within both older and newer professional groups, and hence of enhancing the significance of the possession of managerial assets for members of professional groups in general.

In this chapter we seek to address these issues by examining developments in relation to four groups in three areas – doctors and nurses within the health service, teachers within primary and secondary schools, and social workers within local authority social service departments. While trends towards the 'managerialization' of aspects of professional work in each of these areas have intensified during the 1980s and 1990s, they are not peculiar to this period and need to be situated in their longer-term context.

[. . .] There is a general tendency for the managerial component of established managerial professional roles to increase, and for managerial components to become an increasingly important part of the work roles of most professional groups. However, there are significant variations.

It may be argued that the greatest change is that found in the medical profession. Although some doctors have long had an involvement in management, movement into formal management positions or taking on broader managerial responsibilities has not formed part of the typical medical career. Most doctors have remained practitioners throughout their career, and have been able to secure high status and rewards by doing so. In this respect the medical profession has been atypical, and has been able to retain this position partly because, from the inception of the NHS, doctors have secured (and the state has been prepared to concede) certain of the privileges of employment without concomitant subordination to managerial control. The increasing integration of some doctors into formalized management structures (in a way which has long been common in other professional settings) thus represents an important change, with the development of a significant managing professional role in both Trust hospitals and fundholding practices. The future development of these roles within medicine may depend on the fate of the NHS reforms, but pressures for greater accountability and for control over NHS expenditure are unlikely to abate. In this situation it seems probable that the incorporation of doctors into management will continue as a means of enhancing the control of professional work in ways which are already manifest in other areas. To what extent this represents control *of* the profession and to what extent control *by* the profession is debatable, and the question itself reflects the ambiguity of the role of the managerial professional.

In the other three areas ... career advancement, at least beyond a certain point, has long entailed movement away from practice into a role which is either predominantly managerial in nature or at least involves some combination of management and continuing practice. The trends we have considered in this chapter will, in general, have had the effect of reinforcing this process. This development is perhaps clearest in teaching, where government reforms have shifted the work of those in both the middle ranks and at the top of the school hierarchy in the direction of managerial and administrative tasks. Again, it seems unlikely that developments in the foreseeable future will lead to a significant reversal of this trend. Indeed, processes such as external monitoring and accountability are likely if anything to intensify.

In social work, too, career advancement is likely to become increasingly dependent upon the possession of managerial skills and assets. The increased emphasis on care management will demand such skills from social workers and place managers and supervisors in a situation where their role is increasingly defined in terms of managing and deploying resources. The process of a managerialization of social work activities, initially set in train by the implementation of the Seebohm proposals in the 1970s, will continue.

In nursing, we also see evidence of an increasingly managerial definition of professional work, at least so far as the upper echelon of fully qualified nursing staff are concerned. The division between registered nurses and health care assistants, reinforced by the Project 2000 changes in nurse education, is likely to locate the work of nurses increasingly in the management of patient care and in the overview of the work of those who provide the more basic practical aspects of that care. As this case suggests, the managerialization of aspects of professional work should not necessarily be seen as undermining professional status, but may also serve as a means of enhancing it. However, the erosion of the nursing hierarchy above ward level may impair the scope for movement into more general management roles.

As these examples indicate, the relationship between professional and managerial activities – always more complex than the simple thesis of professional–management conflict implied – has become if anything more complex over time. Processes of marketization and pressures for increased accountability have tended to erode traditional notions of equality of competence on the part of professional employees, and have set up pressures to render professional performance more open to scrutiny. But the very fact that performance of professional tasks rests upon the possession of specialist knowledge or expertise means that those drawn from the ranks of the profession are likely to play a central role in this process (Boreham, 1983). Thus what from one perspective may be seen as a process of managerial control, from another may be seen as a means of retaining a measure of professional self-regulation. Professions are likely to be increasingly characterized by processes of internal stratification, in which both professional identities and sources of authority become more ambiguous in nature. The intra-organizational divisions on which we have focused . . . will be compounded by inter-organizational divisions, both those fostered by the development of quasi-market competition and those based on the growth of external regulation. The growing use of external inspection and audit in a number of areas itself draws upon the expertise of those with professional backgrounds and experience to monitor performance within the areas of professional competence.

In this situation, the status and power of professions may come increasingly to depend upon their ability to cast their goals and objectives in appropriate terms. As we have indicated, the development of a more explicitly managerial definition of the role of the qualified nurse can be seen as part of a strategy to enhance the status of the professional group, and it is not difficult to envisage similar developments in other areas. While 'care management' has been viewed with trepidation by many social workers, one can see how the redefinition of social work in the language of care management could provide a basis for claiming a specialist expertise and an associated professional jurisdiction in the face of threatened encroachment by other occupational groups. Likewise, the increasing involvement of doctors in management may provide scope for the casting of medical goals in the language of markets and competition. In these circumstances managerial and professional discourses are likely to become increasingly fused.

Notwithstanding the interprofessional and intersectoral variations described..., it is clear that the boundaries between professional and managerial work in the public sector are becoming increasingly blurred. The notion of a clear-cut division between managers and professionals – or even between managerial and rank-and-file professionals – is in some respects increasingly unhelpful. Not only will it become increasingly difficult to classify the *functions* of an activity through a simple dichotomy, but comparable problems will also arise in the analysis of the *identities* of those occupying such positions (see Halford and Leonard, 1999).

These conclusions suggest that managerial assets are becoming of increasing importance for career advancement within the professions. To some extent, such assets have always been important in most professions, but their significance is intensifying. For many people engaged in professional activity it may become increasingly inappropriate to ask whether they are a professional *or* a manager, for the essential nature of their work will lie in the combination of both elements.

REFERENCES

Boreham, P. (1983) Indetermination: professional knowledge, organization and control, *Sociological Review*, 31(4): 693–718.

Causer, G. and Jones, C. (1996a) Management and the control of technical labour, *Work, Employment and Society*, 10(1): 105–23.

Causer, G. and Jones, C. (1996b) One of them or one of us? The ambiguities of the professional as manager, in R. Fincham (ed.) *New Relationships in the Organized Professions*, Aldershot, Avebury.

Child, J. (1982) Professionals in the corporate world, in D. Dunkerley and G. Salaman (eds) *International Yearbook of Organization Studies 1981*, London, Routledge and Kegan Paul.

Exworthy, M. and Halford, S. (1999) Professionals and managers in a changing public sector: conflict, compromise and collaboration?, in M. Exworthy and S. Halford (eds) *Professionals and the New Managerialism in the Public Sector*, Buckingham, Open University Press.

Freidson, E. (1994) *Professionalism Re-Born: Theory, Prophecy and Policy*, Oxford, Polity Press.

Halford, S. and Leonard, P. (1999) New identities? Professionalism, managerialism and the construction of self, in M. Exworthy and S. Halford (eds) *Professionals and the New Managerialism in the Public Sector*, Buckingham, Open University Press.

TWENTY-SIX

SUPERVISING PROFESSIONAL WORK UNDER NEW PUBLIC MANAGEMENT: EVIDENCE FROM AN 'INVISIBLE TRADE'

Martin Kitchener, Ian Kirkpatrick and Richard Whipp

Source: *British Journal of Management*, 2000, 11, 3.

Introduction

Contemporary analyses of work supervision (for example, Delbridge and Lowe, 1997; Reed, 1999) devote little attention to developments within UK public services. Ten years ago, Ackroyd, Hughes and Soothill (1989) reported that in this context, professional groups resist the implementation of bureaucratic control strategies. Instead a 'custodial' mode of line management prevailed. This term is used to indicate that the primary concern of supervisors is to: 'preserve and perpetuate customary [professionally determined] kinds and standards of service provision' (p. 603). A cornerstone of this argument is that senior professionals seek to maintain service standards by 'coaching' or mentoring junior colleagues (Scott, 1965). To maintain the collegial relations needed to perform this role, supervisors tend to protect the autonomy of junior staff and restrict the flow of performance data to management information systems (Power, 1997).

Analysts of the 'new public management' project (Hood, 1991) contend that the custodial mode of supervision has been threatened by a political ideology that has been translated into a number of public policy initiatives. These include the development of performance measurement, and attempts to develop a cadre of hybrid 'practitioner managers' who will increasingly monitor and control professionals' work (Exworthy and Halford, 1999;

Ferlie *et al.*, 1996; Kitchener, Kirkpatrick and Whipp, 1999). Whilst there is some evidence of these trends in private-sector professional organizations (Cooper *et al.*, 1996; Greenwood and Hinings, 1993; Hinings, Brown and Greenwood, 1991), no previous study has concentrated upon the trajectory of work supervision in UK public services.

This paper takes the supervision of professional work as the principal subject of study. It has two main aims. The first is to assess the extent to which new public management (NPM) initiatives have influenced the line management of professional work in UK public services. To achieve this, the paper concentrates on the line management of children's homes by the first tier of supervisors within local-authority social services departments (SSDs). The second aim of the paper is to include UK public services in the theoretical discourse on the changing nature of work supervision. This is achieved by using selected concepts from organizational theory and the sociology of the professions to help analyse developments in SSDs. [. . .]

Most of the literature points to how prevailing line-management structures, styles and practices in SSDs have combined to enable a custodial mode of supervision. These arrangements placed serious constraints on management control, although they may have acted to preserve collegial relations between residential staff and supervisors. In the next section, we consider how this situation was challenged in the 1990s, as part of a wider shift towards the new public management.

New public management and the changing nature of professional supervision

During the last twenty years, increasing political attention has been given to the ways in which professional work is organized in UK public services. Across the public sector, concern for the organization of professional work has arisen against a changing political economy that increasingly espouses NPM doctrines such as: consumerism, the attempted reduction of government spending and the introduction of market forms (Hood, 1991). These doctrines form part of a wider political project that was driven initially by the neo-liberal economic theory of 'New Right' Conservative politicians (see for example, Clarke and Newman, 1997). The principal aim has been to 'get more for less' from public services (Hood, 1991).

In this context, the public-service professions were scrutinized from a number of directions. For public choice theorists, the greatest problem was the monopoly power held by established occupational groups. This tended to distort the market and resulted in 'producer capture' of services that were run to promote the interests of the professions rather than users (Alaszewski, 1995: 56–9). By contrast, what might be termed a management critique, was more squarely targeted at the perceived failures of professional bureaucracy as a mechanism for delivering public services. In particular, collegial forms of organization were seen as 'impediments to the development of rationalised managerial control' (Ackroyd, 1995: 6). Professional bureaucracies were criticized for being too operationally driven, their thinking dominated by the provision of existing services and lacking the capacity to respond to change or implement effective strategies. Front-line staff, it was argued, also exercised too much discretion without regard to budgetary constraints or agency priorities.

For advocates of NPM, the solution to this problem was to make professional services more like 'public businesses', with clear goals, corporate strategies and mechanisms for evaluating performance (Farnham and Horton, 1996). In short, it was felt necessary to close off '. . . indeterminate and open-ended features of professional practice, in order to conform with broader corporate goals and resource constraints' (Flynn, 1999: 35). In place of the old custodial management a more bureaucratic form of control needed to be established, one that placed more emphasis on standardizing practice and on establishing clear performance targets for individual professionals (Hoggett, 1996: 13; Pollitt, 1993).

The emerging model of bureaucratic control in SSDs

In personal social services the NPM critique of professional organization centred on issues similar to those found in other parts of the public sector (Langan and Clarke, 1994). The perceived inadequacies of management control systems over front-line practitioners, both in fieldwork teams and residential establishments, were of particular concern. This problem was stressed in a stream of reports for the UK Department of Health (Shaw, 1995). Most recently, a national study by the Social Services Inspectorate concluded that:

> Although all SSDs have developed a range of planning, policy and procedural documents, these were not always followed by staffs . . . We were concerned that front-line managers did not monitor practice . . . The management information systems were poorly developed making effective service planning difficult and were also inadequate in providing managers with the means to ensure effective quality control.
>
> (1998: 3–26)

In the case of children's residential care, a succession of abuse scandals added to political concerns about the failures of management control (Berridge and Brodie, 1996: 184; Social Services Inspectorate, 1993, 1995). The Utting report (1997: 13), for example, famously observed that 'the physical isolation of an establishment from the management structure of its parent body may [still] set it out of mind as well as out of sight'.

To tackle these perceived deficiencies in management, a range of guidance has been produced linked to major legislation – the NHS and Community Care Act 1990 and Children Act 1989. In children's services, this guidance has called for 'tighter managerial control over practitioners, with more emphasis on procedures for child protection...' (Rushton and Nathan, 1996: 372). This has direct implications for the custodial approaches to supervision that we described earlier. In particular, the guidelines suggest a more *bureaucratic* approach towards the control of front line staffs (Packman and Jordan, 1991). To understand what this means it is helpful to return to our three dimensions of supervision: structures, styles and practices (see Table 26.1 for a summary). [...]

In Table 26.1, two 'ideal types' of professional work supervision are synthesized ... Of course, neither schema outlined in Table 26.1 is suggested to reflect exactly the practices of any one supervisor or single SSD. Rather, it is argued that in various ways, and at different speeds, NPM ideas and policies challenge each of the dimensions of the custodial mode to line management that were described earlier. [...]

Research design and methods

The data reported in this paper originate from a two-year Department of Health-funded study of the management of children's homes by local authorities in England and Wales (Whipp, Kirkpatrick and Kitchener, 2000). The project was conducted between 1996 and 1999. It was designed to provide an understanding of the models of management which inform the conduct of SSDs, and their impact on the management of children's homes. The research method employed was largely qualitative in character, as befits the first exploration of the subject in this form. The

Table 26.1 Modes of line management in SSDs

Dimensions of supervision	Custodial mode	Emerging bureaucratic mode
Structure	Residential experience an advantage	Residential experience an asset, but not essential
	Role ambiguity amongst supervisors	Reduced role ambiguity amongst supervisors
	Low levels of financial autonomy for unit managers (UMs)	Increased financial accountability for UMs
Style	High involvement in operational matters	Low involvement in operational matters
	Capacity to provide expert advice	Limited capacity to provide expert advice
Practice	Concern to support autonomous practice of junior staff	Concern to monitor practice and link to agency goals

emphasis was on intensive, comparative examination of 12 local authorities.

[. . .]

Supervising professional work under NPM

Some of the views considered earlier in this paper maintain that NPM should lead to a move away from custodial modes of line management, towards a bureaucratic mode (e.g. Hoggett, 1996). The aim of this section is to draw on our study data to assess how far such change has occurred in SSDs. [. . .]

Changes in supervisory structures

In respect of supervisory structures there was evidence of only a partial shift towards the bureaucratic model described earlier. The area of greatest change was the increasing number of supervisors who did not come from a residential background. Table 26.2 describes the functional background of the supervisors within the case authorities, revealing that less than half the sample (16 out of 34 line managers) had previously worked in residential care. A linked feature was the growing tendency of some senior professionals in SSDs to favour general management skills as the basis for recruitment into supervisory posts. A representative of this view was the Director of Social Services at London 1:

> I think experience is useful but I don't think it's essential by any means. I think there are so many core management functions in terms of looking after and developing staff, supervision, appraisal systems, training, budget management, goal setting, planning, there are some very generic important things as common to all management tasks.
>
> (Director of Social Services, London 1)

The growing importance of general management skills was also reflected in the increased investment by all the case SSDs in management training for middle-ranking professionals, reflecting a wider trend in UK social services (Lawler and Hearn, 1997).

By contrast, there was far less evidence of any marked reduction in role ambiguity of supervisors or any formalization of their responsibilities. It is surprising that only one SSD, Metro 1, produced a document that specified the tasks expected of residential line-managers. The comprehensive Metro 1 document outlines senior management's expectations regarding the role of the children's home supervisor, relevant law and policy, financial arrangements, supervision procedures, departmental personnel policies and

Table 26.2 Background of children's homes' line managers

Local authority	Number of line managers with responsibility for children's homes	Background of children's homes' line managers
Metro 1	7	7 residential
Metro 2	3	2 residential; 1 field social-work
Metro 3	1	1 nursing
Shire 1	1	1 residential
Shire 2	9	3 residential; 6 field social-work
Shire 3	1	1 field social-work
London 1	2	1 field social-work; 1 day centres
London 2	2	2 field social-work
London 3	not applicable	not applicable
Unitary 1	1	1 field social-work
Unitary 2	4	2 residential; 2 field social-work
Unitary 3	3	1 residential; 2 field social-work

information regarding interactions with, for example, parents or clients. The existence of such guidelines in Metro 1 was in stark contrast to the situation in most of the other case SSDs. In these cases, there was no formal document that outlined senior managers' expectations of supervisors' responsibilities, and little sign of any clear reduction in role ambiguity. As a line manager in London 2 explained:

> We are filling a sandwich between the staff team on one level and senior managers on the other because, obviously, the unit managers want one thing, the staff want something completely different and God knows what upper managers and members want. We have got to try and ease the tension and find the middle of the way, as it were – which isn't always possible. Sometimes you have to make decisions, which you don't necessarily agree with because senior managers say they have to be made.
>
> (Line manager, London 2)

[. . .]

Changes in supervisory styles

Looking at supervisory style, a similar picture of slow and uneven development towards a bureaucratic model was evident. For example, in only two SSDs was there any sign that senior managers were encouraging supervisors to adopt a more 'hands-off' approach. In one case, Metro 3, the director saw this as necessary for line managers to become more 'strategic':

one way of solving isolation is to have the line manager often popping in and being almost 'part of the establishment'. I feel there are enormous dangers in that, as well as a loss of use of that line manager's real potential, if they do that. I think you can find systems within the department as a whole that make each team and each establishment feel they are part of a wider department, without it having to be on the basis of 'how often do I see them?' 'how often do our managers call by?'.

(Director, Metro 3)

[...]

In the remaining SSDs, the expectation, both of senior managers and of residential staff, was that supervisors should continue to be closely involved at the operational level. Typical of this view was an ex-residential manager at Metro 2, who stressed that residential experience, empathy, and a willingness to help out in times of crisis were key elements of his line-management style:

The children in the homes know me because I visit them. The staffs in the homes know me. I have been around forever and a day. I have known colleagues for a very long time. Most of the unit managers I have managed elsewhere before their present posts ... So really, in every aspect of the children's homes I have a kind of finger in the pie and a management role ... I can judge a unit based on my experience, what they're doing. I can feel it in the gut. You walk through the door and your gut tells you what the unit's up to. You can feel the atmosphere, it feels good, it feels bad. You've got to understand the concept of residential. I believe it's so unique ... There's no substitute for having that experience around you ... The AD does not have residential experience. I don't know if she's ever been up at 3 o'clock in the morning facing a kid of sixteen with a knife who wants to slash his wrists ... That's the uniqueness of residential care.

(Line manager, Metro 2)

[...] The continued emphasis on line managers being involved in operational details also meant that the supervisor remained, in most cases, the main source of external advice and support for front-line staff. Of course, the extent to which supervisors were able to perform this function depended on their own past experience working in residential care. As was shown in the previous section, this applied to an increasingly small number of managers (see Table 26.2). To deal with this issue, non-experienced supervisors tended to adopt a range of alternative strategies to manage their relationships with staff groups. In Shire 2, for example, one line manager admitted that 'when I came into this job it didn't go down well, that I hadn't got any residential experience...', but she also suggested that she had gained the confidence of staff groups by 'showing an interest' and 'being prepared to fight their corner for them'. What is clear is that support and advice may take on a variety of forms. It may come from a line manager with a long experience in residential care and a detailed understanding of the problems faced. Alternatively, support may take the form of non-expert advocacy and a willingness to listen and empathize with front-line staff.

In only one SSD, Shire 3, had steps been taken to develop a system of advice and support outside the framework of line management. To achieve this, the assistant director had established a professional therapeutic team, made up of ex-residential staff, to offer a range of services to staff groups. According to one senior manager, the aim of this central team was 'to help to absorb some of that "real toxic muck" that supervisors have to manage' and to carry out 'direct work with the group of unit managers, so that they are better facilitated in managing their staff'. Beyond this example, none of the case SSDs had established alternative support mechanisms or any system for separating 'practice' and 'management' supervision (Syrett, Jones and Sercoble, 1996).

Changes in supervisory practices

In this section we assess how far staff supervision in SSDs had changed, from being primarily concerned with maintaining collegial relationships, to a more managerial approach, geared towards monitoring and control. Looking across the 12 cases, there was evidence of only slight change in this direction.

The most obvious shift in practice had come with the new requirement on supervisors to conduct formal, monthly inspections of their residential establishments (referred to as Regulation 22 visits). The aim of these inspections was to evaluate the administration of each home, the general upkeep and the extent to which staff groups were achieving their stated goals. [...]

A further indicator of change in practice was the attempt made in some SSDs to develop a performance–management framework for staff supervision. The aim here was to use supervision sessions in a more systematic way, to appraise staff development and check progress in meeting wider institutional goals. The most developed examples of this were Metros 1 and 3 and Shire 3, all of which had established formal staff appraisal systems and were seeking IIP (Investors in People) accreditation. In Metro 1, for example, a formalized procedure had been established for staff supervision (see above) in which each unit manager was given a 'professional development plan'. Although less developed in Metro 3, there were also plans to set up a more formalized system for assessing and developing staff performance. The aim, according to the director, was to 'achieve the idea of corporate mentalities, the idea of a corporate perspective, making them [unit managers] feel that they're part of the whole and not just a part of something that they don't want to be part of'.

Against these signs of a change in supervisory practice was evidence to suggest continuity with older 'custodial' approaches. For example, whilst it was clear that the supervisory role had become more concerned with formal inspection and regulation, the way in which this was carried out varied immensely between SSDs. In many cases, inspection visits were conducted infrequently and reports were neither fully completed nor passed upwards to senior managers (see Kitchener, Kirkpatrick and Whipp, 1999).

A more general obstacle to change was the way as noted earlier, that a majority of SSDs had not established a clear framework or policy for conducting supervision. Only a minority were moving towards a performance management approach or seeking IIP accreditation. Consequently, in the absence of any central directives, the tendency in most cases was for supervision to continue to emphasize the maintenance of relationships. [. . .]

A further obstacle to change arose from the nature of the work itself. A particular difficulty was faced by inexperienced line managers attempting to impose themselves over front-line operational staff, increasingly under pressure to meet more complex needs with limited resources. For many unit managers, the supervisor's experience in residential care was crucial if he or she was to have any credibility in the eyes of operational staffs. According to an informant in Metro 2, for example:

> . . . it isn't just a job, for many people it's more than just a job it's a vocation. And if you haven't had that experience and you're trying to support and guide and manage people who are in those posts, you don't necessarily understand.
>
> (Unit manager, Metro 2)

In this context, it had become increasingly difficult for supervisors who lacked past experience to adopt a more directive or 'inquisitorial' style. As a result, most tended to avoid conflict by offering support and respecting the autonomy of front line professionals. As a line manager in Shire 2 explained:

> I'm not an expert on everything. Some of them are far better than me in running budgets and rotas and things like that. I let them get on with it. I delegate it. If they can do it better than me, let them do it!
>
> (Line manager, Shire 2)

Conclusion

It is clear that the NPM project has influenced British public-policy initiatives designed to curb the dominance of the custodial approach to the supervision of professional work. Not only have these attempts been concerned with the stated aims of efficiency and accountability but also with imposing bureaucratic control strategies which challenge prevailing patterns of professional organizational power and discretion (Hoggett, 1996; Pollitt, 1993). In this respect, the public sector appears to differ from what many regard as the trend in private organizations towards increased decentralization, flexibility and empowerment (Clegg, 1990; Reed, 1999). In the public sector, the overall thrust of change, many argue, has been to establish a more formalized arrangement for monitoring practice according to agency goals by placing limits on the discretion and autonomy of front-line professionals (Hoggett, 1996; Pollitt, 1993).

[. . .] Looking beyond the context of SSDs, the conclusions presented in this paper have a number of more general implications for our knowledge of the NPM. First, our findings suggest that shifts towards a bureaucratic model of control have been far less dramatic and more contested than is predicted in much of the public management literature. Of course, this is not to ignore the fact that there have been attempts to subject professional work to bureaucratic routines. Rather, our argument is that, at least in the context of SSDs, these changes do not seem to have been so marked. As has been suggested elsewhere (Akroyd and Bolton, 1999), there may be a tendency to understate the difficulty faced by public managers in transforming professional work practices in a context of rising demands on services and declining resources.

The second wider implication of this study is that it points to the importance of understanding professional services as a distinct form of work organization that is robust in the face of management-led change. Of course, a parallel version of this point can be found in the classical literature on professional organizations (Abbott, 1988; Freidson, 1994). It has also been made in a small number of studies on attempts to transform management in contexts such as accountancy (Ferner, Edwards and Sisson, 1995; Hinings, Brown and Greenwood, 1991) and law (Cooper et al., 1996). To date, however, these issues have not received sufficient attention in the context of UK public services. Although concentrating on one under-studied group, this paper has sought to rectify that deficiency. In doing so, it raises questions not only about the obstacles to radical change in supervisory systems but also about whether such change is possible at all.

REFERENCES

Abbott, A. (1988) *The System of Professions: An Essay on the Division of Expert Labour*, Chicago, University of Chicago Press.

Ackroyd, S. (1995) 'The new management and the professionals: assessing the impact of Thatcherism on the British public services', Working Paper No. 24, Work – Organisation – Economy Working Paper Series. Stockholm University.

Ackroyd, S. and Bolton, S. (1999) 'It is not Taylorism: mechanisms of work intensification in the provision of gynaecological services in an NHS hospital', *Work Employment and Society*, 13(2): 369–87.

Ackroyd, S., Hughes, J. and Soothill, K. (1989) 'Public sector services and their management', *Journal of Management Studies*, 26(6): 603–19.

Alaszewski, A. (1995) 'Restructuring health and welfare professions in the United Kingdom: the impact of internal markets on medical, nursing and social work professions', in T. Johnson, G. Larkin and M. Saks (eds), *Health Professions and the State in Europe*, London, Routledge.

Berridge, D. (1985) *Children's Homes*, London, Basil Blackwell.

Berridge, D. and Brodie, I. (1996) 'Residential child care in England and Wales. The inquiries and after', in M. Hill and J. Aldgate (eds), *Child Welfare Services. Developments in Law, Policy, Practice and Research*, London, Jessica Kingsley.

Berridge, D. and Brodie, I. (1997) *Children's Homes Revisited*, London, Jessica Kingsley.

Clarke, J. and Newman, J. (1997) *The Managerialist State*, London, Sage.

Clegg, S. (1990) *Modern Organisations: Organisation Studies in the PostModern World*, London, Sage.

Cooper, D.J., Hinings, C.R., Greenwood, R. and Brown, J.L. (1996) 'Sedimentation and transformation in organisation change: The case of Canadian law firms', *Organisation Studies*, 17(4): 623–47.

Delbridge, R. and Lowe, J. (1997) 'Manufacturing control: Supervisory systems on the "new" shopfloor', *Sociology*, 31(3): 409–26.

Exworthy, M. and Halford, S. (eds) (1999) *Professionals and the New Management in the Public Sector*, Buckingham, Open University Press.

Farnham, D. and Horton, S. (eds) (1996) *Managing the New Public Services*, London, Macmillan.

Ferlie, E., Ashburner, L., Fitzgerald, L. and Pettigrew, A. (1996) *The New Public Management in Action*, Oxford, Oxford University Press.

Ferner, A., Edwards, P. and Sisson, K. (1995) 'Coming unstuck? In search of the corporate glue in an international professional service firm', *Human Resources Management*, 34(3): 343–61.

Flynn, R. (1999) 'Managerialism, professionalism and quasi markets', in M. Exworthy and S. Halford (eds), *Professionals and the New Managerialism in the Public Sector*, Buckingham, Open University Press.

Freidson, E. (1994) *Professionalism Reborn: Theory, Prophecy and Policy*, Chicago, University of Chicago Press.

Greenwood, R. and Hinings, C. (1993) 'Understanding strategic change: The contribution of archetypes', *Academy of Management Journal*, 36: 1052–81.

Hinings, C.R., Brown, J.L. and Greenwood, R. (1991) 'Change in an autonomous professional organization', *Journal of Management Studies*, 28(4): 375–93.

Hoggett, P. (1996) 'New modes of control in the public service', *Public Adminis-tration*, 74: 9–32.

Hood, C. (1991) 'A public management for all seasons?', *Public Administration*, 69(1): 3–19.

Kitchener, M., Kirkpatrick, I. and Whipp R. (1999) 'Decoupling managerial audit: Evidence from the local authority children's homes sector', *International Journal of Public Sector Management*, 12(4): 338–50.

Langan, M. and Clarke, J. (1994) 'Managing in the mixed economy of care', in J. Clarke, A. Cochrane and E. McLaughlin (eds), *Managing Social Policy*, London, Sage.

Lawler, J. and Hearn, J. (1997) 'The managers of social work: the experiences and identifications of third tier social services managers and the implications for future practice', *British Journal of Social Work*, 27: 191–218.

Packman, J. and Jordan, B. (1991) 'The Children Act: Looking forward, looking back', *British Journal of Social Work*, 21(4): 315–27.

Pollitt, C. (1993) *Managerialism and the Public Services: The Anglo American Experience*, 2nd edn, London, Macmillan.

Power, M. (1997) *The Audit Society*, Oxford, Oxford University Press.

Reed, M. (1999) 'From the "cage" to the "gaze": The dynamics of organisational control in late modernity', in G. Morgan and L. Engwall (eds), *Regulation, Risk and the Rules of Corporate Action*, London, Routledge (forthcoming).

Residential Care Association (1982) *Middle Management in Residential Social Work* (The Ollerton Report), London, RCA.

Rushton, A. and Nathan, J. (1996) 'The supervision of child protection work', *British Journal of Social Work*, 26: 357–74.

Scott, W.R. (1965) 'Reactions to supervision in a heteronomous professional organisation', *Administrative Science Quarterly*, 10: 65–81.

Shaw, I. (1995) 'The quality of mercy: the management of quality in the personal social services', in I. Kirkpatrick and M. Martinez-Lucio (eds), *The Politics of Quality in the Public Sector*, London, Routledge.

Social Services Inspectorate (1993) *Corporate Parents: Inspection of Residential Child Care Services in Eleven Local Authorities* (November 1992 to March 1993), London, Social Services Inspectorate.

Social Services Inspectorate (1995) *Interface or Interference?*, London, Social Services Inspectorate.

Social Services Inspectorate (1998) *Someone Else's Children: Inspections of Planning and Decision Making for Children Looked After and The Safety of Children Looked After*, London: Social Services Inspectorate/Department of Health.

Syrett, V., Jones, M. and Sercoble, N. (1996) 'Practice supervision: the challenge of definition', *Practice*, 8(3): 53–62.

Utting, W. (1997) 'People Like Us', *The Review of the Safeguards for Children Living Away from Home*. Summary Report, London, HMSO.

Whipp, R., Kirkpatrick, I. and Kitchener, M. (2000) *A Managed Service*, Chichester, Wiley.

TWENTY-SEVEN

IN PURSUIT OF INTER-AGENCY COLLABORATION IN THE PUBLIC SECTOR: WHAT IS THE CONTRIBUTION OF THEORY AND RESEARCH?

Bob Hudson, Brian Hardy, Melanie Henwood
and Gerald Wistow

Source: *Public Management*, 1999, June, 1, 2.

Introduction: the optimism of collaboration

Inter-agency collaboration in the public sector has been viewed as a self-evident virtue in complex societies for several decades, yet has remained conceptually elusive and perennially difficult to achieve. Paradoxically, these problems have not diminished governmental enthusiasm for it – indeed, if anything, the pursuit of inter-agency collaboration has become hotter. This is particularly so of the United Kingdom, where the 1997 Labour government has been ideologically anxious to jettison the emphasis of the previous administration upon markets and competition. Collaboration – or 'partnership', as the Government prefers to describe it – seemed the ideal alternative. [. . .]

While recognizing that there are other positions, this article takes the normative position that collaboration is generally a 'good thing' – a stance which is consistent with the rather long history of collaboration in organization theory and public administration (Kagan and Neville, 1993). Clearly there are also other variables which are important in securing high quality public services, and effective joint working cannot compensate for services which are simply poor. [...] The main question which we ... seek to answer is 'what increases the probability of collaboration?'

Towards a theoretical framework for collaboration

Our framework accordingly identifies ten stages of *collaborative endeavour*. The notion of 'stages' implies sequential activity, and although such a logic can be identified, it would be wrong to suggest that there is some 'iron law of collaborative endeavour' through which agencies must dutifully progress – some may have made more progress on later stages than earlier ones, or may find themselves losing some of the success they may have gained at any particular stage. The process may need repeated attempts to even begin, and thereafter is likely to be iterative and cumulative rather than merely sequential, with a large element of learning by doing. For these reasons we prefer to refer to 'components' rather than 'stages'. [...]

Contextual factors: expectations and constraints

There is now widespread recognition of the difficulties associated with a fragmented approach to service delivery, and this has led to collaboration being elevated to the status of a desirable – even essential – activity. [...]

THE ACKNOWLEDGED LIMITS OF ORGANIZATIONAL INDIVIDUALISM

Organizational individualism is increasingly seen as an inadequate response to the growth in *task scope* (Alter and Hage, 1993) – that is the degree to which a problem to be solved must be addressed from many perspectives. If greater knowledge persuades us to see problems as multi-faceted, then we will be pushed into more complex kinds of co-ordination mechanisms. [...]

THE PERCEIVED VIRTUES OF COLLABORATION

Notwithstanding the traditional public sector focus, collaboration now tends to be seen as a virtue in both the public *and* private sectors. There is, for example, an extensive literature on how Japanese 'inter-firm networks', such as Toyota, operate. [...] Developments such as these have led to the emergence of a school of thought which emphasizes the positive role of co-operative arrangements between industry participants, and the importance of what Kanter (1994) has termed '*collaborative advantage*' as the foundation of superior business performance. This does not mean that competition is no longer important. Burton's view is that neither a totally adversarial stance on all fronts nor an entirely collaborative approach is necessarily an optimal course of action for any firm, and that the problem lies in deciding upon the right combination of each – what he terms a *'composite strategy'* (Burton, 1995). [...]

Recognition of the need to collaborate

The focus of the first component has been upon the danger of fragmentation and the virtue of collaboration. There is a danger of presenting the debate as a simple conflict between two forces. Although this second component is concerned with recognizing the need to collaborate, it does so with an awareness of the problematic nature of collaboration as a concept. [...]

CONFLICT AS AN ENDURING PRESENCE

...The work of Talcott Parsons focused upon those normative structures which maintained and guaranteed social order, and led him to view conflict as a 'disease' with disruptive, dissociating and dysfunctional consequences (Parsons, 1937). In policy terms it can be argued that a Parsonian perspective has been adopted in which conflict is seen as inherently at odds with the principles of successful management and organization – conflict and collaboration tend to be portrayed as diametric opposites of a single inter-organizational dimension.

Other writers (Distefano, 1984; Alter, 1990) see it as more realistic to view conflict and collaboration as two separate and different dynamics which can occur simultaneously, and therefore propose that conflict needs to be accepted as an unavoidable process in all inter-organizational delivery systems. [...]

COLLABORATION AS A PROBLEMATIC CONCEPT AND POLICY TOOL

As well as acknowledging the existence of conflict, it is important to recognize the problematic nature of collaboration as a concept and as a way of working. [...]

For Warren *et al.* (1974) it is: 'a structure or process of concerted decision-making wherein the decisions or action of two or more organisations are made simultaneously in part or in whole with some deliberate degree of adjustment to each other' (p. 16).

[...]

IDENTIFICATION OF AREAS OF INDEPENDENCE AND INTERDEPENDENCE

Stakeholders need to have an *appreciation* of their interdependence, for without this, collaborative problem-solving efforts make no sense (Gray, 1985). Broadly, collaboration is more likely where organizations have similar *goals*, whereas similar *functions* would be likely to put them in competition. Alter and Hage (1993) use the term *symbiotic co-operation* to refer to relationships among organizations that may have similarities but operate in different sectors, and suggest that these can be intense and stable in nature. This is contrasted with *competitive co-operation* where organizations of the same kind are producing the same product or service. In such circumstances, relationships are predicted to be fragile and insecure. As well as a mutual recognition of *interdependence*, it is also important to acknowledge areas of *independence* – that is, those activities which organizations define as their specialist realm of practice and which they believe can be best undertaken on an intra-agency basis. [. . .]

Identification of a legitimate basis for collaboration

The second component explored some of the tensions surrounding the conflict and collaborative imperatives. and raised the issue of how the two could be reconciled. As has already been noted, collaboration as a policy tool is typically predicated upon altruistic assumptions about individual and organizational behaviour which tend to be unrealistic. Conflict theory, on the other hand, *starts* with what appears to be a mutually beneficial exchange, but then discovers elements of compulsion and exploitation which appear as normative only because the oppressed and exploited do not have the power to resist them (Rex, 1982). One way of reconciling these is to suggest that they apply in different situations – that there are some situations which are orderly and stable (in which collaboration is appropriate) and others which are ridden with conflict and instability. Such an approach belies the reality that collaboration and conflict can co-exist in an inter-organizational relationship, and that the former may help to overcome the latter. . . .

Two interconnected explanations are those of *policy networks* and *exchange theory*. Studies of policy networks endeavour to explore the way in which policy is made within the context of a network of actors and organizations (Rhodes, 1988; Marsh and Rhodes, 1992). Rhodes argues that types of network can be distinguished by their degree of integration. At one end of the continuum are *policy* communities which are highly integrated within the policy-making process, have stable and restricted membership and have a strong sense of shared objectives. At the other end lie *issue* networks which are looser, less stable in membership and with weaker points of entry. Although the concept of a policy network does tend to imply qualities such as stability, trust, shared objectives and the voluntary exchange of resources, Rhodes has also defined policy networks in terms of different structures of dependencies (Rhodes, 1992), and in doing so has linked policy networks with the second perspective of exchange theory.

The basic assumption of exchange theory is that individual and group interests are multiple and divergent, and that the net result is competition, bargaining and conflict. This '*pessimistic*' model is in sharp contrast to the consensual assumptions which underpin the optimistic approach. In answer to the question 'why does collaboration take place?', the answer will be that it is in the self-interest of the organizations (and the individuals who work in them) to do so. Self-interest may not be the only thing which motivates public servants, but it will be a significant factor. [...]

The 'resource dependency' model (Benson, 1975) is ... characterized by three essentials: organizational life is an ongoing struggle to obtain, enhance and protect interests; collaboration is one of the means by which organizations seek to manage their own survival; and collaboration will accordingly only be entered into where there is some mutual benefit to be derived from doing so. The message is not one which is entirely pessimistic about the possibility of collaboration, but it is clear that successful collaboration needs to be rooted in hard-headed deals which seem to promise mutual gain. [...]

Assessment of collaborative capacity

The notion of *collaborative capacity* refers to the level of activity or degree of change a collaborative relationship is able to sustain without any partner losing a sense of security in the relationship. This sense of security encompasses not only the tangible resources which are central to collaborative endeavour, but less obvious matters such as perceived loss of autonomy and perceived change in relative strength. Demands can both overreach or underreach thresholds of capacity: an underestimate can mean that a committed collaborative effort is confined to marginal tasks, while an overestimate can lead to unrealistic expectations of what can be achieved and within what time-scale. A judgement on what is attainable will need to take account of *local* and *national* factors, and may be difficult to make accurately. In such circumstances there will be a degree of 'learning by doing', as new relationships and approaches develop.

[...]

Articulation of a clear sense of collaborative purpose

Most approaches to collaboration take it for granted that an explicit statement of shared vision is a prerequisite to success. In their review of the literature, for example, Mattesich and Monsey (1992) state that collaborating partners should have the same vision, along with a clearly agreed mission, objectives and strategy – although they do suggest that this shared vision may either exist at the outset or develop as work proceeds. They also emphasize that the goals and objectives need to be clear to all partners, and be realistically capable of attainment – goals which lack clarity or attainability will diminish collaborative enthusiasm. [...]

Some writers do acknowledge the difficulty of developing *too* explicit an expression of purpose, at least at the outset. Cropper (1995), for example, argues that collaborative activity can express *purpose* without necessarily declaring *intent*. In similar fashion, Pettigrew *et al.* (1992)

suggest that for a *starting point*, a broad vision may be more likely to generate movement than a blueprint. [. . .]

Building up trust from principled conduct

Trust is often identified as a *sine qua non* of successful collaboration and – conversely – mistrust as a primary barrier, but typically the discussion does not get beyond what Gambetta calls 'irritating rhetorical flabbiness' (Gambetta, 1988: 214). What is often argued to be needed is sufficient trust to initiate co-operation, and a sufficiently successful outcome to reinforce trusting attitudes and underpin more substantial subsequent collaborative activity. Over time, this should lead to what Cropper (1995) terms *collaborative sustainability* – a behavioural quality which connotes *future* persistence, continuity and viability. However, there is a contrast between the emphasis which is normally placed upon trust, and the lack of understanding of the term as either a concept or a working tool. [. . .]

Fundamentally . . . trust is a device for coping with the freedom of other persons (Luhmann, 1979) – their freedom to disappoint our expectations through betrayal, defection and exit. This condition of ignorance or uncertainty about other people's behaviour is central, for there are limits to our capacity ever to achieve a full knowledge of others. In the case of inter-agency collaboration, two ends of a spectrum can be identified. At one end, agencies will *economize* on trust, and at the other, they will *invest* in trust.

[. . .]

Ensuring wide organizational ownership

Reference has already been made to the necessity for, but limitations of, a top-down lead for inter-agency collaboration. A well-developed strategy for collaboration will count for little if links are not made between the macro and micro levels of activity. [. . .]

RECOGNIZING AND NURTURING RETICULISTS

The discussion in managerialist literature of 'champions of change', whose commitment and charisma become crucial to the successful development of collaborative initiatives, bears a strong relationship to the notion of 'reticulists' – those individuals who are skilled at mapping and developing policy networks, and identifying the key resource holders and fellow reticulists in their own and other agencies (Friend *et al.*, 1974). Hardy *et al.* (1992), in their study of joint management initiatives, also noted their key role in developing shared ownership, while Wistow and Whittingham (1988) similarly argue for 'the development of skills in identifying both tactical opportunities for exchange, and the kinds of influence and motivations which shape the behaviour of key individuals in other organisations' (p. 21). [. . .]

Top-down collaborative initiatives need to secure strong links between higher and lower organizational tiers. . . . One of the salient features of welfare agencies is that 'lower level' staff have considerable contact with outside bodies and often enjoy discretionary powers which accord them *de facto* autonomy from their managers (Lipsky, 1980). Although many of their decisions may seem small, in aggregate they may radically redefine strategic policy intention (Hudson, 1993). Questions therefore have to be asked about their incentives to pursue co-operative efforts.

Much of the literature on fragmentation focuses upon inter-*organizational* interfaces, but inter-*professional* rivalries can be equally problematic. Although mutually hostile views have the effect of bolstering group solidarity, they also make co-operative working more difficult, and these issues grow in significance with the shift from *multi*-professionality to *inter*-professionality (Carrier and Kendall, 1995). Multi-professional work is seen as a co-operative enterprise in which traditional forms and divisions of professional knowledge are retained, but there is a willingness to collaborate. More radically, inter-professional work implies a willingness to share and even give up, exclusive claims to specialized knowledge and authority, and integrate procedures. [. . .]

Nurturing fragile relationships

In their study of inter-agency management arrangements in community care, Hardy *et al.* (1992) emphasized the *vulnerability* of the projects they examined. This stemmed from several sources: as organizational forms, they operated on, or outside, organizational boundaries; they can be perceived as unconventional novelties which constitute an administrative inconvenience or even a threat to the *status quo*; and they may prove to be overly dependent upon mutual trust. Their study accordingly showed the need to try to overcome or minimize such vulnerability, and identified four 'key imperatives' – clarity of purpose; commitment and shared ownership; robust and coherent management arrangements; and organizational learning. Much of this is reflected in the framework constructed in this article.

[. . .]

Selection of an appropriate collaborative relationship

Different degrees of collaboration are required for different purposes. Nocon (1994) sees a continuum of collaboration as encompassing three broad options. First, *networks*, involving either a structured or loose system of contacts, but with no specific expectations or commitments to joint working – a different use of the term 'network' to that which is commonly used in the social sciences and which will be referred to in our final component. Second, *coalitional* or *federative* working. This might initially involve only the sharing of information, but could develop into matching separate service plans, producing a joint strategic plan, jointly planning a project and jointly implementing it. And finally, the *unitary* model, with a total pooling of resources to serve a single set of objectives – though this must be limited to partial pooling, otherwise the best description would be *merger*.

[. . .]

Selection of a collaborative pathway

The previous components of this framework have concentrated upon collaborative strategies and collaborative tactics, rather than upon collaborative pathways – different routes to the same destination. Social science literature identifies three such pathways, none of them necessarily mutually exclusive – markets, hierarchies and networks – and each having a general applicability that transcends any particular geographical space or temporal order (Frances *et al.*, 1991). [. . .]

The key feature of networks is that they address the way co-operation and trust are formed and maintained, and in contrast to the other models, co-ordination is achieved through less formal and more egalitarian means. Macneil (1985) has suggested that the 'entangling strings' of reputation, friendship, interdependence and altruism all become an integral part of the relationship, and that the information obtained is thereby both 'thicker' than that in the market and 'freer' than that communicated in a hierarchy. [. . .]

Conclusion

[. . .] This article has sought to bring together strands of theoretical, conceptual and empirical literature from diverse disciplines in order to better understand inter-agency collaboration as a concept and as a process. Although collaborative steps are laid out in a linear, sequential manner, we have emphasized that the process is iterative and requires constant reshaping. In addition, our framework rests upon the interdependency of the components – identifying or responding to only one or a handful of the ten components would give an incomplete picture of the nature of 'collaborative endeavour'. The framework has been pitched at a sufficiently general level to be applied to any public sector interface, both for purposes of retrospective understanding and – where customized – to serve as a developmental tool. [. . .]

REFERENCES

Alter, C. (1990) 'An Exploratory Study of Conflict and Coordination in Inter-Organisational Service Delivery Systems', *Academy of Management Journal*, 13, 3: 478–502.

Alter, C. and Hage, J. (1993) *Organizations Working Together*, California, Sage.

Benson, J.K. (1975) 'The Inter-Organizational Network as a Political Economy', *Administrative Science Quarterly*, 20 June: 229–49.

Burton, J. (1995) 'Composite Strategy: The Combination of Collaboration and Competition', *Journal of General Management*, 21, 1: 1–23.

Carrier, J. and Kendall, I. (1995) 'Professionalism and Inter-Professionalism in Health and Community Care: Some Theoretical Issues', in P. Owens, J. Carrier and J. Horder (eds) *Interprofessional Issues in Community and Primary Health Care*, London, Macmillan.

Cropper, S. (1995) 'Collaborative Working and the Issue of Sustainability', in C. Huxham (ed.) *Creating Collaborative Advantage*, London, Sage.

Distefano, T. (1984) 'Inter-Organizational Conflict: A Review of an Emerging Field', *Human Relations*, 37, 3: 351–66.

Frances, J., Levacic, R., Mitchell, J. and Thompson, G. (1991) 'Introduction', in G. Thompson, J. Frances, R. Levacic and J. Mitchell (eds) *Markets, Hierarchies and Networks: The Coordination of Social Life*, London, Sage.

Friend, J., Power, J. and Yewlett, C. (1974) *Public Planning: The Inter-Corporate Dimension*, London, Tavistock.

Gambetta, D. (1988) 'Can We Trust?', in D. Gambetta (ed.) *Trust*, Oxford, Blackwell.

Gray, B. (1985) 'Conditions Facilitating Inter-Organisational Collaboration', *Human Relations*, 38, 10: 911–36.

Hardy, B., Turrell, A. and Wistow, G. (1992) *Innovations in Community Care Management*, Aldershot, Avebury.

Hudson, B. (1993) 'Michael Lipsky and Street-Level Bureaucracy: A Neglected Perspective', in M. Hill (ed.) *The Policy Process: A Reader*, Hertfordshire, Harvester Wheatsheaf.

Kagan, S.L. and Neville, P.R. (1993) *Integrating Services for Children and Families*, New Haven, CT, Yale University Press.

Kanter, R.M. (1985) *The Change Masters: Corporate Entrepreneurs at Work*, London, Allen and Unwin.

Kanter, R.M. (1994) 'Collaborative advantage: the art of alliances', *Harvard Business Review*, July/August, 96–108.

Lipsky, M. (1980) *Street-Level Bureaucracy*, New York, Russell Sage Foundation.

Luhmann, C. (1979) *Trust and Power*, Chichester, Wiley.

Macneil, I. (1985) 'Relational Contract', *Wisconsin Law Review*, 3: 483–526.

Marsh, D. and Rhodes, R.A.W. (eds) (1992) *Policy Networks in British Government*, Oxford, Clarendon Press.

Mattesich, P. and Monsey, B. (1992) *Collaboration: What Makes It Work?*, St Paul, Minnesota, Amherst H. Wilder Foundation.

Nocon, A. (1994) *Collaboration in Community Care in the 1990s*, Sunderland, Business Education Publishers.

Parsons, T. (1937) *The Structure of Social Action*, New York, McGraw-Hill.

Pettigrew, A., Ferlie, E. and McKee, L. (1992) *Shaping Strategic Change*, London, Sage.

Rex, J. (1982) *Social Conflict: A Conceptual and Theoretical Analysis*, London, Longman.

Rhodes, R.A.W. (1988) *Beyond Westminster and Whitehall: The Sub-Central Governments of Britain*, London, Unwin Hyman.

Rhodes, R.A.W. (ed.) (1992) *Policy Networks in British Government*, Oxford, Oxford University Press.

Warren, R., Rose, S. and Bergunder, A. (1974) *The Structure of Urban Reform*, Lexington, MA, Lexington Books.

Wistow, G. and Whittingham, P. (1988) 'Policy and Research into Practice', in D. Stockford (ed.) *Integrating Care Provision: Practical Perspectives*, London, Longman.

TWENTY-EIGHT

THE ENVIRONMENT OF COLLABORATIVE CARE

Sally Hornby and Jo Atkins

Source: *Collaborative Care: Interprofessional, Interagency and Interpersonal*, London, Blackwell, 2000.

Introduction

In this chapter the authors discuss potential hindrances to collaborative practice at the ground level, unintentionally derived from higher levels of organisational and institutional structures. ... The regulatory mechanisms implied by [demands for quality assurance, clinical audit and clinical governance] are rational and necessary, but the language and focus appear to be concentrated more on the needs of bureaucratic institutions than on the needs of faceworkers dealing with the day-to-day complexities at the user and carer interface. [. . .]

Achieving collaborative integration of care

Individual faceworkers [those who work at the interface with service users, including formal and informal carers] can feel constrained in their ability to meet the needs of users and carers by the broad policies, aims and objectives of their local organisation or agencies, especially when it comes to the distribution of resources. While the faceworker may be able, either alone or as a team, to assess users' and carers' needs and continue to develop the necessary critical thinking and expertise to meet them, they may still fail at the first hurdle of limitations in staffing, lack of time and lack of material resources to meet those needs according to their personal, professional and group standards. One cause of this operational difficulty has already been identified as the failure to link organisational objectives to the resources necessary to achieve them. This failure can be worsened if objective performance criteria, which have been established through processes such as clinical audit, are in place. Unless such audits are managed well they can contribute to a climate of tension and fear of failure in the faceworker.

The security and identities of faceworkers are woven into the familiar and stable order of things within the context of their local and professional organisations. The social organisation in which faceworkers find themselves, including aspects of accepted, embedded power, are made explicit in the natural running of day-to-day systems and processes. Familiar socialisation patterns, illustrated in the use of power in decision-making, policy formation and emergent hierarchies within groups, can be challenged if the expert power of faceworkers' day-to-day monitoring of changing and complex situations is not incorporated into new and adaptable patterns of work.

[. . .]

The faceworker brings their accepted understanding of the organisational contexts in which they work to their first encounter with the users and clients. As soon as they begin to develop a relationship of helping and the process of assessing the users' and carers' troubles they can become aware of the constraints that some organisational contexts exert. The task of feeding information about users' and carers' requirements back into power structures and patterns of work can be difficult, especially when the faceworker needs to challenge the resource power of the decision-makers higher up in the organisation. Faceworkers can feel powerless in the face of existing organisational structures, systems and procedures, especially if what they have discovered at the assessment stages with users and carers suggests a need for organisational change.

[. . .]

Wider organisational influences

As well as problems in making assessments there is an increasing demand for the prediction and monitoring of outcomes in order to establish the relative effectiveness and efficiency of interventions (Muir-Grey, 1998) and present evidence of having met standards through the use of clinical audit (Baker et al., 1999). Both the need to ensure that practice is based on the latest evidence, and that it meets the requirements of quality assurance initiatives and improvement programmes, can be challenging and stressful for faceworkers in the health and social care sectors today even though these demands are perfectly reasonable and rational. This is because they are underpinned by powerful psychosocial components such as the need for social and psychological safety in the group or team and in the organisation.

[. . .]

The obstacle of fear

The obstacle of fear arises from the psychological defences that physicians, nurses, social workers and other members of the multidisciplinary team construct. There are many reasons why such individual defences arise including fear of rejection, fear of powerlessness, fear of social neglect, fear of isolation and fear of failing to deliver adequate services because of time constraints. In instances of team-working these negative forces may be balanced by positive forces such as camaraderie, empowerment and recognition. One way to reinforce the positive and reduce the negative factors includes the use of steps that pose no direct threats to individuals, such as regular meetings to define those processes and outcomes that constitute high quality care, and raise awareness of wider quality issues.

Overcoming defensive behaviours

There are many instances of teams of health care practitioners learning to work together in non-threatening forums. Likewise teams of social care practitioners have learned to do the same. They each work to share their common objectives and to decide on the most efficient use of limited resources. Often they will define their domains of care very carefully with an eye to ensuring that their specific domains are not encroached on, and even offload some aspects of care on to alternative teams or authorities. The following example illustrates how attempts to offload responsibility on to another authority led to three different outcomes, a legal case-law precedent, ground-level collaborative practice that went beyond the current requirements of the law, and an effect on users who did not necessarily benefit from the enhanced collaboration.

Health authorities and social services: who should pay for nursing homes in the community?

In one county social services and the health authority have been increasingly working together to provide services to people with disabilities living in the community. At the same time the health authority had developed stringent criteria for judging when a patient would get needed nursing home care, which was fully funded by the NHS. As a result social services, using means testing, were funding all but a handful. This was very expensive for social services and meant that some very disabled people had to pay for their own care.

In July 1999 the Court of Appeal decided that social services responsibility for nursing care was limited and that health authorities would have to fully fund a substantial proportion of the people who had previously paid for their care or who had been means tested.

The judgement could have led to a rapid move by social services to remove the funding which the decision had indicated they should not have been making. Instead the management kept the matter low key. They did not seek to have the health authority redraft the suspect criteria. They had been working closely with the health authority and saw that if health had to take over payment for a large number of nursing home placements they would have to stop paying for other essential services, which would have caused disruption.

This spirit of partnership had an obvious valuable effect. The other side of it though was that a large number of people continued to be charged substantial sums, which they should not have paid. The close relationship that developed between health and social services prevented disruption, but at a cost to some service users.

Reformulating the boundaries

Several factors in this scenario are worth mentioning. The first is that by some mysterious process the boundaries of both teams had become more permeable and exchanges of perspectives, values, expertise and objectives apparently flowed in both directions across the boundaries. Second, the overall purpose of the authority on one side or the other was managed, presumably through enhanced consultation or negotiation. However, apparently neither the health authority nor social services succeeded in avoiding the team-absorption that tends to create dangers for team-working ... They still failed to meet the needs of some people with disabilities despite their collaborative action. In terms of the rewarding achievements of establishing satisfying relationships, and of meeting a wider set of organisational purposes than the limited perspective of costs, they succeeded: but in terms of the wider goals of user–carer focused care it appears they were not so successful. [. . .]

The impact of organisational structures and dynamics on collaborative care

The current environment of health and welfare services is increasingly affected by internal and external turbulence. The uncertainties that these create will have an impact on the faceworker and the helping relationship at the ground level of practice. They may adversely affect faceworkers' sense of identity and role security and so create a greater need for measures to deal with high levels of stress. Bureaucratic rules and regulations will fail to meet these needs; participative, open management styles might succeed. The perceptions, values and expertise of ground-level faceworkers, including users and carers as central to the helping compact norms, may then be incorporated into decision-making and planning at all levels of the organisation [. . .]

REFERENCES

Baker, R., Hearnshaw, H. and Robertson, N. (1999) *Implementing Change with Clinical Audit*, Chichester, Wiley.

Muir-Grey, J.A. (1998) *Evidence-based Policy Making*, London, Churchill Livingstone.

TWENTY-NINE

CONTRIBUTING AS A MANAGER

Vivien Martin

It is not easy to be a manager in the complex and demanding context of
health and social care. Public services developed with structures and
systems that often operated without clearly designated managers. This
remained the case until the late 1980s, when management ideas were
introduced. There was a perception that services were not responding adequately to the needs of service users and that there was not enough control
to ensure that resources were used efficiently and effectively. These themes
are central to policies concerned with modernising public services and have
led to the widespread introduction of management into services that were
formerly led by professionals and practitioners and served by administrators.

Management is a field of practice and a field of studies. There are many
different views of management, including views from different disciplinary
perspectives concerning the nature of management and which theory may
help us to understand what management is and why it matters. Kallinikos
(1996: 37) suggests that it is helpful 'to make a distinction between management as an overall *world orientation* and management as an ensemble
of *techniques* motivated by and directed towards the nexus of ordinary
problems confronting formal organizations'. He also notes that both of
these aspects need to be considered in making a critical evaluation of management:

> Although perhaps difficult to recognize from the present historical
> horizon, management, as a practice and an academic discipline, is
> closely connected with the overall orientation towards the objectification

and technicalization of knowledge that pertains to modernity. The technical tenor of the industrial world often appears as reasonable, or even natural, and, in this respect, tends to escape the scrutinizing gaze of critical interrogation. At other times it is inappropriately confused with and confined to the actual machinery of industrial production and the processes of transformation of the physical world. However, science, technology and management are allied phenomena and can be interpreted as different manifestations of the same underlying world view (Heidegger, 1977). They constitute a complex tangle of orientations that mark and reproduce an attitude whereby society and nature are looked on as if they were things to be made and remade, changed and transformed, corrected, amplified, destroyed, reconstructed, etc. This broad orientation towards objectification and mastery is implied by, or even intrinsic to, management. It lies at the heart of the compartmentalization of the material and social world, the growth and academic institutionalization of administrative techniques, and also the constitution and reproduction of particular sets of beliefs, priorities and ideas that help define the basic orientations of contemporary human beings (see also Derrida, 1982).

(Kallinikos, in French and Grey, 1996: 37–8)

Thus management is linked with science, technology and industry. This association with science has supported a belief that it is possible to carry out change within the boundaries of a particular setting. This belief has gained such interest and support that most organisations in the western world use management as one of the central mechanisms with which they attempt to manage change and transformation.

Management of change is a core role for managers in public services. Change is inevitable in public services that are re-configuring to respond to ever-more demanding expectations of high quality, efficiency and effectiveness. Policy changes seek to reflect public opinion and perceived need, but change is also initiated from direct experience of practice, particularly when things go wrong. Alterations in the ways in which services are configured bring structural changes within organisations and within multi-agency service provision. There is pressure on all staff to be more flexible and to develop new roles, including roles as leaders and managers in these changing structures. We might criticise the social conditions that seem to reduce organisations and parts of organisations to compartmentalised units in which objectives for the outcomes of change might be set and achieved. This is, however, the world in which a manager has to align personal values and beliefs with a role that has the power to influence the working conditions of colleagues and the quality experienced by service users.

The range and ambiguity of explanations of management can make it difficult for people who are both practising as a manager and studying management. Managers as learners often encounter both the theory that directly underpins activities as a manager and also the theory that attempts to develop an understanding of the implications of management as a phenomenon within a social setting.

Some managers dismiss the idea that theorising about management is of any importance and claim that management is only a set of processes and techniques. As Grint remarks:

> Theory in management studies, perhaps more than almost any other academic context, arrives at the management student's door laden with moral and political baggage: theory, according to some anti-theoretical accounts, is apparently irrelevant to the 'real world' of management where decisions are taken on the basis of facts or rationality or whatever happens to be the anti-theoretician's particular animus.
>
> (1995: 4)

Much of the theory in management is presented as a rational approach and includes techniques, processes and theories intended to inform practice. For example, there are techniques that can be used to structure teamwork and there is a substantial theoretical domain of research and theory development about teams and work in teams. For many managers these 'theories of practice' are enough to inform them about their management role and they may not question why they do what they do beyond the observation that it seems to work in the context of their workplace.

The workplace context is key to management. A convenient summary of the purpose of management in public services might be that it is to ensure that services are delivered in the way that is intended and within the resources available. This demonstrates one of the characteristics of management – it is essentially about carrying out the purposes of the organisation in which a manager works. Becoming a manager includes taking on a responsibility for furthering the direction of the organisation that employs you. Hales examines the close relationship between management and the processes within organisations:

> The starting point and the basis for the theoretical framework is the proposition that the management process – the process of planning/decision-making, allocating, motivating, coordinating and controlling work – has become separated from work itself, and has amalgamated with ownership functions to form a distinct extended 'management' function which is dispersed, through a management division of labour, and is institutionalised into organisational arrangements

and mechanisms. Hence the management of work is attempted through organisation. Different approaches to organisation of work may then be compared and contrasted in terms of the mechanisms which they use to try to manage work and the people who do it.

(1993: xviii)

The view presented by Hales is of management as an approach to organisation of work and only one of a range of possible mechanisms. Different approaches to the way in which work is organised will cause differences in both management and organisations. This begins to explain why the experience of being a manager can be very different in different organisations.

Some would say that management is a neutral term for the approaches, techniques and skills that can be applied in the practice of management. Others would say that no individual can be neutral and that management is not a neutral activity because of the degree of political and position power that is assumed along with the title of manager. Assumption of the role of manager does bring both power and responsibility within an organisational context. It follows that if you broadly agree with the purpose and direction of your organisation it is easier to feel comfortable about being a manager than if you disagree with these things. Similarly, it is more comfortable to be a manager in an organisation that has values that you agree with and enacts these values through its policies and processes.

Managers often choose to work in public and voluntary services because they want to contribute to the provision of high-quality services that really meet the needs of service users. Many managers talk about having the opportunity to 'make a difference'. This does not, however, always mean that management ideas and approaches are welcome in health and care services. Sometimes people question why managers are needed and they may suggest that people in these roles are more concerned about finance and enforcement of regulations than they are about caring for service users. Others think that their time is best spent on working directly with service users and prefer to leave responsibility for resource management, finance and regulation to managers. Sometimes professionals and practitioners resist taking on management roles if they fear that their values or practice will be diluted or reduced. Others may take on the role of a manager with the intention of continuing to act in a way that is consistent with personal values and in a way that respects the values of colleagues. One of the roles of a manager is to facilitate efficient and effective working and this is often approached by trying to create an environment in which staff are committed to the purpose of the organisation and in broad agreement about how to work together to achieve the objectives.

It is widely believed that effective management is essential to the provision of high-quality care. Those who adopt management roles can develop a management practice that enhances both the quality of care and the quality of working life. A manager has the opportunity to contribute to high-quality service delivery and to improvement of services. Whether an individual comes into management of care from a professional or other background, there is an opportunity to influence the working conditions of all those who contribute to delivering services. Therefore the work of a manager can have a direct impact on the experience of a service user.

Although there are many similarities in the work of managers in different types of organisations, the context is very important in shaping the nature of a manager's work. Stewart (1991: 14–18) suggests that any manager's job is defined and limited by demands and constraints. Demands are the things that a manager must do and constraints are the limits that define what the manager cannot do. For example, a manager in a drop-in advice centre for young homeless people may have considerable flexibility in deciding how to deliver the service within the direction set by a management board. A nurse manager in an operating theatre would have very little freedom to make choices as there are many protocols and regulations that constrain flexibility in the role. There is increasing regulation of health and care services and most managers will have responsibility for ensuring that standards of performance are achieved. Many managers will also find that there are not always sufficient resources to ensure that standards are achieved. In order to meet the demands of the job, managers often have to make choices within the constraints to try to maintain the quality of service provision. Much of the stress experienced by managers arises from jobs in which there is little scope for flexibility and where demands on services are greater than the service is resourced to meet. In this situation, a manager might identify and clarify the problem and then involve more senior managers in considering how the situation might be improved, rather than assuming that the responsibility lies entirely with themselves because of their role as a manager in that situation.

While some pressure can be positive and stimulating, if a person is under so much pressure that they become stressed, this can be harmful. Handy (1993: 72–3) identifies five common causes of stress in organisations:

- responsibility for the work of others,
- innovative functions,
- integrative or boundary functions,
- relationship problems,
- career uncertainty.

Most managers have to attempt to reconcile competing or conflicting objectives when these differ for individuals, groups and areas of work. Innovation and change are often stressful if there is resistance. Those taking co-ordinating roles often have to act without clear authority or adequate resources. In services where change is significant, there are usually relationship problems and often career uncertainty.

In addition to these general causes of stress, Handy (1993: 68–71) proposes that there are four role problems that managers may experience that can be sources of tension, low morale and communication difficulties. These are:

- role ambiguity (when the role is not defined clearly),
- role incompatibility (when a manager's expectations of his or her role are significantly different from those of his or her staff and colleagues),
- role conflict (when someone has to carry out a number of different roles and some of these have conflicting features),
- role overload or underload (when a manager's job includes either too many or too few roles, so that the individual feels either overworked or undervalued).

As in many other problem areas, once these issues are identified as causing stress that is damaging quality of life and work, it becomes easier to consider ways in which the problem might be addressed and to find the support and authority to make improvements.

There are many opportunities as a manager to contribute to improvement of services. Clarke (Reading 23, this volume) poses the question of whether the management claim of attempting to 'do the right thing' was self-referential. Who does know what 'the right thing' might mean in any particular set of circumstances? Managers often have the role of creating processes through which many different voices and perspectives can be heard and processes through which discussion can lead to agreement about a way forward. He also asks whether it is 'possible to develop a conception of management as stewardship, responsible for the preservation and enhancement of the public realm rather than management as entrepreneurialism chasing the next big transformation?' (p. 202). It is. Managers are individuals who make choices about how they will balance the demands, constraints and stresses of their work. Managers can be stewards acting as facilitators in identifying collective visions of 'better services' and supporting developments in the agreed direction.

Managers are not a special breed – they are people with values, experience and personal concerns and interests who take on management roles. There are opportunities in a management role to influence the way in which work is organised and carried out so that staff and service users are empowered to contribute to creating the improvements that the community want and will commit to achieving.

REFERENCES

Clarke, J. (2003) 'Doing the Right Thing? Managerialism and Social Welfare', this volume, pp. 195–203.

Grint, K. (1995) *Management: a Sociological Introduction*, Cambridge, Polity Press.

Hales, C. (1993) *Managing Through Organisation*, London, Routledge.

Handy, C. (1993) *Understanding Organizations* (4th edition), London, Penguin Books.

Kallinikos, J. (1996) 'Mapping the Intellectual Terrain of Management Education', in R. French and C. Grey (eds), *Rethinking Management Education*, London, Sage.

Stewart, R. (1991) *Managing Today and Tomorrow*, Basingstoke, Macmillan.

THIRTY

IDENTIFYING AND IMPLEMENTING PATHWAYS FOR ORGANIZATIONAL CHANGE – USING THE *FRAMEWORK FOR THE ASSESSMENT OF CHILDREN IN NEED AND THEIR FAMILIES* AS A CASE EXAMPLE

Jan Horwath and Tony Morrison

Source: *Child and Family Social Work*, 2000, 5.

Social workers and their managers operate in a climate of relentless change. As the Chief Inspector for Social Services in England stated, managing changes to policies and procedures, although never easy, can be done relatively quickly. However, achieving cultural change requires a more complex change management approach (SSI, 1999). In the late 1990s those employed in child welfare organizations in a number of countries have been recognizing and coming to terms with a cultural change in child care practice. This change, known as 'Reshaping' or 'Refocusing' in England, refers to a change in emphasis from an investigative approach to safeguarding children from significant harm to both safeguarding and promoting the welfare of children through a more balanced approach between preventative and tertiary interventions. [. . .]

In England, national guidance has been introduced to develop and support practice to reshape children's services. One key element is a document that focuses on assessment which is seen by the Department of Health to be crucial in terms of promoting better outcomes for children (Gray, 1999). This document, *Framework for the Assessment of Children in Need and their Families* (Department of Health, 1999a), is based on findings from a range of research studies, theories from a number of disciplines and lessons learned from policy and practice. However, its successful implementation not only depends on professionals recognizing the need to both safeguard and promote the welfare of children but also requires an attitudinal shift away from a procedurally driven system to one based more on the use of professional judgement within a framework of procedures (Department of Health, 1999a).

As with most changes, the guidance is not being introduced in isolation. Its introduction is part of a broader government agenda to promote the welfare of children (Department of Health, 1998a, b). [...] These other initiatives also act as drivers for change in terms of the implementation of the Assessment Framework. For example, funding from 'Quality Protects' is available to assist social services departments with the implementation of the new framework. By contrast other factors can act as barriers to change. These include the impact and range of other changes which agencies are having to address at the same time, as well as the integration of the new Assessment Framework in terms of current organizational culture. In addition to the sheer burden this places on the agency's capacity and energy for change, these other changes may or may not be consistent in philosophy or intent with each other. A major challenge is therefore how to distil and reconcile these different agendas into a coherent set of strategic plans, not just for the lead agency, but also for other agencies on whose cooperation the lead agency is dependent if the change is to be achieved.

The task facing senior managers is therefore to manage the introduction of the change, using the drivers for change that exist within and outside their organization and identifying and addressing the barriers to change. If this is to be done effectively, two key steps will be required: an audit of organizational readiness for change and the development of a strategy for managing the change (Smale, 1998). We shall consider ways in which these processes can be undertaken using two models that have been adapted from practice: the *Framework for the Assessment of Children in Need and their Families* and the Protchaska and DiClimenti model of change which has been used in work with people with drug and alcohol problems (Protchaska and DiClimenti, 1982) and in cases of child protection (Morrison, 1998). These models complement each other. The adapted Assessment Framework provides a structure to assess the readiness of the organization for change. The model of change provides a framework for planning, implementing and reviewing the introduction and operation of the change. We will use the introduction and implementation of the new Assessment Framework as an example of the way in which the models can be used to undertake a major organizational and inter-agency practice change.

A model for organizational change

The model for change offers practical guidance for engaging staff effectively in a major shift of professional attitudes and practice. . . .

Protchaska and DiClimenti's model (1982) is based on the idea that change is a matter of balance. Therefore change occurs when there are more motivational forces in favour of change than in favour of the status quo. Thus, motivating people to change involves increasing the motivators for change, whilst removing or decreasing barriers to change, whether they are material, environmental or psychological. The model also emphasizes the role that ambivalence plays in the change process, acting like a tide, in which surges of motivation may be followed by withdrawal and disengagement. . . . Motivation for change is therefore seen to reside not in individuals per se (Miller and Rollnick, 1991) but in the interaction between the person and their environment, or in an organizational context, the worker and their agency.

The original model describes six possible stages in a change process: (1) pre-contemplation → (2) contemplation → (3) determination → (4) action → (5) maintenance → (6) lapse or relapse.

[. . .]

Adapted model of change

The basic concepts around change can be adapted to the context of organizational change as shown in Figure 30.1. Ten stages of organizational change are presented in stepwise format together with how they relate to the original Protchaska and DiClimenti model. Each of these 10 stages will be expanded upon below, outlining useful organizational strategies to consider for each stage.

PRE-CONTEMPLATION

This represents denial of, and resistance towards, the need to change. Whilst this rarely reflects the totality of the agency's response, resistance may be located in parts of the agency or in other agencies whose cooperation with a change is required. It is very important therefore that the mandate for changes in professional attitudes and practice is clear and as unambiguous as possible. The role of central government guidance at this stage, both as to the clarity and the status of new policies and the implications for other agencies whose assistance is required to deliver the policy goals, is therefore very significant. For instance, in relation to the draft document *Framework for the Assessment of Children in Need and their Families* (Department of Health, 1999a) the role and mandate of non-social services agencies remains unclear.

. . . Gaining ownership of the change process is the next step and the beginning of the contemplation process, outlined in stages 1–5 of Figure 30.1.

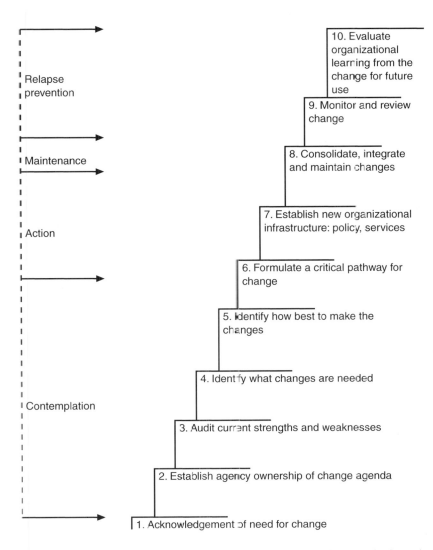

Figure 30.1   Organizational model for change based on concepts from Protchaska and DiClimenti (1982).

1 Acknowledge the need for change

It is important that the ownership of the change process is located at the right level. Assuming that the external mandate for change is established, step 1 is to ensure that the agenda for change becomes located at a strategic level within the relevant agencies. For instance, the need for change in practice is often identified by specialists within the agency but their capacity to manage organizational or inter-agency change is limited.

A second early task is for the lead agency, usually social services in the context of child welfare work, to identify the other key agency stakeholders, including elected members, who need to be brought on board. At a practical level, step 1 might see the identification of a senior manager to act as the commissioner or lead manager for the change work, in each of the key agencies, and the setting up of a project team to drive forward the next stages of the change process. [. . .]

One point to consider is timing for the inclusion of other agencies in the change process. Where, as is the case with the new Assessment Framework, there is clearly a lead agency, social services, it can be premature to open up an inter-agency debate if the lead agency is confused and unclear about its thinking and direction. Too early exposure to inter-agency debate can result in intra-agency confusion widening to inter-agency confusion. Conversely, failure to engage the other agencies early on in the process can leave them feeling excluded and consequently unwilling to engage in the change process.

2   Establish agency and inter-agency ownership of the change agenda

Change cannot be properly managed if different agencies hold divergent opinions as to the rationale and desired outcomes of any change. For instance, it has not been uncommon in the authors' experience to discover that levels of understanding of key research underpinning the new framework such as *Child Protection: Messages from Research* (Department of Health, 1995) has been very varied and occasionally quite poor even amongst key managers in social services departments. In order to increase agency understanding and to provide a wider professional context for the changes, a research and policy briefing or seminar for a small 'driver' group can be helpful to ensure that the rationale, research and underpinning professional issues are understood. [. . .]

A communication strategy is important to alert and signpost staff about the changes that are coming, identify who are the lead officers, and how agencies will communicate with staff as things progress. . . .

3   Assessing current strengths and weaknesses

. . . It is necessary to lay the foundations for change by undertaking an organizational audit of the readiness for change. This can be done by identifying existing strengths, good practice, the nature of the changes and the impact they are intended to have on practice (Smale, 1996).

Audit of readiness for change: An organizational audit in many ways mirrors an assessment of a child and family. In both cases the purpose is to identify what is currently going on: what needs to change; current drivers that will promote and support change and barriers that need to be addressed. The *Framework for the Assessment of Children in Need and their Families* has three domains which can be adapted to provide a framework for organizational readiness for change:

- child's developmental needs,
- parenting capacity,
- wider family and environmental factors.

...There are a number of organizational factors that need to be considered, which mirror the three domains referred to above. These are shown in Figure 30.2.

- Practitioners' needs: these are the professional and organizational needs of the front-line staff who will be responsible for the assessment process.
- Agency capacity: this describes the capacity of the organization to meet the needs of the practitioners.
- Collaborative arrangements: this domain describes external relationships with other agencies and community networks which are required by the practitioners.

The assessment task for practitioners working with children and families is to complete an assessment of the developmental needs of the child and to identify the capacity of the parents/carers to respond to these needs. In the same way an audit of an organization should consider the needs of practitioners in light of the changes that are to be introduced and the agency's capacity to provide the organizational infrastructure to enable high-quality assessment practice. [...] Direct consultation often refines the picture gained from paper-based analysis and provides essential insights not only to the degree of congruence between policy and practice, but also about

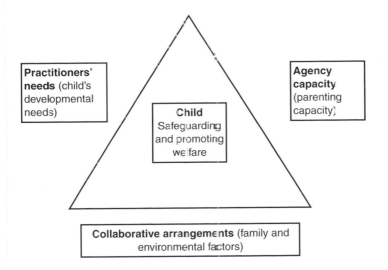

Figure 30.2   Triangle for auditing organizational readiness for change.

underlying professional attitudes and responses to change. In addition, consultation engages staff at an early stage in the process of shaping the road ahead. [. . .]

4 Identify what changes are needed

The emphasis at this point is on 'what' rather than 'how', with the focus on identifying from the previous stage what changes to policy, resources, services, structures, attitudes, skills and practice are required. Often having identified good local practice the challenge is how to bring all practice up to the standards of the best. Pilot projects may have shown the way and the task is how to integrate their achievements in a range of different work and practice contexts throughout the agency (or agencies). However, creating attitudinal changes to practice is complex, not least because what workers believe in the sanctity of a training course is not necessarily how they may think under pressure at the coal-face. Intellectual and emotional belief systems can be very different. This points to the critical importance of policy, resource and practice changes being framed within an explicit rationale and value base, and the specification of key success criteria against which changes will be measured. Such criteria need to include both *output*-based measures (for example, proportion of assessments of children in need completed within agreed timescale) and *outcome*-based criteria (for example, the degree to which assessments resulted in the delivery of services that met a child's needs).

5 Identify how best to make the changes

In many ways this is the most difficult part of the contemplation process. The task here is to work out how staff can be engaged in a meaningful manner in the change process, without which changes may be either partial or superficial. The engagement strategy is therefore dependent on the quality of analysis undertaken in steps 3 and 4. It is also useful to consider how changes have been managed in the past. As with service users, previous experiences and history can be a significant indicator of future capacity for change, as can the number of other competing demands currently facing an individual or organization. Our own experiences in assisting a wide range of social care and health agencies to address change suggests that responses to change can be described along a continuum: (i) denial → (ii) quick fix → (iii) partial/temporary → (iv) integrated.

The main features of each are now delineated taking as an example agency and inter-agency initial responses to the refocusing or reshaping of children's services as described at the beginning of the paper. [. . .]

i *Denial or delay.* Senior management appear suspicious or cynical towards the specific change, sometimes due to a lack of information. As a result there is no formal response to refocusing which may be rationalized in terms of 'we're doing this already'. . .

ii *Quick fix*. Here management's response to change is simply at a pro-cedural level. Thus the response to refocusing is a managerial require-ment for a reduction in the number of children on child protection registers so it appears that the problem is solved. . . . There is little or no involvement of front-line managers or staff or any serious develop-mental work on improving services to children in need. The change process becomes an exercise in rationing rather than providing.

iii *Partial*. This may take a number of forms:

(a) There may be some constructive initiatives on the ground, for instance establishing a family support resource in one area, but in a vacuum of strategic thinking and planning. So change remains isolated.

(b) A social services department is overwhelmed with a high volume of complex and difficult child protection cases, perhaps in an area of high deprivation. Whilst there is a commitment to develop more needs-led services, and to develop staff skills and knowledge, pressure of work, high staff turnover, and occasional Part 8 reviews undermine and derail genuine attempts to refocus services.

(c) A social services department makes significant changes but fails to engage the other agencies.

In all three of these scenarios the danger is that the progress made in one part of the system may be undermined by the lack of attention to the system as a whole and to the strategic issues of policies, priorities, services and training.

iv *Integrated*. Here the change is managed at both strategic and opera-tional levels, and at both departmental and inter-agency levels. The task is addressed as a major piece of inter-organizational development work led from the top but involving all staff. Change is underpinned by: a user-focused ethos at senior management level; high-quality man-agement information to guide the process; policy review and develop-ment; widespread training; mapping of user needs; redirecting of resources; and a proactive involvement of front-line staff to maximize ownership of the change process.

One important message is that the prospects for successful implementation of change, for instance the new Assessment Framework, need to take account of the way in which other related organizational and professional changes have been handled. The better these changes have been handled, the more prepared and willing staff will be to adapt to further change. Conversely it can be seen that the prospects for change in a 'quick-fix' environment are much more problematic.

Identifying potential drivers and barriers to change, be they political, policy, professional, resource or personnel based, will be helpful. Who will be the winners and losers as a result of the changes? [. . .]

6 Formulate a critical pathway for change

This simple and practical activity involves mapping out a sequence of individual steps over a time period that together achieve the goals. The pathway provides a strategic plan for change based on steps 4 and 5. However, the pathway also needs to incorporate other changes and imperatives facing the key agencies in order to anticipate what demands are likely to be placed on which staff, or resources, at what points. For instance, in creating a mandatory staff training strategy for a new Assessment Framework, it would be necessary to consider whether other training will be competing for staff time during the same period. Awareness of other changes such as Quality Protects Management Action Plans is also important in being able, as far as possible, to integrate different but related changes within an over-arching strategic plan.

The pathway enables progress to be monitored against key delivery points (for example, a new policy). This will enable momentum to be maintained and plans to be modified if necessary. This helps to keep complex change processes on track, and to maintain managerial commitment when other crises arise and threaten to derail the whole project. . . .

Disseminating the plan is necessary too. It may well be from the practitioner's perspective that a considerable period of time has elapsed since they first heard that changes were in the wind. They may feel disconnected with the agenda, or have concluded that nothing is going to happen. The work involved in steps 1–6 may well have been conducted by a small inner group with only limited involvement from others. The staff need to be re-engaged in the change process if the next steps are to be successful.

7 Establish organizational infrastructure for improved practice

This step focuses on creating the changes identified in step 6 through work on values, policies, structures, resources, services, priorities, standards, skills and practice. It is likely that parallel work will be required on inter-agency policies, structures and in particular eligibility criteria and threshold levels for intervention and services. [. . .] Maximizing the involvement of staff at this stage in creating new policies, devising new thresholds or piloting new assessment and recording frameworks both engages staff in the process and increases their ownership of the changes. This reduces the degree to which training is asked to deliver changes that are unmanageable or professionally unacceptable.

8 Consolidate, maintain and integrate changes

The task now is to embed and integrate work undertaken on policy, etc. throughout the agency (or agencies). Successful pilot programmes need to be translated into application throughout the agency. [. . .] A public launch or 'going live' event can assist in bringing staff together both to mark the implementation of change and to instil a sense of shared responsibility for the change process. An implementation plan based on the critical pathway is essential but must be followed up by monitoring and review (step 9).

9 Monitor and review changes

Maintaining the kinds of complex change that have been described is perhaps one of the most difficult tasks of all. The continual bombardment of change, budgetary constraints, unforeseen crises, and the very nature of large organizations combine to make the task of staying on track with change very tricky indeed. [...] The monitoring process may combine management information, file auditing, user feedback as well as seeking feedback from a variety of stakeholders both internal and external to the agency.

The monitoring process may also identify unintended effects of the changes or unforeseen gaps (for instance in training) and may highlight areas where the new policies or practices are not working or are at risk of failing or lapsing. This allows remedial or relapse prevention action to be taken rather than waiting for a more serious failure which might threaten the rest of the changes. An example of a serious failure might be a child death in which a new assessment process was judged to have failed to identify clear risks of abuse, thus jeopardizing the whole Assessment Framework. If there has been a thorough review of the implementation process, then any individual 'failure' can be evaluated in the context of overall standards of practice, thus reducing the threat that a single failure will compromise all the other improvements made.

Finally, monitoring compliance with policy must incorporate identifying and celebrating successes, an experience which staff have all too infrequently.

10 Evaluate organizational and inter-agency learning from the changes for future use

Writers such as Wasdell (1997) have focused on the difference between first-order and second-order change and learning. First-order change refers to managing change at the level of tasks, systems and outputs. Second-order change involves change at the level of underlying attitudes, paradigm and culture. Both can occur at the same time. Second-order change occurs when the organization is able to learn how it learns and applies that knowledge to future changes. [...]

Conclusion

We have offered two models which are designed to assist agencies in implementing change. The adapted model of change provides a guide to the *process and management* of the implementation task. The triangle (see Figure 30.2) provides three dimensions along which to assess the organization's *readiness* to implement change. The models are not offered as a 'quick fix' or panacea for rapid change. Rather they seek to distil from experience a number of building blocks to assist busy and overstretched managers in implementing a wide range of changes.

REFERENCES

Department of Health (1995) *Child Protection: Messages from Research*, London, HMSO.

Department of Health (1998a) *The Quality Protects Programme: Transforming Children's Services*, London, Department of Health.

Department of Health (1998b) *Modernising Health and Social Services: National Priorities Guidance*, London, Department of Health.

Department of Health (1999a) *Framework for the Assessment of Children in Need and their Families* (Consultation Draft), London, The Stationery Office.

Department of Health (1999b) *Working Together to Safeguard Children* (Draft), London, HMSO.

Glissen, C. and Hemmelgarten, A. (1998) The effects of organisational climate and interorganisational coordination on the quality and outcomes of children's service systems. *Child Abuse and Neglect*, 22: 401–21.

Gray, J. (1999) Getting the whole picture, in *Quality Protects Newsletter*, London, Department of Health.

Miller, W. and Rollnick, S. (1991) *Motivational Interviewing*, London, Guildford Press.

Morrison, T. (1993) *Staff Supervision in Social Care*, Harlow, Longman.

Morrison, T. (1998) Partnership, collaboration and change under the Children Act, in *Significant Harm*, 2nd edn, M. Adcock and R. White (eds), Croydon, Significant Publications.

Pedlar, M., Boydell, T. and Burgoyne, J. (1989) Towards the learning company, *Management Education and Development*, 20: 1–8.

Protchaska, J. and DiClimenti, C. (1982) Transtheoretical therapy: towards a more integrative model of change, *Psychotherapy: Theory, Research and Practice*, 19(3).

Smale, G. (1996) *Mapping Change and Innovation*, London, HMSO.

Smale, G. (1998) *Managing Change through Innovation*, London, The Stationery Office.

SSI (1999) *Modern Social Services: A Commitment to Development*, The 8th Annual Report of the Chief Inspector of Social Services, London, SSI.

Wasdell, D. (1997) Consulting and advanced learning, in *Developing Organisational Consultancy*, J. Neumann, K. Kellner and A. Dawson-Shepherd (eds), London, Routledge.

THIRTY-ONE

SOCIAL WORK MANAGEMENT: A SYSTEMS CASE STUDY

Andy Bilson and Sue Ross

Source: *Social Work, Management and Practice.*

... [There are] a number of principles to be considered when attempting to adopt a systems approach to social work management. This chapter describes ... a systems approach to helping a manager deal with a particular and difficult problem. [...] [This] example [is] being put forward not as [a] model for others to slavishly follow, nor because the strategies being described were uniquely successful in bringing about positive change. What [it] raises are some of the issues encountered when applying systems ideas to real life managerial situations.

Case study

The ... case study concerns the use of information to deal with a problem in an organisation. In this case the managerial action is not focused directly on the provision of services, but on the internal 'politics' of the organisation. The issue was raised by a home help manager at an in-service course for managers in a social work agency which was led by one of the writers. The course ... was aimed at giving managers skills in creating patterns from management data.... The course also focused on presenting the patterns in ways that 'make a difference'. In addition to data drawn from the agency's client information system, participants were encouraged to bring along information which they regularly handled in their jobs. This included client information as well as budget statements and budget monitoring reports. It should be noted that whilst managers in social work are increasingly expected to be able to use information systems, few have had even basic training in this area.

The participants on the course were asked to share a problem that they had in the use of information. A home help manager was concerned about absence monitoring (the collection of information on the proportion of staff being absent due to sickness in a given period). The agency was facing a possible overspend on its budget and senior managers were looking for savings. At the same time figures had been published which showed that the social work agency had a particularly high rate of staff absences. A prominent local politician had raised the heat on this issue in the media, berating the senior managers for not dealing with this problem whilst they were looking to cut services to make budget reductions.

In view of this background it was not surprising that the management had decided to scrutinise this element of expenditure. All departmental managers were given instructions on dealing with this problem; information was provided on the crude rate of absences split down to the level of individual budget holders; and where this reached a particular threshold the responsible manager was called in to headquarters to be interviewed by the director and other senior managers.

The home help manager had been called to an interview which was to take place after the course. She raised this as a problem she would like to focus on and brought along the details of her staff absences. She had taken over the management of the service only six months earlier and felt that she had done a lot to improve things. However, looking at the overall figures that were being used by the senior managers it appeared that the problem had become worse during the time she had been in charge.

Thus the problem she faced was how to deal with the 'interview' which, from rumour in the department (which may or may not have been true but was believed), would effectively consist of her being given little chance to explain and being dressed down for failure to take the issue on. The senior management of the department had recently had industrial action taken by managers focusing on a restructuring which had initially been dealt with in a very authoritarian way and the approach to the problem of sickness leave also suggested that they were operating within an epistemology based on power – i.e. that problems could be solved by issuing directives and taking managers who did not comply 'to task'. Any attempt at dealing with the home help manager's position needed to take this into account and should also be aimed at helping to move them from this epistemological position.

The home help manager was understandably nervous at the thought of having to defend herself in an interview as a relatively new and junior member of staff. Also it was difficult for her to see the situation other than from within the same epistemology. [. . .]

On discussing the situation with her it became clear that she had been taking the issue of staff absence seriously. Fortunately she had collected her own information on staff absences and from this it was possible to create a more complex pattern which carried a very different meaning. The figures showed that the overall pattern of absence amongst her staff was low, with the exception of two home helps who had been absent for the majority of the time she had been in charge. Both these staff members had had poor sickness records over a long period under the previous manager who had taken no action. Since taking over she had taken formal action following the procedures of the agency and the contracts of both staff members were soon to be ended due to their inability to carry out their duties. This pattern thus showed her to be managing the problem. She had also set up support systems for her other home carers, arranging group meetings and supervision to provide them with support and reduce the risk of unnecessary stress.

Whilst this data gave her a good case there was a real danger that if the managers acted as it was predicted it may not be heard. She had to get the opportunity to present it and to do it in a way which would make a difference. As well as feeling worried at being called to the meeting, she was also angry that she was being 'punished' for a problem which she had taken seriously and which she was close to solving. She also felt powerless because of her position. In addition, having to pay the staff during their absence had meant that she had been forced to reduce the service in her area to keep within her budget. This was in contrast to some other areas which were over-spending. There was the danger that, even if she could convince the senior managers that she had solved the sick-leave problem, she would still face a budget reduction on the basis that she could continue to provide the same level of service once the two absent staff were no longer employed, thus saving their wages.

Any strategy thus had to deal with the problems of the epistemology of power. In the first instance this meant helping the home help manager to move out of this as it left her feeling 'powerless'. Drawing parallels between what the senior managers were trying to do and her own actions in combating the absence records of her own staff, helped her to reassess the situation and providing a new framework for understanding the situation (the systems framework...) gave her the ability to see different options for action and to devise a strategy.

If her input was to be heard she would have to get a fit with the senior managers. This was difficult because of her feelings at being summoned there. The approach she decided to use was what in family therapy is called a 'yes and...' approach. She would agree with the managers at the seriousness of the current situation regarding sick leave in her area. This would give her the opportunity to join with them and show her genuine concern at the problem. She would then show how the problem was worse than they thought because the reduced service caused by the absences was negatively affecting the lives of service users, increasing their risk of entry to residential care which they did not want, and would lead to greater expenditure by the agency.... [T]rying to address problems of epistemology through logical argument is unlikely to succeed. It was important to engage them in reflecting on the impact of their actions. She needed to engage them emotionally before giving more rational arguments. To do this she would use case examples demonstrating the very real impact of her decisions to temporarily reduce service levels on service users. She would then give some brief figures demonstrating the pattern identified in the sick leave and showing how this would be resolved in the next monitoring period. The important thing here was to present in a way which had an impact. As is often the case with managers in such situations, the home help manager wanted to present very detailed information, but she had limited time and it was important to get her point across quickly, stressing the differences between her analysis and the crude figures being used for monitoring. The writer helped her to devise a tightly focused presentation which could quickly demonstrate the issues. In this way she would not only put across her own case but also expose issues about an approach based on crude information.

Following her 'interview' the home help manager reported that things had gone well. Not only had she been praised for the work she had done on monitoring, but there had also been no cuts in her budget, allowing her to reinstate the precious level of service.

Using a systems approach had enabled the home help manager to deal successfully with a situation in which she had previously felt powerless and oppressed. The example shows the importance of avoiding being drawn in to view problems through the epistemology of power and how systems approaches can help managers to look for different ways of tackling difficult situations. [. . .]

PART IV

MANAGING FOR A LEARNING AND DEVELOPING ORGANISATION

Janet Seden

INTRODUCTION

This Part includes readings about the manager's role as a facilitator of learning. Clarke and Stewart suggest that, in order to respond to the 'wicked' issues of social care, by which they mean complex problems with no easy solutions, management should be based on recognition of the need for learning. This is not just about individuals but also about organisations, communities and government being open to new ideas. Learning is needed at all levels of care activity to create change.

Managers learn by doing. Importantly, they learn from service users, colleagues, research and training events. The frontline manager's responsibilities include the appraisal and the professional development of themselves and others. The concept of the manager as controller/director/leader of activities sits alongside ideas about the manager as enabler and staff developer, within a learning organisation. Once these ideas might have seemed contradictory. A holistic response to managing to learn suggests that the manager who understands the developmental needs of the organisation enables workplace learning without making artificial distinctions between work tasks and professional development. This creates an environment for learning in the organisation.

Clarke and Stewart set the context by identifying that new solutions to complex problems require flexible, holistic and participatory approaches. These include understanding that organisations newly working together to deliver services will need to learn together. This involves people with care, education and health backgrounds amongst others.

It is puzzling that, despite what is known and often reiterated as good practice, such knowledge is not always utilised in the workplace. Obholzer's reading presents a particular perspective on this. He theorises from psychodynamic, human relations approaches. Is it the unconscious at work? Do the defences of practitioners against the anxieties of their jobs block their learning experiences? The reading explores how defences against anxieties may block best outcomes in practice. Obholzer argues for a psychologically informed management to take account of such human tendencies.

What is classical management theory? The next readings from Mintzberg, an engineer turned management expert, explores from 20 years of research the relationship between management theory and practice. This piece gives a flavour of this work, highlighting managers' roles. Twenty years ago, perhaps more managers were he than she. Here the manager is referred to as 'he', so it is important to flag up that managing is not a gender specific role, especially in the frontline of social care, where many managers are women.

There is a large body of theory on leadership, and approaches vary over time. Hartley and Allison provide an analysis taken from established concepts and their research study in local authorities. They reflect on how models of leadership are updated to respond to new challenges, and examine the manager's influence across organisational boundaries in network arrangements.

Learning involves drawing from past experience and from research to make applications in new contexts. At the same time, listening to current service users and practitioners to inform management actions as the practice environment changes is essential. There is a rich literature on supervision in the helping professions, and its role in professional development. The issue here is about what is neglected through the pressure to act. Practitioners often lack consistent supervisory support. Public inquiries over the years have highlighted the need to raise the profile of consistent, effective management practice. The Victoria Climbié inquiry (2002) highlights this again. The Sawdons' work covers much of what is said about the usefulness of the supervisory process in caring work and addresses some issues of power inequality. They argue persuasively that supervision is the place where societal, user, practitioner and agency agendas meet. This is where dilemmas and challenges can be explored and strategies for improvement discussed. Supervision provides opportunities for management, support, education, mediation and appraisal if agency supervision policies are embedded in workplace routines.

Sadly, learning in care settings can come painfully, through mistakes. Ayre argues that professionals can both learn from inquiries and the recommended changes in policy, while also developing proactive approaches to informing and using the media, thus challenging the blame culture that media handling of care issues can generate. Managers can avoid promising the public unrealistic outcomes and thereby setting the service up to fail. They can also use the media to inform the public about what practitioners can realistically do. In a world where managers of care are subject to media scrutiny, a proactive approach to educating the media about the real world of social care is probably overdue.

Using new ways of communicating, with new information media and technologies, has been a steep learning curve for many people in care work. Now that e-communication is expected from government and between agencies, there is much to learn about using these tools effectively. Bates recognises that good information is essential to effective practice and draws from a research study to explore some of the opportunities and threats such technologies bring. He explores some of the issues for the training and development of practitioners and also the implications for the agency.

There are, then, many ways in which managers of care settings learn and facilitate the learning of others. People grow through experience, feedback from service users, training courses and supervision to develop professionally. The concept of the 'learning organisation' has been something of a buzzword in organisational and management writing. Gould focuses not so much on defining what a learning organisation is, but rather on identifying how learning happens. Bringing the rhetoric of learning in organisations into reality is a challenge. In this reading, literature is reviewed, and a grounded theory approach taken to examine a particular setting.

Managers can work with individuals, their organisations and partners to link activity and learning in a diversity of ways. Throughout this Reader, it has been suggested that there is no blueprint for managing in the complex and fast changing world of care. It has also been argued that there is much to draw on from a range of disciplines and approaches to find ideas and models for managing. This Part brings together some writing about managing to learn and develop which may provide ideas for practice, or a springboard for further exploration. In learning, as in the daily events of practice, managers are always in the front line.

THIRTY-TWO

HANDLING THE WICKED ISSUES

Michael Clarke and John Stewart

Source: Discussion paper, School of Public Policy, Birmingham, 1997.

What are the 'wicked issues'?

The idea of the 'wicked issue' has become part of the contemporary currency of public administration and management. The words are used to refer to a variety of policy challenges. The sense they convey is of something different to the conventional issues of public policy which are solved or, at least are capable of solution, by a mixture of common sense and ingenuity. They suggest a special class of policy problem; one without an obvious or established (or even common-sense) solution, defying normal understanding – and often not sitting conveniently within the responsibilities of any one organization. . . .

Why are some issues called 'wicked'? The word is used, not in the sense of evil, but as a crossword puzzle addict or a mathematician would use it – suggesting an issue (or problem) difficult to resolve. The phrase seems first to have been used by Horst Rittel and Melvin Webber in the USA. They wrote of wicked problems:

> We are calling them 'wicked' not because these properties are themselves ethically deplorable. We use the term 'wicked' in a meaning akin to that of 'malignant' (in contrast to 'benign') or 'vicious' (like a circle) or 'tricky' (like a leprechaun) or 'aggressive' (like a lion, in contrast to the docility of a lamb).
>
> (Rittel and Webber, 1973: 160)

Wicked problems are distinguished from tamed problems, some of which may themselves have been wicked before they were tamed. A tame problem is one which one can be readily defined and for which a solution is easily found.

Wicked problems, on the other hand, are those for which there is no obvious or easily found solution. They seem intractable. . . . There can be hope that wicked problems will be solved over time, but that requires learning of the nature of the problems and of their causes. They require a capacity to derive and design new approaches for their resolution and to learn of their impact. They are likely to be resolved not directly but through an iterative process – learning, trying and learning. [. . .]

Almost by definition, wicked problems cannot be dealt with as management has traditionally dealt with public policy problems. They challenge existing patterns of organization and management. Organizations are usually structured by – or themselves structure – problems and defined solutions. For the wicked problems there is no accepted solution; what is required is a learning approach which must not be confined and should be prepared to think and accept the unthinkable. Where there is a tamed problem there is a solution or a set of known skills that are required to solve the problem. People can then be trained to find and apply the solution; they can be fitted into an appropriate organizational context.

Wicked problems cannot be dealt with like that. The issues need to be framed and reframed. The problems are not fully understood and solutions have to be searched for in uncertainty. The skills required are often not fully appreciated. The problem is unlikely to belong to any one organization; in all likelihood it will implicate many. Indeed, awareness of the wicked nature of the problem is often associated with the fact that the problem cannot be fully understood by any one organization, never mind solved by it. . . .

However, it is important to recognize that it is not just the fact that issues overlap organizational or even conceptual boundaries which makes them wicked. The inclination to confuse the wicked with the corporate or overarching strategic issues is a mistake. The latter will usually include the former, but not vice versa. . . . The resolution of wicked issues will almost inevitably require action not by government alone but by many individuals and organizations. The wicked issues by their nature will be enmeshed in established ways of life and patterns of thinking; they will only be resolved by changes in those ways of life and thought patterns. If society is wasteful and polluting the earth's resources, it will be because it has supported particular ways of living; these have to change if sustainable development is to be achieved. Equally, a healthy society will seem a welcome objective to all, but its achievement will require changes in the way many people live.

Trying to resolve the wicked issues will mean working through people. The changes required will be such that they are unlikely to be imposed by legislation or regulation alone; nor would such legislation be passed or regulation be accepted without public acceptance of what is required. The wicked issues are likely only to be resolved by a style of governing which learns from people and works with people. The wicked issues require a participatory style of governing because the changes have to be owned by people.

Underlying the tackling of the wicked issues is recognition that the task is not the government or management of certainty, where clearly identified problems are faced, with understood causes and for which there are accepted solutions. Rather, the task is the government or management of uncertainty. It may not be clear what the problem is – at least in the sense of understanding its causes – and it will certainly not be clear what the solution is. Politicians and officials have to respond without necessarily knowing how to respond.

Theorists and commentators have often defined government as being about learning. In tackling the wicked issues the need is to create a learning government. Such an approach starts from a recognition of uncertainty, both about the issues and how they should be handled. This means that management should be based on a recognition of the need for learning. Ways and means have to be plotted – not so much as the path to a certain destination but for an exploration in imperfectly known territory. Policy-makers may move forward – but with reflection and ready to learn and to adapt to that learning.

Tackling wicked issues therefore requires:

- holistic not partial or linear thinking, capable of encompassing the interaction of a wide variety of activities, habits, behaviour and attitudes;
- a capacity to think outside and work across organizational boundaries;
- ways of involving the public in developing responses;
- embracing a willingness to think and work in completely new ways. While most people will come to this trapped or constrained by conventional organizations, labels and assumptions, what is needed is willingness to entertain the unconventional and pursue the radical.

This implies:

- a new style of governing for a learning society.

Holistic – not linear or partial – thinking

. . . This is thinking capable of grasping the big picture, including the inter-relationships of objectives and the interaction of activities and different objectives. By their nature, the wicked issues are imperfectly understood and so the placing of boundaries upon analysis and thought may lead to what is important in handling the wicked issues being neglected. . . .

Recognizing interrelationships (of issues, organizations and people) and breadth of attention are necessary to holistic thinking. There is a need to be inclusive, not exclusive, in the search for connections and to resist the traps of the organization perspective, of limited experience and of reducing the complex to the simple. The problem is the constant inclination – because of the dominance of linear modes of thinking – to confine analysis within a framework of neat certainty. Not to do so is uncomfortable. This problem is exacerbated by the fact that, inevitably, we use formal organizations to tackle public policy issues – and most organizational design is premised on the need to focus, simplify and order; and, in contemporary vogue, to operate efficiently and economically as well as effectively. We do not dispute the value of such an approach for problems easily identified and to which solutions are easily found; the danger lies in its dominance. Organizations in the public domain need a capacity to work in different ways. They need a capacity for holistic thinking both within and across organizations, as well as for linear thinking within.

Thinking and working across organizational boundaries

A crucial part of handling wicked issues involves crossing organizational boundaries and drawing many organizations into the frame. The need to think and work across organizational boundaries raises issues both between organizations and within them. Organizations cannot work effectively together if they do not work effectively within themselves. Inter-organizational working will be limited by the inadequacy of intra-organizational working. Again it is important to think in a holistic way. In seeking to build inter-organizational working between levels of government or agencies and parts of government the focus easily becomes limited.

For example, a concern for building a healthy society tends to concentrate on those whose contribution is most obvious. This is most clearly seen at the local level with a focus on the social services department and the health agencies. Such a focus does not realize the full potential of local authorities for building a healthy society. Functions as diverse as education, housing, planning and leisure services all have a contribution to make. Then there are contributions from a wide range of agencies, across levels of government and from individual citizens which need to be taken into account. Neglect of such contributions reflects linear thinking, limiting involvement to the obvious, rather than taking a holistic view. Too narrow a focus will fail to encompass the potential contribution to be made by many services and agencies to a healthy society. Similarly, limited vision will ignore the contribution the health agencies can make to dealing with other wicked issues such as urban and rural deprivation, poverty, public safety, the environment and the like. [...]

Developing a capacity to work across both internal and external boundaries raises a number of people issues. The need to raise awareness of the importance of a wicked issue(s) *implies a commitment to development and training*. These activities should be designed, in part, to give knowledge and to build understanding of the issue. But they should, equally, be used to draw on the understandings, experience and knowledge of the staff of the organization. After all, problems of the environment, of health, of discrimination or of safety can impinge on many activities and on many staff. Drawing them in builds ownership of the issue. It also recognizes that these are issues in which the understanding given by any one perspective is limited, even when those perspectives claim to embrace the whole of the issue. Organizational and personal development and training can be part of a strategic search as groups explore the interrelationship between their own activities and the issue. Training can then itself be part of organizational learning. The culture of the organization should encourage holistic thinking, and training should nurture it.

Development and training have to be reinforced by *communication*. A focus on the wicked issues, with the imperative of crossing internal and/ or external organizational boundaries, requires openness, debate and information. If the wicked issues are to be understood and tackled – and an appropriate culture developed – they have to be sustained by communication sideways, upwards and downwards. . . .

Part of building the capacity for thinking and working across boundaries is the need to identify and promote particular *skills and style*. Thinking laterally and not being constrained by linear models or trapped by experience or organization is important; equally, the ability to span organization boundaries is vital. Some people will be better at these things than others. However, training, development and varied experience and career progression will play their part. Senior managers and officials will need to be especially adept at these things as they should play a key role in identifying, exploring, defining and handling wicked issues. While the position inevitably varies from government organization to government organization, many will probably suffer from a deficit in these skills and competences. Correcting this will be a key contribution to public policy, given our suggestion that the wicked issues are not only more important but will increasingly dominate the public policy agenda. A starting point would be identification of the skills required and then an audit of the organization.

Involving the public

An important part of handling many wicked issues will be finding ways of drawing in the public. Many of the traditional processes of representative democracy are inadequate in this context, because they have tended to assume the passive citizen. In these processes the role of the citizen is often reduced to no more than that of the elector making a choice between competing parties every few years. The process of representation has been reduced to the passive roles of electing or being a representative rather than involvement in an active process of deliberation between the representative and those represented. It is all too easy to see the handling of wicked issues as a top-down process. Learning and problem-solving may come as well – or better – from the bottom up. . . .

There are two problems here, and both have to be tackled. On the one hand increasing amounts of governmental activity and public policy formation and delivery take place at a distance from the representative democratic institutions of Westminster and town hall; and, on the other, too little has been done to surround the traditional institutions of democracy with ways of involving the public other than through the ballot box. More needs to be done to develop means of accountability and to open up opportunities for debate and involvement.

These are serious issues. Wicked issues require the involvement of citizens for two reasons. Because the wicked issues represent intractable problems imperfectly understood, it is important that they are widely discussed, both to deepen understanding and to draw upon *the experience of those who face these problems* at their point of greatest impact. The voices of those who live in crime-ridden areas, of those who know discrimination, or of those who face poverty, have to be heard if the reality of the issues is to be understood.

Second, many of the wicked issues, as we have said, require *changes in the way people behave*. Those changes cannot readily be imposed on people. Thus the changes that may be required to meet the threats to the environment will require ways of life that are less wasteful of non-renewable resources or that cause less pollution. Behaviour will be changed only if issues are widely understood, discussed and owned. Public participation is a necessary part of gaining this and so of handling the wicked issues.

Both of these things remind us of the importance of handling wicked issues at the local level. It is here that it is much easier to involve people – both for them to learn and for public policy to learn from their experience and involvement. It is, of course, the local level which also most readily lends itself to experiment and the development of a variety of approaches – a necessary part of trying to handle and solve uncertain and intractable issues. . . .

Conclusion: a new style of governing

Handling the wicked issues requires a new style of governing. It involves a capacity to work across organizational boundaries, to think holistically and to involve the public. However, underlying these requirements must be a recognition of the intractability of the issues faced. As we have repeated, the wicked issues are imperfectly understood, their causes are far from clear and the responses to them are uncertain. This does not make the task of governing impossible, but it cannot be based on certainty of responses.

The style of governing should not be based on the assumption that a clear and final programme of action will quickly become obvious or that the management task is to carry out such a programme as effectively and efficiently as possible. Such is the task of managing tame issues and the government of certainty. Here the task is the government of uncertainty.

Equally, it should not be assumed that action is impossible, that nothing can be done and that problems are intractable in an absolute sense. Action is possible and initiatives should be encouraged. But government cannot assume it knows the answers to the problem. Comprehensive plans will be inappropriate. . . .

The style is not so much that of a traveller who knows the route, but more that of an explorer who has a sense of direction but no clear route. Search and exploration, watching out for possibilities and interrelationships, however unlikely they may seem, are part of the approach. There are ideas as to the way ahead, but some may prove abortive. What is required is a readiness to see and accept this, rather than to proceed regardless on a path which is found to be leading nowhere or in the wrong direction. There will be a need, too, to ensure that wicked issues are not crowded out by the more routine and mundane.

This suggests that what is required in dealing with the wicked issues is a style that encourages initiative, but recognizes the need for learning – not merely in government but in society. Public learning should underlie the initiatives, which should be about expanding understanding, opening the working of organizations, policy-makers and public to research, and to views and ideas. Learning should guide the process of exploration. . . . Handling the wicked issues of public policy requires different modes of thinking and action to dealing with the tamed ones (and that goes even for the tame ones which require inter-organizational working). It means different ways of:

- *understanding* which recognize that understanding is partial at best; seeing from a variety of perspectives; being wary of apparent certainty and accepting uncertainty;
- *thinking* which pursue the holistic and are not being seduced by the linear; looking for the interactions and interrelationships;

- ■ *working* which refuse to be trapped by the obvious and conventional; tolerate not knowing; and accept different perspectives, approaches and styles;
- ■ *involving* which are inclusive, drawing in as wide a range of organizations and interests as possible and open to public participation. 'Outsiders' will bring new insight and thinking and many wicked issues will involve new attitudes and behaviours as well as government action;
- ■ *learning* about the issues and about the responses, encouraging experiment and diversity and requiring reflection. Learning government is a prerequisite for handling wicked issues.

These different ways of working make a crucial point. Wicked issues are handled by government through and between organizations. Here is a paradox. Most organizations are designed – and find it easier – to handle linear thinking and tame problems. Perspectives can be more limited, routines more readily accepted and focus more closely set. The wicked issues demand that these things are set aside. As we have shown, organizational means are needed, but organizational form and experience must not be allowed to subvert. Issues which are improperly understood cannot be handled by organizations which assume understanding. Holding on to that paradox is at the heart of the challenge to government in handling the wicked issues. Organizations which seem instinctively more comfortable with the conventional and the secure need to be able to espouse the unconventional and the radical.

REFERENCE

Rittel, H.W.J. and Webber, M. (1973) 'Dilemmas in a General Theory of Planning', *Policy Sciences*.

THIRTY-THREE

MANAGING SOCIAL ANXIETIES IN PUBLIC SECTOR ORGANIZATIONS

Anton Obholzer

Source: *The Unconscious at Work: Individual and Organizational Stress in the Human Services*, Obholzer, A. and Roberts, V. Z. (eds), London, Routledge, 1994.

It is hard to avoid the conclusion that what is wrong in our public services (or public sector organizations) today has to do with management. Article upon article, broadcast after broadcast, inform us that financial criteria have not been adhered to, that workers have too much power, that working practices are outmoded, that we are not as successful a country as we might be. The implication is that we are too soft: we need firmer management based on sound economic principles, and we need less consultation and more action. [. . .]

Management, structure and organization are not unimportant – in fact, they are vital. Nor is the emphasis on money inappropriate: financial constraint is a reality. In my experience of consulting to institutions, however, I regularly find that no attention whatsoever is paid to social, group and psychological phenomena. Consequently, by neglect, the factors that should be an integral part of good management become the very factors that undermine the venture.

As an example, it is common knowledge that any group numbering more than about twelve individuals is ineffective as a work group, incapable of useful debate and effective decision-making. Yet a great many committees are made up of many more than twelve people. [. . .]

Besides group size, other factors necessary for groups to be effective include clarity of task, time boundaries and authority structures. And yet it is quite common to receive the agenda for a so-called work group too late for it to be of any use in preparing oneself, for meetings not to start on time, and not to be clearly chaired. Not only are groups frequently too large for work, but it is also common for their membership to be so inconsistent as to make work impossible: if one representative cannot come, another is sent instead. [. . .]

The recent emphasis on 'tighter' management and control is a response to these kind of processes. The previous systems of public sector management are understandably written off, but the new concept seems to be based on a lack of understanding of what went wrong in the earlier scheme. So we have repeated re-organizations, each equally uninformed and unsuccessful. These changes, directed at improving organizational effectiveness, come from . . . 'purposive systems thinking', which focuses on input–transformation–output processes. However, effective management also requires 'containing systems thinking'. This focuses on how people's needs, beliefs and feelings give rise to patterns of relations, 'rules' and customs which often continue unaffected by structural changes (Grubb Institute, 1991).

Institutions as containers of social anxieties

Here, I use the term 'institution' to refer to large social systems such as the health, education and social services. Each of these, besides providing for specific needs – health care, schooling and so forth – through its primary task, also deals constantly with fundamental human anxieties about life and death, or, in more psychoanalytic terms, about annihilation. . . . The individual who is prey to these primitive anxieties seeks relief by projecting these anxieties into another, the earliest experience of this being the mother–baby relationship. If all goes well, the mother processes or 'metabolizes' the baby's anxieties in such a way that the feelings become bearable; we then say the anxieties have been 'contained' (Bion, 1967). It is this process of containment that eventually makes possible the maturational shift from the paranoid-schizoid position, which involves fragmentation and denial of reality, to the depressive position, where integration, thought and appropriate responses to reality are possible. In an analogous way, the institutions referred to above serve to contain these anxieties for society as a whole.

Health care systems

In the unconscious, there is no such concept as 'health'. There is, however, a concept of 'death', and, in our constant attempt to keep this anxiety repressed, we use various unconscious defensive mechanisms, including the creation of social systems to serve the defensive function. Indeed, our health service might more accurately be called a 'keep-death-at-bay' service. [. . .]

In some countries, there is a national health service which is used as a receptacle for the nation's projections of death, and as a collective unconscious system to shield us from the anxieties arising from an awareness of illness and mortality. To lose sight of the 'anxiety-containing' function of the service means an increase in turmoil, and neither its conscious nor its unconscious functions are served adequately. Consider, for example, the outrage in developed countries when advanced medical technologies cannot be made available to all; or the unfounded hopes placed in experimental treatments; or the tendency to feel duped when interventions fail. In all these situations, both individuals and society at large are quick to blame, as if good-enough medical care should prevent illness and death. Patients and doctors collude in this to protect the former from facing their fear of death and the latter from facing their fallibility. [. . .]

Defensive structures in public sector organizations

For the container to have the best chance of containing and metabolizing the anxieties projected into it, it needs to be in a depressive position mode . . . which means it has a capacity to face both external and psychic reality. For organizations, this requires not only agreement about the primary task of the organization, but also remaining in touch with the nature of the anxieties projected into the container, rather than defensively blocking them out of awareness. In order for a system to work according to these principles, a structured system for dialogue between the various component parts is necessary. This depends on all concerned being in touch with the difficulties of the task, and their relative powerlessness in radically altering the pattern of life and of society.

The present position of many public sector organizations, however, is quite a different one. The new style of management is to give managers more power and to eliminate consultation as 'inefficient'. It has become a top-down model, with dialogue and co-operation between the different sectors seen as old-fashioned, and care staff increasingly excluded from policy- and decision-making. This style of management could be described as 'paranoid-schizoid by choice', fragmenting and splitting up systems instead of promoting collaboration. The splitting up of functions makes it more comfortable for managers to make decisions.

For example, in health care systems, managers are kept at a distance from the clinicians and the patients. The structure thus enables managers psychologically to turn a blind eye to the consequences of their actions. In the short term, this gives an impression of effective change; in the long term, the consequences are disastrous. Meanwhile, the caring that has, so to speak, been 'leached out' of the management system is precipitated into the carers, who in turn have left their administrative/financial-reality side in the managers. [. . .]

What effect does the existence of this psychic configuration have on doctors? It makes for the creation of a system, strengthened by group and institutional processes, that fosters individual and professional omnipotence, a system in which weakness, doubt and distress are seen as undesirable qualities and where failure can be attributed to uncaring managers and insufficient resources. An integral part of the unconscious social system that is intended to shield us all from death is the requirement that the office-bearers of the system – in this case the doctors – be as powerful as possible. As a result of the widening gap between the management and clinical sectors of the health service, doctors have become more vulnerable than ever to the projection into them of societal fantasies of their omnipotence, caught up in an unconscious social projective system in which the capacity to do heroic things is imputed to them, and they are expected to perform. Yet it is hard for the system and its functioning to be questioned, for both doctors and the public have a vested interest in keeping it in place. Any tampering with the system creates a great deal of anxiety and resistance on all sides.

Facing psychic reality

In a management climate such as this, in which contact between the various component parts is at a minimum, it is easy for doctors to fall into a state of mind believing that much more would be possible in the fight against death if only more money were available. The shared fantasy between doctors, the public and the media seems to be that we could have eternal life, if only there were unlimited health funds.

Within the hospital, too, the staff need to protect themselves from the reality of illness, pain and death. [. . .] This flight from reality happens gradually and largely unconsciously. In the process of inducting new members, the group unconsciously gives the message, 'This is how we ignore what is going on – pretend along with us, and you will soon be one of us.' It can be called settling down, or it can be called institutionalization. In fact, it is a collusive group denial of the work difficulties.

Another way of protecting oneself against what is unbearable is to organize the work in ways that ward off primitive anxieties, rather than serving to carry out the primary task. A great deal of what goes on is not about dramatic rescue but about having to accept one's relative powerlessness in the presence of pain, decrepitude and death. Staff are ill-prepared for this in their training, and in their work practice there is often no socially sanctioned outlet for their distress. . . . This then expresses itself as illness, absenteeism, high staff turnover, low morale, poor time-keeping and so on. [. . .]

At a seminar, top health service managers were asked to name their own worst personal anxieties. They mentioned death, debilitating illness, divorce, insanity, abandonment, loss of employment and so on. All of these are of course central to the work (and the workers) of the health service and, indeed, all our public sector services. They viewed their task as one of management, and stressed that the only requirement legally laid down was for them to live within their allocated budgets. It clearly was too painful for these managers to be in touch with the needs of the patients and the consequences of their actions, and psychologically more comfortable to focus on budgets – a classic example of splitting used to avoid depressive-position pain. A great deal of the disorganization, time-wasting on and off committees, bureaucracy and the like is a way of avoiding face-to-face contact with patients and their ailments.

Similar processes occur in our other public sector services: it is contact with pain – the clients' pain and our own – that regularly puts us in touch with our feelings, our impotence and the inadequacy of our training and of our professions. Many of our so-called administrative or managerial difficulties are in reality defence mechanisms arising from the difficulty of the work. Furthermore, a system of financial reward for 'effective' management further bolsters this defensive style of functioning. From a psychoanalytic point of view, we then have a system in which the caring depressive-position functioning of managers and management systems is penalized, and the defensive paranoid-schizoid component is rewarded.

Implications for management

Our public sector institutions can usefully be thought of as comprising three sub-sectors: the public and its consumer representatives (patients, pupils and their parents, etc.); the care sub-sector (the staff of the services); and the administrative system (representing government). So far, we have looked at the anxieties that are being defended against. There are, however, other factors at play of an intergroup nature. These take place within the sub-sectors, and have to do with a rivalry between various professional and administrative sub-groups. They have always been there, but in a climate of increased pressure and, therefore, of increased splitting and projective identification, they are obviously exacerbated.

In the caring sector, the result is more strife between the various professional disciplines and heightened competition for resources. [. . .] Within the administrative sector, it is also not uncommon to find massive divisions between the various departments. This of course hinders competent management and encourages a technique of playing one group off against the other. In order for any organization to function at its most effective, certain guidelines, based on group relations understanding and sound management principles, need to be laid down.

For *all* members of the organization, be they cleaner or managing director, there is the need for:

- clarity about the task of the organization;
- clarity about the authority structure;
- the opportunity to participate and contribute.

In addition, for those in authority there is a need for:

- psychologically informed management;
- awareness of the risks to the workers;
- openness towards the consumers;
- public accountability.

Clarity about the task of the organization

As an example, cleaning contracts in the health service now go out to tender. It is clear from the contracts that no account is taken of the fact that while cleaners are there to clean, they are cleaning in a hospital with patients bearing anxiety and pain. The human contact is important for both patients and cleaners. Cutting out the commitment to the overall task is done to the detriment of all.

Clarity about the authority structure

Clear lines of authority make for accountability and therefore for the possibility of changing work practices into more appropriate ones. [. . .]

The opportunity to participate and contribute

Contract labour does not make for good staff morale or effective organization, first because contract labour does not have institutional allegiance, and, second, because of the ill-will created in the permanent staff. At one stage, more than half the secretaries in the health service were temps because they could get much better salaries that way than as permanent members of staff. An organization run on a *Gastarbeiter* ('guest-worker' – being a euphemism for disenfranchised staff) principle is not a good idea.

Psychologically informed management

This would include awareness of group and social factors that might interfere with the task of the organization. Such awareness can enable managers to take measures to combat anti-task phenomena. For example, most meetings not only do not start on time, but, more surprisingly, do not have a designated ending time. . . . Decisions are therefore made on the basis of grinding down, rather than by working through. Decisions made on the basis of out-manoeuvring or wearing down the opposition do not lead to successful management; they are often Pyrrhic victories.

Awareness of the risks to the workers

For any organization to function effectively the managers must take into account the stresses on the staff as a result of the work they are doing. They need also to make adequate provision for dealing with staff distress, and to ask themselves whether seemingly unrelated anti-task phenomena might not be manifestations of this. It is crucial that a climate is created in which the stress of the entire system can be acknowledged openly, with an awareness of the particular risks to the workers from the nature of the particular task they are performing. [...]

Openness towards the consumers

Given the defensive tendency in the health service to push patients and what they so painfully stand for aside, it is not surprising that patients are, by and large, forgotten. It is much easier to deal with diseased organs than with a person who has a complaint.... Similarly, senior health service managers may think and talk in terms of populations, again as a defence against the pain of thinking about individuals.

Public accountability

It is a moot point whether the public have a right to know via the media that their local hospital has no beds available for emergencies. Administrators are loath to inform the media of relevant local or national issues.... It seems that the authorities are accountable to those further up the line, and that public information and opinion count for very little. However, the authority for running public sector services derives ultimately from the public (the electorate), and accountability to the public needs to be held in mind and built into the system.

Conclusion

Looking at the various defensive patterns described – whether between institutions and their environment, or inter-institutional, or interpersonal – we can see how a style of work that is essentially and consistently defensive is bad not only for the work but also for individual workers. To be constantly out of touch with many aspects of psychic reality at work puts individuals at risk of being out of touch with themselves as a result of a combination of work defences and personal vulnerabilities. There is then an increased tendency to take no alcohol, sedatives, sleeping tablets and so on. This brings the further risk of endangering marital and family mental health. The pattern can influence the behaviour of children and their reactions to stress, and therefore perpetuate itself. The chances of developing stress-related diseases are also increased. We therefore come to the end of the road – an unhealthy mind in an unhealthy body in an unhealthy organization.

Groups and institutions accept newcomers and mould them to the institutional ways of doing things, including joining into their particular version of institutional defences. Eventually, the individual to a large extent loses his or her capacity to be detached and to 'see' things from an outside perspective. Yet, to maintain some outside perspective is essential if one is to retain a capacity for critical thought and questioning. Without these, our institutions are doomed to operate more and more on a basis of denial of reality – the reality that they exist to help people cope with pain, unfulfilled hopes, sickness and death. The more this is denied, the less effective the systems become, and the greater the toll on those involved in them.

REFERENCES

Bion, W. (1967) Attacks on Linking in *Second Thoughts: Selected Papers on Psychoanalysis*, London, Heinemann Medical (reprinted, London, Maresfield reprints, 1984).

Grubb Institute (1991) *Professional Management Notes*, prepared by the Grubb Institute on concepts relating to professional management.

THIRTY-FOUR

THE MANAGER'S JOB: FOLKLORE AND FACT

Henry Mintzberg

Source: *Harvard Business Review*, 1975, July–August.

Just what does the manager do? For years the manager, the heart of the organization, has been assumed to be like an orchestra leader, controlling the various parts of his organization with the ease and precision of a Seiji Ozawa. However, when one looks at the few studies that have been done – covering managerial positions from the president of the United States to street gang leaders – the facts show that managers are not reflective, regulated workers, informed by their massive MIS systems, scientific, and professional. The evidence suggests that they play a complex, intertwined combination of interpersonal, informational, and decisional roles. The author's message is that if managers want to be more effective, they must recognize what their job really is and then use the resources at hand to support rather than hamper their own nature. [...]

Back to a basic description of managerial work

[...]

The manager's job can be described in terms of various "roles," or organized sets of behaviors identified with a position. My description, shown in Figure 34.1, comprises ten roles. As we shall see, formal authority gives rise to the three interpersonal roles, which in turn give rise to the three informational roles; these two sets of roles enable the manager to play the four decisional roles.

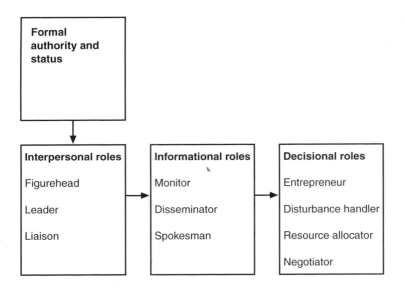

Figure 34.1   The manager's roles.

Interpersonal roles

Three of the manager's roles arise directly from his formal authority and involve basic interpersonal relationships.

1   First is the *figurehead* role. By virtue of his position as head of an organizational unit, every manager must perform some duties of a ceremonial nature. The president greets the touring dignitaries ... and the sales manager takes an important customer to lunch.

[...]

Duties that involve interpersonal roles may sometimes be routine, involving little serious communication and no important decision making. Nevertheless, they are important to the smooth functioning of an organization and cannot be ignored by the manager.

2   Because he is in charge of an organizational unit, the manager is responsible for the work of the people of that unit. His actions in this regard constitute the *leader* role. Some of these actions involve leadership directly – for example, in most organizations the manager is normally responsible for hiring and training his own staff.

In addition, there is the indirect exercise of the leader role. Every manager must motivate and encourage his employees, somehow reconciling their individual needs with the goals of the organization. In virtually every contact the manager has with his employees, subordinates seeking leadership clues probe his actions: "Does he approve?" "How would he like the report to turn out?" "Is he more interested in market share than high profits?"

The influence of the manager is most clearly seen in the leader role. Formal authority vests him with great potential power; leadership determines in large part how much of it he will realize.

3   The literature of management has always recognized the leader role, particularly those aspects of it related to motivation. In comparison, until recently it has hardly mentioned the *liaison* role, in which the manager makes contacts outside his vertical chain of command. This is remarkable in light of the finding of virtually every study of managerial work that managers spend as much time with peers and other people outside their units as they do with their own subordinates – and, surprisingly, very little time with their own superiors.

[. . .]

As we shall see shortly, the manager cultivates such contacts largely to find information. In effect, the liaison role is devoted to building up the manager's own external information system – informal, private, verbal, but, nevertheless, effective.

Informational roles

By virtue of his interpersonal contacts, both with his subordinates and with his network of contacts, the manager emerges as the nerve center of his organizational unit. He may not know everything, but he typically knows more than any member of his staff.

Studies have shown this relationship to hold for all managers, from street gang leaders to U.S. presidents. [. . .]

The processing of information is a key part of the manager's job. In my study, the chief executives spent 40% of their contact time on activities devoted exclusively to the transmission of information; 70% of their incoming mail was purely informational (as opposed to requests for action). The manager does not leave meetings or hang up the telephone in order to get back to work. In large part, communication *is* his work. Three roles describe these informational aspects of managerial work.

1   As *monitor*, the manager perpetually scans his environment for information, interrogates his liaison contacts and his subordinates, and receives unsolicited information, much of it as a result of the network of personal contacts he has developed. Remember that a good part of the information the manager collects in his monitor role arrives in verbal form, often as gossip, hearsay, and speculation. By virtue of his contacts, the manager has a natural advantage in collecting this soft information for his organization.

2   He must share and distribute much of this information. Information he gleans from outside personal contacts may be needed within his organization. In his *disseminator* role, the manager passes some of his privileged

information directly to his subordinates, who would otherwise have no access to it. When his subordinates lack easy contact with one another, the manager will sometimes pass information from one to another.

3   In his *spokesman* role, the manager sends some of his information to people outside his unit – a president makes a speech to lobby for an organization cause, or a foreman suggests a product modification to a supplier. In addition, as part of his role as spokesman, every manager must inform and satisfy the influential people who control his organizational unit. . . . Consumer groups must be assured that the organization is fulfilling its social responsibilities and government officials must be satisfied that the organization is abiding by the law.

Decisional roles

Information is not, of course, an end in itself; it is the basic input to decision making. One thing is clear in the study of managerial work: the manager plays the major role in his unit's decision-making system. As its formal authority, only he can commit the unit to important new courses of action; and as its nerve center, only he has full and current information to make the set of decisions that determines the unit's strategy. Four roles describe the manager as decision-maker.

1   As *entrepreneur*, the manager seeks to improve his unit, to adapt it to changing conditions in the environment. In his monitor role, the president is constantly on the lookout for new ideas. When a good one appears, he initiates a development project that he may supervise himself or delegate to an employee (perhaps with the stipulation that he must approve the final proposal).

[. . .]

2   While the entrepreneur role describes the manager as the voluntary initiator of change, the *disturbance handler* role depicts the manager involuntarily responding to pressures. Here change is beyond the manager's control. He must act because the pressures of the situation are too severe to be ignored: a strike looms, a major customer has gone bankrupt or a supplier reneges on his contract.

It has been fashionable, I noted earlier, to compare the manager to an orchestra conductor, just as Peter F. Drucker wrote in *The Practice of Management*:

> The manager has the task of creating a true whole that is larger than the sum of its parts, a productive entity that turns out more than the sum of the resources put into it. One analogy is the conductor of a symphony orchestra, through whose effort, vision and leadership individual instrumental parts that are so much noise by themselves become the living whole of music. But the conductor has the com-

poser's score: he is only interpreter. The manager is both composer and conductor.

(1954: 341–2)

Now consider the words of Leonard R. Sayles, who has carried out systematic research on the manager's job:

> [The manager] is like a symphony orchestra conductor, endeavouring to maintain a melodious performance in which the contributions of the various instruments are coordinated and sequenced, patterned and paced, while the orchestra members are having various personal difficulties, stage hands are moving music stands, alternating excessive heat and cold are creating audience and instrument problems, and the sponsor of the concert is insisting on irrational changes in the program.
>
> (1964: 162)

In effect, every manager must spend a good part of his time responding to high-pressure disturbances. No organization can be so well run, so standardized, that it has considered every contingency in the uncertain environment in advance. Disturbances arise not only because poor managers ignore situations until they reach crisis proportions, but also because good managers cannot possibly anticipate all the consequences of the actions they take.

3   The third decisional role is that of *resource allocator*. To the manager falls the responsibility of deciding who will get what in his organizational unit. Perhaps the most important resource the manager allocates is his own time. Access to the manager constitutes exposure to the unit's nerve center and decision-maker. The manager is also charged with designing his unit's structure, that pattern of formal relationships that determines how work is to be divided and coordinated.

Also, in his role as resource allocator, the manager authorizes the important decisions of his unit before they are implemented. By retaining this power, the manager can ensure that decisions are interrelated; all must pass through a single brain. To fragment this power is to encourage discontinuous decision making and a disjointed strategy.

There are a number of interesting features about the manager's authorizing others' decisions. First, despite the widespread use of capital budgeting procedures – a means of authorizing various capital expenditures at one time – executives in my study made a great many authorization decisions on an ad hoc basis. Apparently, many projects cannot wait or simply do not have the quantifiable costs and benefits that capital budgeting requires.

Second, I found that the chief executives faced incredibly complex choices. They had to consider the impact of each decision on other decisions and on the organization's strategy. They had to ensure that the decision would be acceptable to those who influence the organization, as well as ensure that resources would not be overextended. They had to understand the various costs and benefits as well as the feasibility of the proposal. They also had to consider questions of timing. All this was necessary for the simple approval of someone else's proposal. At the same time, however, delay could lose time, while quick approval could be ill considered and quick rejection might discourage the subordinate who had spent months developing a pet project.

[. . .]

4   The final decisional role is that of *negotiator*. Studies of managerial work at all levels indicate that managers spend considerable time in negotiations: the president of the football team is called in to work out a contract with the holdout superstar; the corporation president leads his company's contingent to negotiate a new strike issue; the foreman argues a grievance problem to its conclusion with the shop steward. As Leonard Sayles puts it, negotiations are a "way of life" for the sophisticated manager.

These negotiations are duties of the manager's job; perhaps routine, they are not to be shirked. They are an integral part of his job, for only he has the authority to commit organizational resources in "real time," and only he has the nerve center information that important negotiations require.

The integrated job

It should be clear by now that the ten roles I have been describing are not easily separable. In the terminology of the psychologist, they form a gestalt, an integrated whole. No role can be pulled out of the framework and the job be left intact. For example, a manager without liaison contacts lacks external information. As a result, he can neither disseminate the information his employees need nor make decisions that adequately reflect external conditions. (In fact, this is a problem for the new person in a managerial position, since he cannot make effective decisions until he has built up his network of contacts.)

[. . .]

To say that the ten roles form a gestalt is not to say that all managers give equal attention to each role. In fact, I found in my review of the various research studies that

. . . sales managers seem to spend relatively more of their time in the interpersonal roles, presumably a reflection of the extrovert nature of the marketing activity;

...production managers give relatively more attention to the decisional roles, presumably a reflection of their concern with efficient work flow;

...staff managers spend the most time in the informational roles, since they are experts who manage departments that advise other parts of the organization.

Nevertheless, in all cases the interpersonal, informational, and decisional roles remain inseparable.

REFERENCES

Drucker, P.F. (1954) *The Practice of Management*, New York, Harper & Row.

Mintzberg, H. (1973) *The Nature of Managerial Work*, New York, Harper & Row.

Sayles, L.R. (1964) *Managerial Behavior*, New York, McGraw-Hill.

THIRTY-FIVE

THE ROLE OF LEADERSHIP IN THE MODERNIZATION AND IMPROVEMENT OF PUBLIC SERVICES

Jean Hartley and Maria Allison

Source: *Public Money and Management*, 2000, April–June.

'Leadership' is a common word in recent policy and academic papers on the modernization and improvement of public services ... (DETR, 1998), ... (DETR, 1999a); ... (DfEE, 1998). The debates about new political arrangements for local authorities, including the role of elected mayors, are built on arguments about strong, visible and accountable leadership. Local authorities are to be given new powers and responsibilities for community planning, based on strengthening their community leadership role....

It is not just local government which has been charged to show greater leadership in order to modernize public services. In central government, the Sunningdale discussions among permanent secretaries in late 1999 identified leadership as a key theme in aiming for innovation and excellence (Cabinet Office, 1999). In the health sector, there is an increased concern to ensure that managers are also leaders, for example, through the forthcoming NHS Leadership Programme.

Why is leadership seen to be significant in the development of 'modernized' governance and 'improved' public services? Is it simply a mantra or is there some logic to the promotion of leadership in public services? We examine these questions in the context of leadership in local government.

The national policy context for local government

The Government's modernization agenda argues for an increased role for local authorities in leading their communities and being responsible for the social, economic and environmental well-being of the locality.... (DETR, 1998b, section 2.4).

[...]

Leadership is proposed as significant for modernization and improvement, but is often alluded to without definition. There are at least two levels of analysis in the concept of leadership. In the first, leadership is the behaviours and actions of individuals, sometimes acting in concert but primarily as solo figures. For example, the proposal that an elected mayor or a head teacher will bring about 'strong' leadership is based on this. The second approach has the local authority organization as the unit of analysis. Here a focus on community leadership is by the local authority as a whole, working with other agencies in the locality, and having particular responsibility for voicing and addressing the needs and aspirations of local communities. This approach includes the role of individuals, but as part of organizational functioning.

Leadership and influence

What is leadership? First, we distinguish the concept of leader from that of leadership. It is helpful to distinguish between the person, the position and processes. These may in practice co-exist, but it is important to distinguish them conceptually.

The person

There has been a lot of academic research on the personal characteristics of leaders (see Yukl, 1994 for a review). It tends to focus on skills, abilities, personality, styles and behaviours (for example Avolio, 1999; Burns, 1978) of individual leaders. The role of individuals in shaping events and circumstances at certain times is clear. A difficulty can be that such approaches can lionize individuals, assuming that they have pre-eminent capacity and power. This ignores both so-called 'followers' and also organizational and community constraints.

The position

Leadership is sometimes used to refer to a formal position in an organization for example, Leader of the Council or Chief Executive. Some commentators (for example Rost, 1998) argue that such formal positions give authority, though not necessarily leadership. Leadership requires more than holding a particular office or role. Heifetz (1996) distinguishes formal from informal leadership, arguing that each may tackle issues through different processes.

The processes

A third approach is to regard leadership as a set of processes or dynamics occurring among and between individuals, groups and organizations. Here, leadership is concerned with motivating and influencing people, and shaping and achieving outcomes. Burns (1978) distinguishes between transformational and transactional leadership and this has been widely used in conceptualizing leadership. The approaches are complementary. Transformational leadership is characterized by inspirational motivation (the ability to create and build commitment to goals); challenging current reality and established patterns of thinking; and individualized consideration (fair but individual treatment of group members). Nadler and Tushman (1990) describe these as envisioning, energizing and enabling. Transactional leadership, on the other hand, is concerned with embedding actions in a substantial way through the use of systems and rewards which support the objectives.

The idea of leadership as a set of processes concerned with influencing people and achieving goals and outcomes is reflected in the key definition of leadership by Heifetz (1996) as 'mobilizing people to tackle tough problems'. This is very different from the conventional view of leadership of providing solutions to problems. The role of leadership is to work with people to find workable ways of dealing with issues for which there may be no known or set solutions (Heifetz and Sinder, 1988).

Benington (1997) argues that community leadership is based upon three inter-related assumptions. Each has an impact on conceptions of leadership:

- The first is that the purpose of a local authority is not simply to deliver, manage and/or commission services but also to govern and lead the local community. This includes not only representing the needs but also developing the diverse voices and interests in the local community. Leadership in local government therefore includes capacity building, empowerment and representation.
- Second, the local council cannot govern the local community on its own, but needs to do this in partnership with the public, private and voluntary sectors. This requires not just leadership and management of local authority staff, budgets and services but also leadership beyond the boundaries of the organization. This may have to be through influence, persuasion, negotiation and coalition-building, as well as through command.
- Third is the recognition that within such inter-organizational partnerships and networks, the local authority has a unique and distinctive

role to play because of its democratic mandate to reflect and represent the needs of the whole community rather than just its diverse and separate parts. In addition, it needs to plan for the needs of future generations as well as current users. Here, the role of political leadership in balancing competing interests is particularly important. But leadership has to mobilize and involve local communities and gain their active consent. Political leadership has to be won not only through the ballot box, but also through policies, actions and development processes in which local communities have reasonable confidence.

Consortium research on leadership and the management of influence

Our research on leadership and the management of influence has been conducted with the Warwick University Local Authorities Research Consortium, as part of the Local Government Centre's research programme on organizational and cultural change The research aims to build knowledge about how leadership and influence are exercised in the pursuit of key changes by local authorities, and to transcend traditional models of leadership (which tend to focus on individual action and are often applied without question from the private sector).

The research is based on case studies in four local authorities (here referred to as Eastern County, Western County, Metropolitan, and District). The case studies were chosen as local authorities which are innovating in ways of leading their local communities. Each is engaged in major organizational and cultural change aiming at strengthening democratic local governance or to achieve more citizen-centred services. Our case studies therefore concentrate particularly on the community leadership role, and the use of influence across internal boundaries and across inter-organizational networks.

The case studies cover a variety of organizational change:

- Using information and communication technologies to develop citizen-centred services.
- Developing a community information programme for economic and social regeneration.
- Restructuring the organization to enhance responsiveness to local communities.
- Developing and strengthening relationships between county and district councils.

The four cases include different types of authority (county, metropolitan and district); include primarily rural, primarily urban and mixed geographical areas; range from large to small; and have varied political control (Liberal Democrat, Labour, Conservative and no overall control).

The research team, consisting of both academics and practitioners using co-research methodology (Hartley and Benington, 2000), visited each organization for two days to conduct interviews. These were undertaken with a range of stakeholders so that the different contributions to and perceptions of leadership by political leaders, senior officers, managers, staff, trade union representatives, and community, voluntary and private sector partners could be examined. In total, 75 in-depth interviews were carried out and five focus groups with staff. Observations and documentation were also included in the analyses.

Key findings

There is clearly a leadership role for particular individuals in shaping visions of the future and encouraging the local authority to look beyond immediate pressures. These were primarily, but not exclusively financial (in the wake of local government reform, economic decline and social exclusion). In each of the case studies, we can discern key individuals who act as leaders, shaping debates and actions about change.

However, there are two interesting features. First, it was not always the person at the political and/or managerial apex. While the role of political leaders and chief executives is clearly crucial, we found that they do not always lead from the front but that some empower nominated others to foster and promote change in the organization. They also create a climate of innovation. Innovation is nurtured rather than mandated. Leadership which 'grows' development, rather than 'pulls levers', was commented on among those we interviewed. This is either a different kind of leadership or a different dimension of leadership than is sometimes assumed from the debates about 'strong' leadership, which often imply more of a command and control approach to leading organizations.

The second interesting issue about individuals is that there is a temporal dimension to leadership which can mean that the leadership role is passed from one individual to another in different time periods with their different leadership challenges. For example, in Metropolitan, leadership has spread out from the corporate centre and is now also being carried by some middle managers and staff.

Leadership may also, from our case studies, provide a different approach to 'the vision' (traditionally an achievement of leaders). The local authorities were concerned to develop transformational change, but much of this cannot be clearly specified in advance. For example, the establishment of the community information programme in Metropolitan, or electronic access to services in Eastern County, requires working with private sector partners on advanced information and communication technologies where the social and organizational implications and outcomes cannot be fully predicted. The customizing of Internet technologies and software by and with people with learning difficulties at a day centre in Metropolitan was not foreseen at the outset of the change. Another example took place in Western County where the vision for greater joined-up working between the District and the County led to the development of partnership committees, although this has taken quite different trajectories in the seven committees.

Each of the case study local authorities was addressing complex, shifting changes, which were dynamic. Both the political and managerial leaderships addressed this not only by plans and schedules but by creating a framework and a vision, within which new developments can be encouraged and sustained to grow organically. Leadership in part may involve empowerment of staff within the organization to take forward change and to work with communities to achieve this. For example, in District Council organizational restructuring has led to the development of a strategic team to address key cross-cutting priorities for the locality. This is about providing the conditions for citizen-centred services rather than specifying them through command and control (though there is still a place for this in some services and some circumstances).

Leadership is therefore no longer (if it ever was) solely about command and control from the 'top' of the organization. Many interviewees reported the role of politicians and managers in encouraging the active engagement of others at all levels and locations in the organization. We observed in our case study research where the active engagement among some groups of politicians, managers and staff contributed to community leadership, helping the authority to exert influence beyond its boundaries. If leadership is taken to be helping people to mobilize resources (Heifetz, 1996), then this is evident at several levels. For example, the library assistants in Metropolitan see themselves as outreach workers, leafleting cafés and talking to people in the street in order to encourage poorly educated people to 'have a go' with computers to access information and jobs. The front-line professionals, such as social workers, educational managers and [others in] different departments and agencies who work with children with a disability have constructed alliances, support, systems and a collaborative culture for inter-agency working. We describe such initiatives as distributed leadership, because it is dispersed across the organization.

Leadership and influence at the corporate and strategic level (by both elected members and managers) have been concerned not only with the organization (the local authority) but also with leadership between organizations. Here, leadership is concerned with building alliances, links and networks with and between several organizations to achieve synergies, integration and joint outcomes. This may be with the private sector (Metropolitan and Eastern County), with district councils (Western

County and Eastern County), with health agencies (Western County, Eastern County) and/or with the voluntary sector (all case studies).

Inter-organizational leadership, however, is a further challenge. As an example, Western County is a local authority with dispersed and diverse communities, which has established and is nurturing seven partnership committees with other levels of local government (district and in some cases parishes), and with some other agencies. This requires not only understanding the context of each organization but also their complex inter-relationships and changing dynamics. Such complexity is taken for granted by some politicians but is a major challenge for political and managerial leaders, even where they are well steeped in local conditions and contexts. From our interviews, it requires responsiveness to changing conditions as well as deep understanding of histories.

Leadership is not only about influence. The role of formal power through a directive style can also be important. The role for politicians, managers and project directors to unlock sticking points through the use of authority and power at times was also evident. For example, a project director at Eastern County explored engaging the local districts and other agencies in using the capacity of the call centre and told them all when the opportunity to join the project with potential private sector contractors would close.

The existence of both influence-based leadership and authority, through formal structures and positions, created some tensions in all four case studies. The use of lateral influence and networks (across services, across departments, across organizations, drawing in appropriate partners according to contribution rather than position) is different from the vertical, hierarchical relationships which are fostered in structured organizations providing services on a large scale. Not everyone finds the interface between the lateral and vertical modes of organizing easy. For example, in Western County there were seen to be two organizational logics of formal and informal authority, centralized and decentralized budgets, resources and power, and lateral as well as vertical systems of influence. In addition, in all the organizations there were differences between those who were engaged in new forms of organizing across boundaries and those who felt shut out or switched off. Trade unions also report finding it hard to organize around citizen-centred services and joined-up government, given that their membership base and organization is largely departmental.

Leadership through influence means that a larger number of politicians and managers work in boundary locations. Managers are no longer buried inside the organization but like politicians, have to work in multiple arenas, locations and with groups with different identities, cultures and histories. We still do not know enough about how to organizationally support politicians, managers and staff in these roles, which are at the points of intersection between different arenas – partly inside and partly outside the organization, working with elected members and with officers, with staff and with communities, within the local authority and with other agencies.

Conclusions

Overall, the four case studies have provided a rich picture of inter-organizational leadership and influence. The role of leadership and influence in such complex networks of inter-relationships between organizations moves beyond traditional models of leadership, which tend to emphasize individual action. The case studies highlight both the potential and the risks of distributed leadership throughout the organization and the importance of inter-organizational leadership. All four case studies also demonstrate the immense changes in internal work organization, cultures, behaviours and processes which are needed for community leadership.

The implications for the debates about modernization and improvement of public services and local governance are substantial. First, the case studies demonstrate distributed leadership throughout the organization, from apex to front line. By contrast some of the implementation of the new political arrangements can be read in terms of concentrating political leadership at the apex of the organization. Although new political arrangements are intended to strengthen community representational roles, much of the intellectual and emotional focus from politicians concerns the role of the executive. To what extent are distributed and concentrated leadership roles compatible, and if so, in what ways? How can they be combined?

Second, much of the debate about modernization and improvement is focused on internal leadership to achieve change. Yet, community leadership takes place not only in the organization but also at the cross-roads of different cultures and organizational forms – for example, at the cross-roads between political and managerial activities, with local groups as well as with the internal organization, in different geographical areas, working with senior managers and front-line staff. The modernization debate has taken insufficient account of this complexity and its consequences for roles, structures, cultures, accountabilities, training and development.

Third, the emphasis from central government has often been about individual leaders (head teachers, elected mayors, chief executives), occasionally about collective leadership (cabinets or corporate teams) but rarely about organizational leadership other than in very broad terms. Our research shows that inter-organizational leadership is complex and requires developmental and influence skills, as well as traditional hierarchical skills.

Fourth, we defined our research in terms not only of leadership, but also the management of influence, to emphasize that the skills of shaping directions, shifting resources and achieving outcomes requires directive types of leadership together with the subtle skills of influencing and negotiating. This implies a different model of leadership.

Finally, leadership of modernization and improvement is taking place in conditions of increasing complexity and uncertainty, where outcomes cannot always be specified in advance. Leadership therefore is not about directing a steady state organization where the problems and the solutions are largely known, but leadership takes place in a context of change, flux and uncertainty (Hartley, 2000). This requires an approach which is not only about 'implementation' of pre-specified policies but the 'enactment' (Weick, 1995), or emergence (Allison and Hartley, 2000) of outcomes. Innovation cannot be pre-specified and therefore part of the role of leadership is to provide a framework and to observe, nurture, shape and reflect as well as to implement. Models of leadership in the UK public sector urgently need updating to reflect this.

REFERENCES

Allison, M. and Hartley, J. (2000) *Generating and Sharing Better Practice: Reports of the Better Value Development Programme Workshops*, London, DETR.

Avolio, B. (1999) *Full Leadership Development*, Thousand Oaks, Sage.

Benington, J. (1997) New paradigms and practices for local government: capacity building within civil society, in Kraemer, S. and Roberts, J. (eds), *The Politics of Attachment*, London, Free Association Press.

Burns, J.M. (1978) *Leadership*, New York, Harper and Row.

Cabinet Office (1999) *Report to the Prime Minister from Sir Richard Wilson, Head of the Home Civil Service*, London, Cabinet Office.

DETR (1998a) *Modernizing Local Government: Local Democracy and Local Leadership*, London, The Stationery Office.

DETR (1998b) *Modern Local Government: In Touch with the People*, London, The Stationery Office.

DETR (1999) *Local Leadership, Local Choice*, London, The Stationery Office.

DfEE (1998) *Teachers Meeting the Challenge of Change*, London, The Stationery Office.

Hartley, J. (2000) Leading and managing the uncertainty of strategic change, in Flood, P., Carroll, S., Gorman, I. and Dromgoole, T. (eds), *Managing Strategic Implementation*, Oxford, Blackwell, pp. 109–122.

Hartley, J. and Benington, J. (2000) Co-research: a new methodology for new times. *European Journal of Work and Organizational Psychology* 9, 463–76.

Heifetz, R. (1996) *Leadership without Easy Answers*, Cambridge, MA, Harvard University Press.

Heifetz, R. and Sinder, R. (1988) Political leadership, in Reich, R. (ed.), *The Power of Public Ideas*, Cambridge, MA, Harvard University Press.

Improvement and Development Agency (1993) *Benchmark of the 'Ideal' Local Authority*, London, IDeA.

Nadler, D. and Tushman, M. (1989) Leadership for organizational changes, in Mohrman, A., Mohrman, S., Ledford, G., Cummings, T. and Lawler, E. (eds), *Large-Scale Organizational Change*, San Francisco, Jossey Bass.

Rost, J. (1998) Leadership and management, in Hickman, G. (ed.), *Leading Organizations: Perspectives for a New Era*, Thousand Oaks, Sage.

Weick, K. (1995) *Sense-Making in Organizations*, Thousand Oaks, Sage.

Yukl, G. (1994) *Leadership in Organizations* (3rd edn), London, Prentice Hall.

THIRTY-SIX

THE SUPERVISION PARTNERSHIP: A WHOLE GREATER THAN THE SUM OF ITS PARTS

Catherine and David Sawdon

Source: *Good Practice in Supervision*, Pritchard, J. (ed.), Jessica Kingsley, 1995.

[...]

Central and marginal

...move from the margin to the centre.

(hooks 1991)

Supervision is both central and marginal to the practice of social work. It is central because 'the most vital social work resources are the personal resources of the workers' (Payne and Scott, 1982), and they need to be controlled and fostered in the interests of effective service delivery. It is marginal in that in practice its purposes and functions are often confused, and its potential efficacy undervalued and undermined by low commitment. Marginality thus leads to unhelpful criticisms that the impact of supervision on practice outcomes cannot be measured, therefore it is of questionable value. A net result is that supervision in terms of regularity, content and outcome is patchy and variable in quality.

This ambivalence about the value of supervision is reinforced by the current political context and its increasing influence on the nature of practice. [...] One purpose of supervision is therefore clear, 'to establish the accountability of the worker to the organisation' (DHSS, 1978). Unfortunately, emphasis on one purpose risks disturbing the fine balance with the other, 'to promote the worker's development as a professional person' (DHSS, 1978). As the two purposes are seen as 'practically and conceptually interwoven' (DHSS, 1978), disruption in practical application leads either to simplistic one-dimensional prescriptions, or confusion, and ultimate ambivalence and resistance. This is not to deny that the two main purposes of supervision have not always been in tension. The challenge has been to wrestle creatively with that tension, and to recognise that each of the three core functions of 'managing', 'teaching', and 'supporting' require a place on the stage as part of the whole, rather than to give one purpose assumed or explicit priority over the other.

[...]

Functions and sources of authority

It is salutary to read the early texts on supervision if only to appreciate that the theories and principles have not actually changed much since first articulated in a social work context by Virginia Robinson in 1930 (Richards et al., 1991). Pettes (1967) draws on Towle (1963) to highlight the three core functions of 'administration', 'teaching', and 'helping'. Kadushin (1976), Westheimer (1977), and Payne and Scott (1982) adjust these labels to incorporate 'managing' (administration) and 'supportive' or 'enabling' (helping). More recently, Richards et al. (1991) and Morrison (1993) have added a fourth, 'mediation', to reflect the pace of change and the need to work in partnership with other agencies, particularly in work concerned with child protection.

Current emphases on the assessment of competence in social work education (Evans, 1990) and performance appraisal in subsequence practice (Sawdon and Sawdon, 1991) suggest that a fifth function, 'assessment', may now be to the fore where previously it has tended to be subsumed within the core three. It can be seen as a potential driving force, geared to producing measurable outcomes and improved effectiveness through a focus on staff performance. The literature on appraisal (e.g. Harrison, 1988; Stewart and Stewart, 1977) draws intrinsic connections with the practice of supervision whether the motivation is towards improved profits and service delivery or staff care and development. The pace of introduction of staff appraisal schemes within social services seems likely to quicken.

[...]

The majority of those who use scarce training and education opportunities to explore the meaning of supervision competence, recognise in theory and practice a willingness to achieve a balance of interrelated functions. They want to be able to tolerate the ambiguities and tensions involved. Such a stance reflects what they experience in terms of their own expectations and the demands of those they supervise. Their often expressed sense of loss and bewilderment, far from being a pathological indicator of weakness, appears to stem more directly from imposed reductionist structures which do not want to recognise either the complex nuances of responsibility or individual strengths and needs. Statements of this order often attract the criticism of 'whingeing' and invitations to leave the heat of the kitchen. Continuous restructuring, permanent instability and resource constraints are recognised features of social work agencies and it seems that we all have to learn to work with them. Our argument, knowingly repeated, is that to fail to recognise such essential staff resources makes the task impossible to manage, wasteful, and dull.

We would, therefore, endorse the three principles proposed by Richards *et al.* (1991) that permeate the work of a competent supervisor:

- to be more proactive *v.* being purely reactive
- to attempt to become a good role model for practitioners
- to develop personal effectiveness.

Sustaining aspirations through learning

These three principles have the quality of aspirations, and to remain alive require sustenance. Each reflecting practitioner collects and refines an eclectic toolbag of workable practice theories which make the journey possible. Commonly quoted theoretical constructs which have potential relevance to supervision are *adult learning* models (Rogers, 1969; Freire, 1972; Knowles, 1978; Reynolds, 1965; Kolb and McIntyre, 1979; Haring *et al.*, 1978); transactional analysis (Berne, 1964); and counselling and therapy models (Shohet and Hawkins, 1989; Heron 1975, 1990). Many of these are concisely summarised by Morrison (1993). [. . .]

As we have implied earlier, the first and most obvious connection made by writers in this field is that the health of the organisation and the quality of service delivered will depend considerably on the learning and development of its main resource: *the staff*.

Understanding how people learn, facilitating and indeed accelerating these processes, is critical and underpins the educative function of supervision. Knowles (1978) and Freire (1972) and before them Rogers (1969) invite us to challenge objective pedagogic models of teaching and to consider androgogy 'the art and science of enabling adults to learn'. The teacher/supervisor is seen as facilitator, joining the learner/supervisee in a process of enquiry, and mutual challenge rather than an expert transmitter of knowledge.

Knowles' concept of androgogy is based on four assumptions about the characteristics of adult learners. These are:

1   as a person matures, his self concept moves from one of being a dependent personality towards self direction;

2   he accumulates a growing reservoir of experience that becomes an increasing resource for learning;

3   his readiness to learn becomes oriented increasingly to the developmental tasks of his social roles;

4   his time perspective changes from one of postponed application of knowledge to immediacy of application, and accordingly his orientation towards learning shifts from one of subject centredness to one of problem centredness.

This model is student/supervisee centred, with an emphasis on problem-focused learning which takes account of prior experience and developing needs. Such an apparently creative and open model of learning is clearly connected with Payne and Scott's desired 'democratic and egalitarian approach' (1982) and has been influential in developments in practice teaching and social work education in general.

[. . .]

Developing skills

John Heron's work (1975) offers one model for building in some practical analysis of what actually happens in supervision, and refining the core skills, language, and behaviour that contribute to effective practice. His counselling and psychotherapeutic perspectives may seem outmoded for some in the current organisational context of social services. Yet counselling outside social work would now appear to be a growth industry! In our view, such skills are directly transferable and can offer an important sense of stability within an apparent sea of chaos. Shohet and Hawkins (1989) indicate for example how workers who become supervisors may abandon initially their very useful practitioner skills, yet ultimately draw strength from revaluing them, albeit in a new context and role. Instead of rejecting these skills, there is a clear case for celebrating them.

Heron's thesis, put simply, is that all helping interventions can be divided or reduced to six categories. We thus have the possibility of a framework which can assist supervisors in becoming aware of the different interventions they use. Retrospective analysis of language and behaviour using the framework can reveal 'valid' and 'degenerate' intervention, with the prospect of applying this understanding towards skill improvement and a potentially wider repertoire of choice. Crucially, the categorisation also enables us to examine the dynamics of power and authority within the supervisory partnership. This dimension is central, whether one is concerned with issues of control, accountability and effectiveness, or personal learning and development. This can be expressed diagrammatically in Figure 36.1.

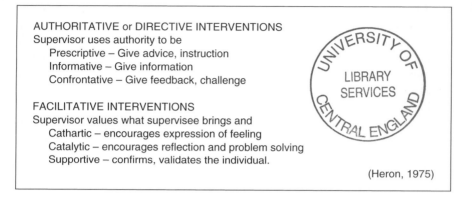

AUTHORITATIVE or DIRECTIVE INTERVENTIONS
Supervisor uses authority to be
    Prescriptive – Give advice, instruction
    Informative – Give information
    Confrontative – Give feedback, challenge

FACILITATIVE INTERVENTIONS
Supervisor values what supervisee brings and
    Cathartic – encourages expression of feeling
    Catalytic – encourages reflection and problem solving
    Supportive – confirms, validates the individual.

(Heron, 1975)

Figure 36.1 A framework for helping interventions

These six types of intervention only have meaning if they are rooted in care and concern for the individual supervisee. Most of us manage to be both valid and degenerate. Occasionally, some supervisors may regrettably lapse into 'perverted' use which is to be deliberately manipulative or malicious. One final note of caution. Heron's counselling-specific terms can for some be off-putting. Jargon terms in this case are worth struggling with, as each reading seems to present further insight. Furthermore, one needs to remember to place this person-centred approach within the context of a locally and nationally accountable context.

The effective supervisor does not deny her/his power and authority but uses it to ensure with the supervisee that s/he is clear about what is required and how they are meeting or not meeting those requirements together. The effective supervisor does not lean over backwards nor abrogate power and authority. S/he shares the responsibility for dealing with the pain and complexity of vulnerable life situations in a manner which promotes the supervisee's own sense of worth and personal authority. Anecdotal evidence from recent workshops for a significant sample of manager/supervisors at different levels suggests that it is the facilitative interventions which tend to be absent or poorly practised at the higher levels of hierarchical management structures. 'Moral patronage', 'smiling demolition', and 'sweet syrup' to use some of Heron's degenerate terms tend to evoke distrust, limited respect and downright suspicion, especially amongst potentially oppressed groups. Training to enhance the use of facilitative intervention skills tends not to be seen as a priority for senior management work. One result may be a vacuum or disparity between what most supervisees actually want and the preparedness or ability of some supervisors to deliver.

What seems to be important to recognise here is that individual skills are placed within context through the supervisory partnership. This can help to ensure that the wider functional needs of the agency do not deny that everyday social work is still about deploying those individual skills effectively on behalf of service users or clients. Opportunities to receive feedback on these skills in a relatively safe atmosphere of mutual respect should not be something that ends with qualifying training. Like driving, we all slip into poor practice. Supervision should be the central reflective tool for us to remind ourselves of personal standards as individual 'professionals', as well as the agency's preference for monitored service delivery.

Problem solving

A keen thread extending through all the models put forward is the need and desire to solve problems. Andragogic approaches offer more perspectives through pooling, enquiry, and mutual challenge but Humphries (1988) warns us that traditional common sense ways of tackling problems may need to be unlearned rather than simply 'unfrozen'. She argues that a more radical concept of problem solving is necessary – one which allows a re-evaluation of past experience, and a preparedness to confront commonly held assumptions, stereotypes, and the view that 'one's values are one's own private affair'. This argument seems more than pertinent in relation to the continuing 'political correctness' debate, and the progress towards a reality rather than just a rhetoric of anti-oppressive practice. Confronting the bias and prejudice which support the 'isms', as Jean Kantambu Latting (1990) demonstrates, requires more than exhortation and information, 'Only those who already agree with the values expressed are likely to be influenced by the arguments presented' (Latting, 1990). It is also a myth that social workers and their employing agencies are critical exponents of anti-racist, anti-discriminatory, anti-oppressive practice. Any sample of older people in residential care, or people with disabilities using day care, or black people with mental health problems would quickly dispel any such myth. Although many grass roots workers aspire to improved practice in these areas, the evidence of senior management support is far less available.

Addressing such wider issues should be part of the stuff of supervision. They tend, however, to be rapidly sidelined by the pressure to focus on the micro detail of cases. The time for interactive debate and the development of 'cognitive sophistication' (Gabelko and Michaelis, 1981) or critical thinking skills is rarely deemed to be available. Such skills, first promoted in education and training contexts, enable us to be free to question our own and other's immediate reactive thinking processes. Whilst acknowledging the time factor and the felt pressure, we would ask what other opportunities for critical questioning and reflection-in-action (Schön, 1987) actually exist outside supervision? The occasional quality training programme and/or the pursuit of post qualifying credits (e.g. Approved Social Worker, Child Protection, or Accredited Practice Teacher Training) may well trigger and help to consolidate new awareness and knowledge. Quality is variable, however, and any learning derived usually requires agency commitment, reinforcement and support. Regular effective supervision offers opportunities for both supervisor and supervisee to draw on such experiences, build on them and sustain a critical approach to practice.

[...]

Managing self

One of the recurring 'problems' in relation to being a supervisor is the business of self-care when arguably most time is spent giving out to or being alongside others. We all know most of the strategies for dealing with stress and self-care, at least at an intellectual level, but at one time or another most of us fail to follow our own good advice. Much has been written of the areas of stress and burnout (e.g. McDerment, 1988; Dainow and Bailey, 1988) and the concerned reader will either have addressed this area already or will be able to pursue these and other sources.

Given the child protection focus of much social work practice, the contribution of Richards *et al.* (1991) seems particularly accessible and useful for both members of the supervisory partnership. They remind us how situations faced by social workers can evoke quite primitive and painful feelings, and that 'the most ordinary and natural response to pain is to try and avoid it'. Strategies for avoiding pain, previously outlined by Kadushin (1976) are cited again so that most of us can recognise when we have been in 'denial' or 'professionally distant' or become 'obsessive' about adherence to laid-down policies or procedures. We can ultimately spend more time and energy avoiding pain and conflict than may be necessary to deal with it direct. The image of a head swathed in bandages to block the senses is very powerful. As always, care must be taken not to polarise the causes for stress as either solely extrinsic – 'it's them' – or internalise the reasons and accept oppressive pathologising.

[...]

The whole is greater than the sum of the parts

[...]

Each member of the partnership ... has to recognise their own vulnerability and capacity to make mistakes as human beings still needing to and being open to learn. The process of engaging and setting a mutually beneficial working contract or agreement, whilst sounding formal, cannot be overestimated here. Morrison (1993) also suggests the development of a Staff Care Statement and a Self Care Plan for supervisors and supervisees which many teams might usefully adopt. The difficulty with such 'plans', valuable as they are as statements of good intent, is that they often represent a counsel of perfection. In other words, we rarely achieve the high and demanding standards that they set, and in trying and failing, we run the risk of injury or increasing the stress they were designed to prevent. Thus, Morrison's tenth point – 'Accept that you cannot anticipate all stress' – is timely, as is the selected quote from Erica Jong (1978), urging us to:

> Renounce useless guilt
> Don't make a cult of suffering
> Live in the now, or at least in the soon...
>
> (How to Save Your Own Life)

Self care extends to supervisors as well. Their needs for stimulation, support and development as well as being accountable are equally valid.

These ideas ultimately lead us to more fundamental philosophies and strategies for living, and responding to complex, sometimes life-threatening situations. Our own different perspectives as a white man and woman find some complementarity within our partnership, but as training consultants, supervisors and practitioners we have different styles which rest significantly upon differences of gender, class and other socially constructed characteristics. [...]

Final thoughts ...

The supervisory partnership is, in current jargon, good value for money. It is not a sort of liberal free thinking left over from the 1960s, but offers a radical opportunity for developing and monitoring good standards of practice. Crucially for those directly engaged and prepared to make the time, it opens up ways of working positively with power and difference in the context of unremitting change. We believe that it is a central part of the survival tool bag, and can ensure that front line practitioners experience positive role models for providing an effective service.

REFERENCES

Berne, E. (1964) *Games People Play*, Harmondsworth, Penguin.
Dainow, S. and Bailey, C. (1988) *Developing Skills in People*, New York, Wiley.

DHSS (1978) *Social Services Teams: A Practitioner's View*, Parsloe, P. and Hill, M. (eds), London, HMSO.

Evans, D. (1990) *Assessing Students' Competence to Practise*, London, CCETSW.

Freire, P. (1972) *Pedagogy of the Oppressed*, Harmondsworth, Penguin.

Galbelko, N.H. and Michaelis, J.U. (1981) *Reducing Adolescent Prejudice: A Handbook*, New York, Teachers College Press.

Haring, N. *et al.* (1978) *The Fourth R*, Columbus, Ohio, Merrill.

Harrison, R. (1988) *Training and Development*.

Heron, J. (1975) *Six Category Intervention Analysis*, University of Surrey.

Heron, J. (1990) *Helping the Client*, London, Sage.

hooks, b. (1991) *Yearnings. Race, gender and cultural politics*, London, Turnaround.

Humphries, B. (1988) 'Adult learning in social work education: towards liberation or domestication?', *Critical Social Policy*.

Kadushin, A. (1976) *Supervision in Social Work*, Columbia University Press.

Knowles, M. (1978) *The Adult Learner: A Neglected Species*, Englewood, NJ, Prentice Hall.

Kolb, D. and McIntyre, J.M. (1979) *Organisational Psychology: An Experiential Approach*, Englewood Cliffs, NJ, Prentice Hall.

Latting, J.K. (1990) 'Identifying the "Isms": Enabling social work students to confront their biases', *Journal of Social Work Education*.

McDerment, L. (1988) *Stress Care*, Social Care Association.

Morrison, T. (1993) *Staff Supervision in Social Care*, Harlow, Longman.

Payne, C. and Scott, T. (1982) *Developing Supervision of Teams in Field and Residential Work*, National Institute for Social Work.

Pettes, D. (1967) *Supervision in Social Work*, London, Allen and Unwin.

Reynolds, B.C. (1965) *Learning and Teaching in the Practice of Social Work*, New York, Farrar and Rinehart.

Richards, M. *et al.* (1991) *Staff Supervision in Child Protection Work*, London, NISW.

Rogers, C.R. (1969) *Freedom to Learn*, Columbus, Ohio, Merrill.

Sawdon, D.T. and Sawdon, C. (1991) *Developing Staff Supervision and Appraisal in the Probation Service*, Humberside Probation Service.

Schön, D.A. (1987) *Educating the Reflective Practitioner*, San Francisco, Jossey Bass.

Shohet, P. and Hawkins, R. (1989) *Supervision in Helping Professions*, Buckingham, Open University Press.

Stewart, V. and Stewart, A. (1977) *Practice Performance Appraisal*, Aldershot, Gower.

Towle, C. (1963) 'The place of help in supervision', *The Social Service Review*, 38, 4.

Westheimer, I. (1977) *The Practice of Supervision in Social Work*, London, Ward Lock.

THIRTY-SEVEN

CHILD PROTECTION AND THE MEDIA: LESSONS FROM THE LAST THREE DECADES

Patrick Ayre

Source: *British Journal of Social Work*, 2001, December, 31, 6.

Summary

During the 1970s, 1980s and 1990s, sensationalist coverage of a series of celebrated child abuse scandals in England and Wales resulted in the repeated vilification in the mass media of those child welfare agencies deemed culpable for the deaths of the children involved. This chapter explores the contribution of the media to the creation of the climate of fear, blame and mistrust which seems to have become endemic within the field of child protection. It suggests that damaging distortions have been introduced into the child protection system as a result of the defensive responses of the relevant authorities at both national and local level to the media onslaught. A more strategic approach to understanding and managing media coverage of this difficult field is outlined.

Influences on the development of services in England and Wales

Those involved in devising and delivering child protection services in England and Wales over the last three decades will have observed a gradual but inexorable increase in the scope, complexity and sophistication of the child protection system and of the associated legislation and guidance. However, though more and more resources were invested in the system for most of this period, public confidence in it remained stubbornly and alarmingly low. Developments in services and in public attitudes may be seen to have been influenced primarily by three interrelated factors (Ayre, 1998a). [. . .]

Increasing awareness of abuse, a conflict-oriented legal framework and public and professional responses to headline grabbing scandals were important both in setting the general climate for developments in child protection and in influencing directly the pattern and character of the services which were created. Whilst these factors had the potential to contribute positively to the development of a more careful and accountable service, they also display considerable potential for introducing unhelpful biases and misplaced emphases. In particular, it may be helpful to explore their influence on the emotional context within which child protection work is undertaken and how they contributed to the creation of a climate of fear, a climate of mistrust and a climate of blame.

A climate of fear

The increased public awareness of abuse has been important in creating a more protective environment for our children and much of the coverage of this field in the media has been very helpful in this respect. Informative and supportive messages have been carried in adult fiction, in children's fiction and in the features or editorial output of the print and broadcast media. The influence of the news media has been much less helpful. [. . .]

For example, as Kitzinger and Skidmore (1995) found, media coverage has increased public awareness of sexual abuse but, for most people, the concept tends to be associated strongly with 'stranger danger' and the likelihood of abuse or abduction by an unknown assailant. There is usually little awareness of the much more likely contingency that children will be abused by someone well-known to them. Gough (1996) points out that the news media 'tend to report rare hazards rather than commonplace events but in dramatising such extreme adversities as child murder, sex rings and social workers abducting children into care, encourage the development of moral panic, which over-sensitises people to the risks involved'.

It is important to recognize that the climate of fear is not confined to the general public, but extends also to the policy makers and professional groups most closely involved. Close scrutiny of developments in child protection in England and Wales over the last two and a half decades may suggest that the allocation of resources during this period has been driven primarily by the desire of politicians and senior managers to avoid featuring on the front page of the tabloid press following the latest celebrated child abuse scandal (Aldridge, 1994; Ayre, 1998b; Franklin and Parton, 1991a). The development of services offering a balanced and confident professional response is not promoted by the fear of seeing your picture on the cover of a mass circulation daily above the headline 'Sack her, child abuse doc must go' (The *Sun*, 7 July 1987).

A climate of mistrust

Whilst increased awareness of abuse undoubtedly has some impact on our general level of trust in our friends, neighbours, associates and fellow citizens in general, I wish to pay particular attention to trust between the general public, politicians and policy makers on one hand and the professionals working in child protection on the other. As we have seen, considerable tension is thrown into relationships by the adversarial character of the child protection system. The climate of mistrust can only be increased when the values underpinning the selection of news stories inevitably emphasize drama and conflict. [. . .]

Such messages can do little to generate public confidence in child protection services which come across as sometimes too weak, sometimes too strong but never to be trusted. The notion that professional practice in this field is generally unreliable and unsafe seems to have had a powerful influence not only on the perceptions of the general public but also on policy makers and managers at all levels of national and local government and may clearly be seen reflected in the patterns of service which have developed.

A climate of blame

Over the past three decades, a climate of blame has come to be characteristic of child protection services in England and Wales. This may be seen, in part, as arising from the development of an influential discourse which centres on the responsibility of professionals for the abuse which they are attempting to prevent. The media have played an important part in creating and maintaining this discourse. As Hall *et al.* (1997) perceptively point out, child abuse stories were once represented in the news media primarily as crime stories and, accordingly, reporting followed the standard formula for this genre: discovery of crime, arrest and charge, trial, conviction and sentence. This mode of presentation still seems to hold sway in much press reporting in continental Europe and North America. However, in recent years a further concluding element which concerns itself with the attribution of blame and 'how was this allowed to happen?' has begun to be added routinely to story lines in the British press.

When looking for explanations for the fault-oriented bias which characterizes child abuse reporting, it seems to have become conventional within the professions most associated with child abuse to place responsibility primarily on the news media and on the agendas and imperatives which drive them (Aldridge, 1994; Franklin and Parton, 1991a; Illsley, 1989). However, a little reflection on the role played by the child protection system itself in the generation of this situation may be appropriate.

The promise to protect

[. . .]
Unfortunately, the rather rash promise to keep children safe implicit in the name of the service was made still more rashly explicit during the 1970s, 1980s and early 1990s. During these decades, unremitting pressure on local government to reduce its expenditure seems to have induced senior managers to play on the climate of fear already described by deploying the argument that if the resources devoted to child protection services were reduced, children would die. Whilst many newspaper stories continued to reflect and create the 'incompetent service' discourse throughout this period with headlines such as, 'Social workers failed to save battered baby' (*Daily Mail*, 21 June 1990), we can detect in other reports of the same incident the influence of the 'cash = safety' discourse reflected in story lines such as, 'Cash cuts linked to child's death' (*Daily Mirror*, 21 June 1990) and 'Cash curbs played part in abused girl's death' (*Independent*, 21 June 1990).

The inevitable but unwelcome corollary of child protection managers' emotive argument for continuing generous funding was an expectation on the part of the public, the politicians and the press that if sufficient resources were devoted to the service, children would no longer die as a result of abuse. Yet of course they did, because no amount of expenditure can ever render human behaviour totally predictable nor totally eliminate error, incompetence or folly, whether corporate or individual. To this extent, it ill becomes those of us engaged in child protection to criticize the media for pointing out when we fail, sometimes in dramatic fashion, to deliver what we are perceived to have promised.

The deprofessionalization of child protection

[. . .] The deprofessionalization of the social work services in the field of child protection may be seen to some degree as falling within a more general movement taking place within public services in Britain and elsewhere in the English speaking world in the last quarter of the century (Deem, 1989; Dressel *et al.*, 1988). We have seen in most public agencies widespread shifts of culture and function associated with the advent of managerialism (Brewster, 1992), McDonaldization (Ritzer, 1993) and the audit culture (Grayson and Rogers, 1997). The trend towards management by externally defined objectives, standardization, routinization and the attitude that 'if you can't count it, it doesn't count' is exemplified by the advent of the National Curriculum and examination league tables for schools, and of comprehensive nationally defined standards and perform-ance targets in health care, policing and the Probation Service.

We may surmise that the feeling, reflected in these developments, that the professions cannot be trusted to behave sensibly unless they are given very firm guidance about what to do, might be particularly prevalent in the sphere of child protection, where there has been so much emphasis on what has gone wrong. It is an entirely natural management response to address problems which have arisen by writing new guidance and proce-dures. In doing so, we may hope to achieve two particularly desirable objectives. Not only are we helping our staff to act more appropriately next time, but also, and perhaps more importantly, we are shifting the level of responsibility one level down the line. National government writes guidance for local authorities which then write guidance and procedures for their managers who in turn write detailed instructions for their staff. If anything then goes wrong, each can say 'I told you what to do and you failed to comply; the fault is yours'. In the blame oriented culture charac-teristic of child protection, this can be very comforting. [. . .]

During the 1970s, 1980s and 1990s, legislative change, statutory guid-ance, lengthy recommendations from public enquiries and research find-ings relevant to child protection (Department of Health, 1991; Reder *et al.*, 1993; Warner, 1996) proliferated at such a rate that it was difficult for ordinary competent practitioners and managers to feel confident that they were aware of all the important guidance relevant to their work. [. . .]

The idea that we can control child protection and render it safe by writing increasingly detailed procedures describing right action is unfortu-nately fundamentally flawed. It rests heavily on the notion that if we could just get the system right, all would be well. However, we are here straying again into the territory covered by the 'myth of predictability'. Unpre-dictability is of the essence of human behaviour, both that of abusers and that of the professionals who work with them. [. . .]

We may predict that over-reliance on feedforward controls and the con-sequent proceduralization and technicalization of child protection is likely to have two important adverse effects. First, workers may come increas-ingly to lack confidence in their own judgement and to be dependent on being told the right thing to do. Second, the system may become so wrapped up in process and procedure that it loses sight of objectives and outcomes. When those involved at all levels are asked to explain why certain actions were taken, they are likely to respond in terms of com-pliance with procedures and technical requirements. They are much less likely to speak, or perhaps even to think, about what they were trying to achieve for their clients. Participants in recent English research into decision making in child protection (Ayre, 1998a) suggested that they found these characteristics to be so widespread within their local child protection services that they might be regarded as typical.

Specialization in child protection

One of the most unfortunate consequences of the pressures outlined in this chapter has been the opening up of a widening gulf between child protection and more general child welfare. The risks and complexities of child abuse work in this hazardous environment seemed to require that child protection services and the workers who offered them become highly specialized. In response to the generally hostile and challenging environment in which they found themselves, such services inevitably developed sets of priorities and survival strategies distinct from those found within other child welfare services where the workers felt less vulnerable. The fear of missing something vital encouraged practice so defensive that it seemed, at times, primarily calculated to protect the system rather than the child. Fear of public vilification led to a preoccupation with the acute and the dramatic. Services were configured to focus on physical and sexual abuse at the expense of neglect and emotional abuse and on the identification and elimination of danger at the expense of preventive or therapeutic responses (Audit Commission, 1994; Department of Health, 1995). This contrasts sharply with developments in continental Europe where child welfare workers in France and Italy were placing much more emphasis on the provision of on-going supportive services for families aimed at the prevention of abuse (Caffo, 1983; Girodet, 1989).

[. . .] It is, then, unsurprising that a series of influential and important recent studies have suggested that too many families were being drawn into the scrutiny of the child protection system and further that services in the field of child and family welfare have come to concentrate so narrowly on child protection investigation that little time and money is left for anything else (Audit Commission, 1994; Department of Health, 1995). These findings are having a profound effect on the realignment of child-care services in England and Wales, but the perception of child protection as a particularly hazardous activity and its enduring appeal to the media as a source of front page headlines inevitably place constraints on the rate of change.

Learning lessons

When we reflect on the role of the news media in contributing to the pressures impinging on child protection in England and Wales over the last three decades and on the distortions in the system which have been created by the responses of managers and policy makers to these pressures, it seems appropriate to draw out some of the lessons which we can learn from this experience. All too often the media are regarded as essentially and inevitably hostile to child protection services and the only strategic approach deployed is avoidance at all costs. In its simplest form, this strategy has consisted of non-co-operation with press enquiries about specific incidents, refusal to comment and failure to provide background information or to make credible spokespersons available for interview. This is essentially a hazardous approach, leaving the media with a story which they want to tell but large gaps in the narrative. In the absence of any contribution from official sources, they are forced to rely on the one side of the story they have, which is usually highly critical of the authorities, and to plug the holes with contributions from 'rent-a-quote' commentators with well-known, and often controversial, positions but no knowledge of the case in question.

At a slightly more sophisticated level, avoidance involves failure to maintain a routine, on-going media strategy. Such a strategy should involve agencies in promoting the successes and socially valued aspects of their services and in forming enduring relationships with journalists such as features writers who work in sectors of the media less driven by the hard-edged imperatives of news reporting (Aldridge, 1994). [. . .]

Better then to abandon avoidance as a strategy and to become more sophisticated in our understanding of the media and of how news is created. Fully to learn the lessons which are there to be learned, we must move beyond the conventional wisdom prescribing better management. Certainly, more effective handling of the media would yield useful results. [. . .]

If we want to be truly effective in developing our services and their public image, we must understand and work constructively with the deeper forces. First, we must understand how discourses are created and maintained and what makes one discourse more influential than another. We must then apply this understanding to the way we represent our services. We must recognize in particular the relationship between the generation of discourses affecting our work and discourses in the wider socio-economic milieu. Shifts in the prevailing paradigm applied at any time to our services are more likely to occur if they conform to powerful external political discourses (Burke, 1996). Thus, the 'incompetent service' discourse in child protection became prominent in the United Kingdom when public services were under attack in the political arena. We need to note that this discourse was never extended to child protection work undertaken by voluntary agencies such as the NSPCC, which seem to have retained their very positive public image throughout the general onslaught. An understanding of precisely which aspect of our services was fundamentally being attacked, in this case that they were exemplars of the reviled public services, might have allowed us to respond more effectively and proactively. Instead, we, for the most part, simply bought into and addressed the superficial manifestations of a negative discourse being created for us by those with little sympathy for the public sector.

We must also be more effective in the creation and promotion of our own preferred discourses. Clearly, we must avoid sending out messages which will ultimately prove damaging to us by, for example, seeming to promise to keep children safe from abuse in exchange for generous funding. More generally, we must recognize that, whilst the approved set of professional understandings enjoys an impressive degree of acceptance across the multi-agency community in the field of child protection in England and Wales, it has limited impact within the wider community. Whatever marketing strategies may be developed, it seems likely that the degree of penetration of the professional discourse will only be improved when it can be aligned with wider, stronger and more influential political and social currents within the body politic.

The drive on the part of the present government of the United Kingdom towards the elimination of social exclusion by means of 'joined-up government' represents just such a current. Child protection services in England and Wales have much to do to rectify the poor public image under which they have toiled for the last three decades. Their success in doing so may depend crucially on their ability to align themselves with the thrust against social exclusion. They are already doing much to shake off their preoccupation with the more dramatic and sensational forms of abuse and to find a distinctive role within the general struggle to promote child welfare. If they are able to maintain progress in this direction despite the pressures towards narrowness and rigidity outlined in this chapter, they may soon find themselves in a position to begin to re-establish their standing and reputation.

REFERENCES

Aldridge, M. (1994) *Making Social Work News*, London, Routledge.

Audit Commission (1994) *Seen But Not Heard*, London, HMSO.

Ayre, P. (1998a) 'Significant harm: Making professional judgements', *Child Abuse Review*, 7: 330–42.

Ayre, P. (1998b) 'The division of child protection from child welfare', *International Journal of Child and Family Welfare*, 3(2): 149–68.

Brewster, R. (1992) 'The new class? Managerialism and social work education and training', *Issues in Social Work Education*, 11(2): 81–93.

Burke, R. (1996) *The History of Child Protection in Britain: A theoretical reformulation*, Leicester, Scarman Centre for the Study of Public Order.

Caffo, E. (1983) 'The importance of early intervention for the prevention of child abuse', in Leavitt, J. (ed.), *Child Abuse and Neglect: Research and innovation*, The Hague, NATO AS1 Series, Martinus Nijhoff Publishers: 75–82.

Deem, R. (1989) 'Educational work and the state of education', *Work, Employment and Society*, 3(2): 249–60.

Department of Health (1991) *Child Abuse: A study of inquiry reports 1980–1989*, London, HMSO.

Department of Health (1995) *Child Protection: Messages from research*, London, HMSO.

Dressel, P., Waters, M., Sweat, M., Clayton, O. and Chandler-Clayton, A. (1988) 'Deprofessionalisation, proletarianization and social welfare work', *Journal of Sociology and Social Welfare*, 15(2): 113–31.

Franklin, B. and Parton, N. (eds) (1991a) *Social Work, the Media and Public Relations*, London, Routledge.

Franklin, B. and Parton, N. (1991b) 'Victims of abuse: Media and social work', *Childright*, 75: 13–16.

Girodet, D. (1989) 'Prevention and protection in France', in Davies, M. and Sale, A. (eds), *Child Protection in Europe*, London, NSPCC: 13–14.

Gough, D. (1996) 'The literature on child abuse and the media', *Child Abuse Review*, 5(5): 363–76.

Grayson, L. and Rogers, S. (eds) (1997) *Inlogov Informs on Performance Management 2*, Birmingham, University of Birmingham, Institute of Local Government Studies.

Hall, C., Srangi, S. and Slembrouck, S. (1997) 'Narrative transformation in child abuse reporting', *Child Abuse Review*, 6(4): 272–82.

Illsley, P. (1989) *The Drama of Cleveland: a Monitoring Report on Press Coverage Between 23 June 1987 and 31 July 1987 of the Sexual Abuse of Children Controversy in Cleveland*, London, Campaign for Press and Broadcasting Freedom.

Kitzinger, J. and Skidmore, P. (1995) 'Playing safe: Media coverage of child sexual abuse protection strategies', *Child Abuse Review*, 4(1): 47–56.

Reder, P., Duncan, S. and Gray, M. (1993) *Beyond Blame: Child abuse tragedies revisited*, London, Routledge.

Ritzer, G. (1993) *The McDonaldization of Society*, Newbury Park, California, Pine Forge.

Warner, N. (1996) 'Social work today: inquiries overload', *Community Care*, 31 October 4.

THIRTY-EIGHT

AN EVALUATION OF THE USE OF INFORMATION TECHNOLOGY IN CHILD CARE SERVICES AND ITS IMPLICATIONS FOR THE EDUCATION AND TRAINING OF SOCIAL WORKERS

John Bates

Source: *Social Work Education*, 1995, 14, 1.

Introduction

As the need increases for agencies and individual social workers to manage and disseminate information more efficiently, the potential for use and abuse of information technology (IT) expands. In this context, IT can be seen to be crucial in supporting and maintaining social work's role within a rapidly changing social and economic environment. Technology has now advanced to the point that computers can be used by anyone although their potential for intensifying the structure of domination – economic, political and cultural is evident (Downing, 1991). For social work educators and trainers, it is vital to understand the processes by which we can begin to train workers who are equipped to deal with this revolution so that they may play a full and active part in its positive use. These processes may demand a re-evaluation of curriculum methodologies as well as a clearer understanding of the ways in which adults learn and make sense of new skill demands. In order to begin this process, it was thought helpful to ascertain the situation with regard to the current practice of computer usage amongst qualified social work practitioners and their perceptions of this innovation. [. . .]

The approach of this exploratory study was to ascertain the views and perceptions of the authority's child care workers following initial discussion with the authority's computer staff. The sample of workers chosen was based on the premise that the child care workers were significant users of computers and, also, because this group had the highest expectations placed upon them of accurate recording and dissemination of information through the computer system. The results of this enquiry are discussed and the implications for IT teaching on qualifying training courses are considered.

The authority examined is geographically mixed with the population focused in two predominantly urban centres. The authority began its computerisation in 1990 with the introduction of CRISSP (Care Records in Social Services Package) and currently has 170 terminals connected around the county feeding off a main frame based at the county headquarters. CRISSP is a standard client information and retrieval system. Plans are currently on line for integrating CCLAWS (Child Care Law and Systems) within the authority's computer package. CCLAWS is discussed more fully later in this paper. [. . .]

The debate around the relevance and efficacy of computers within the human services is not a new one. In 1972 there appeared an article by Abels (1972) who posed the intriguing question 'Can computers do social work?' A similar debate was taking place in both education and the health service against a background of government encouragement to adopt the new technology, as a failure to adapt would result in the loss of the country's competitive edge. The debate was taking place against an astonishing rate of technological change as computers became smaller in size, more complex and accessible to a mass market.

By the beginning of the 1980s the majority of local authorities had some computer usage within their social services departments (LAMSAC, 1982). By 1991 a survey found that 23% of departments had a fully computerised client index (Streatfield, 1991). [. . .]

Often, the reasons for introducing IT into social services departments seem obscure and ill defined (Sharma and Hunter, 1992). It may be that the decision was taken in order to improve a functional task or to achieve an additional task like the monitoring of community care statistics. On the other hand, it may be more to do with exercising control over internal operational procedures like monitoring car mileage expenditure.

The social work profession has indeed been slow to embrace the technological revolution. Research continues to show widespread computer illiteracy (Cnaan and Parsloe, 1989; Reinoehl and Hannah, 1990; Ezell et al., 1991; Reinoehl and Mueller, 1991). There is some evidence that this illiteracy is becoming costly in terms of program development, administration, research and practice innovation (Mutschler and Hoefer,

1990). Social workers seem to be more negative or resistant than other professional groups in adapting to IT usage (Zuboff, 1983; Barnes, 1984; Nurius *et al.*, 1989). Negative attitudes clearly will have an impact on the ultimate usage of computers within social work. This is borne out by Nurius and Nicoll (1989) and Finn (1989). Perhaps the seemingly cold and detached processes of data gathering and keyboard manipulation are felt by some social workers as being at odds with fundamental social work values creating a fear that the human processes implicit in the social work act may somehow be compromised and that clients are being reduced to mere statistics. For women, of course, the issue is compounded by the fact that men mystify machinery because they have the power to make the rules. For example, distinctions are made between word processing and computing although the machinery may well be the same. Women will tend to be the 'word processor operators', men the computer operators. The fact that women are the primary users of technological devices in the home has not enabled them to exploit this advantage in the workplace.

Cockburn (1991) suggests it is partly because of:

> the national scarcity of women with IT qualifications. That absence itself, however, has to be seen as generated partly by the masculine appropriation of technology and its associated skills, a cultural exclusion of women effective in both training and employment.
>
> (Cockburn, 1991: 157)

The voluntary sector in the UK has, however, been proactive in encouraging women to demystify computers by organising agencies like the Women's Computer Centre which provides training courses for women and gives information on training and computer related issues. Searching the literature for similar innovations for black people provided little in the way of studies or information on the subject, apart from a few government sponsored schemes involving the training of black young people in word processing and spreadsheet skills. The conclusion must be drawn that, for many black people, access to computers remains discriminatory. As Reamer (1986) argued, however, the competent and appropriate use of information technology could have the potential to liberate and to empower both practitioners and their most oppressed service users alike. Its success will depend on whether or not the expanding use of computers within the social services continues to mirror the private sector with predominantly male dominated, large management information functions that provide little return for the social worker or service user. There are few signs, as yet, that equal opportunities issues are being addressed to the use of computers within statutory agencies.

Method

[...]I used a guided or 'focused' interview, as described by Marriot (1953), using a given set of topics in a systematic way, namely:

1   level of IT knowledge;
2   regularity of IT usage in practice;
3   exposure level and perceived value of IT training;
4   perceived competency level in using available software;
5   an indication of the prospective value of an IT module on qualifying training courses.

Using this approach it was hoped to avoid the inflexibility of more formal methods and yet give each interview a structure and form that would ensure that all the topics were covered. The respondents would be free to develop their views at length and I would be able to explore and probe within the framework imposed by the topics. Despite the obvious scope in such an approach for bias to creep in, it is counterbalanced by the advantage of being able to obtain a richer understanding of the workers' views and attitudes, resulting in a fuller and more rounded picture. [...]

Findings

All of the respondents were most constructive and helpful during the interviews. Many of the dialogues were refreshing and stimulating and the fact that some interviews were done individually and some as a group did not seem to affect the quality or the frankness of the discussions. The information was disseminated under headings previously referred to.

Level of knowledge

The level of knowledge of IT was shown to be minimal. For example, there was a general inability to access the word processing part of the on-line software. Only three workers (two men and one woman) had their own personal computers (PCs) at home and only one of those was genuinely computer literate in that he was able to access a PC and find his way around the system. Only one of the group had heard of CHIAC (Child Abuse Information and Computers), although all the clerical staff had! [...]

Regularity of IT usage

The majority (16) of the social workers interviewed alleged CRISSP to be a complex and unfriendly program. Currently, as it is only used as a client information and retrieval system, a significant number of workers (13) were suspicious of its value, thus usage was limited. Over half (14) admitted they found the process a chore: '. . . it's not social work', '. . . what are they doing with all the information at Headquarters?', '. . . there are so many blocks in the system with restricted access it drives you mad', '. . . sometimes you have to wait half an hour to access the bloody thing'.

There was an overwhelming lack of interest in using the system, despite growing management pressure to keep information up to date. For a number of workers (11) it was seen as yet another pressure in a rapidly changing and devalued profession. One team leader admitted that if she could avoid touching 'the thing' for weeks at a time she was happy. A majority of the workers (13), however, would feel more positive about the system if programs had more relevance to their jobs, like a welfare benefits package, or CCLAWS (Child Care Law and Systems). This program is an interactive data base which allows users to access the complete range of child care legislation. It provides three basic modules of a Legal Commentary on child care legislation in force, a Sources module summarising the principal Acts, Guidance and Regulations and a glossary of terms that have a specific meaning within the text. Subjects covered include adoption, care and supervision orders, family law proceedings, regulations and local authority monitoring procedures. [. . .]

Exposure level to IT training

The majority (14) of the workers had attended the one day training courses at the authority's headquarters, although there were four still avoiding it despite the fact there was officially no option.

All those who attended agreed it was insufficient and only succeeded in leaving them more nervous and less competent. [. . .]

Perceived competency level in using available software

All of the teams visited were delighted with achieved competency levels of their clerical support staff! Only two of the social work staff interviewed (both men) regarded themselves as 'competent' in using the systems available. Much of the obligatory usage of CRISSP was handled by the clerical support staff, although it is a tool designed as much for social work practitioners to use. Those workers that did make use of the computers relied heavily on their support staff to get them out of trouble which seemed to be a fairly regular occurrence.

An indication of the value of an IT programme on qualifying training

Despite the general unease and mistrust of the authority's computerisation programme, all of the respondents accepted its inevitability. They articulated the emotional barriers to engaging with the computer; the 'unsympathetic' way the project had been introduced and their lack of involvement in planning its introduction.

Several felt their lack of knowledge left them vulnerable to exploitation by the way systems are introduced. When the discussions widened to talk about the potential advantages to social workers in child care, most (15) accepted that it was a dimension they had not considered or been aware of. [. . .]

All of the respondents enthusiastically supported vigorous IT training on qualifying courses and many lamented the lack of it on theirs, although several (6) of the respondents also commented on the fact that they felt using IT within social services departments was as much a management issue as a training one. Several (7) workers articulated the point that their involvement in the original inception of the project had been minimal, and also that the information needs of managers and social workers are fundamentally different. This point is highlighted by Williams and Forrest (1987) when they stress the importance of involving all of the social work staff in implementing technological changes as well as recognising the essential differences in information needs of social workers and managers. They point out that, for managers, the information needs are essentially statistical for planning, monitoring and evaluation purposes. Social workers, however, are more interested in the immediate, pragmatic details of individual clients and care episodes.

Discussion

This brief analysis has highlighted a number of important factors which may be pertinent although it is acknowledged that the respondents to this part of the study cannot be considered representative of child care workers throughout the UK; [. . .] Some implications and impressions for teachers, trainers and practitioners can, however, be recorded.

The interviews revealed most forcibly that the subjects of this study wanted to know about information technology and its positive use for social work, supporting the view that social workers are not necessarily technophobic but, as Flynn (1993) suggests 'the applications of computing have not largely been seen as personally applicable or helpful'.

[. . .]

Clearly, this is an area that demands further detailed study, but it is interesting to note that in the department studied, many social workers' first introduction to computing was with the client information system, CRISSP. The introduction of these innovations are, by their very nature, problematic. They are expensive to set up and maintain, and data is seldom reliable enough to use (Stewaert, 1993). Many of the client information systems produced by software houses have their origins in the commercial world where the processing of information takes on a quite different form. It is often a straightforward operation to posit a clear articulation of the problem to be addressed, define the goals and plan the methods to deal with the problem but, for a social services department rooted firmly in a 'messy' and shifting social policy framework, this necessity to provide a clear articulation of goals is virtually impossible.

Implications for practitioners

As Thompson (1990) argues, social work functions in an environment of uncertainty influenced by conflicting values, political uncertainties and inaccurate theoretical constructs. Schön (1983) describes this environment as a 'swampy lowland' in which social workers have to operate and make sense of ambiguity and affective uncertainty. For social services departments beset with the intractable problems of poverty, relationship difficulties and the victims of oppression the logic of the commercial world does not dovetail easily. In other words, however competent and well trained are end users, the 'garbage' on the information system will increase if the interaction required with the computer is at odds with the end-users' perception of their role within the agency. This brief study revealed, however, that the social workers wanted to play an active part in bridging the professional/technological gap but lacked the skills and knowledge to engage in the debate. [. . .]

Although in-service training will provide for existing staff it will undoubtedly be necessary for IT skills to be a feature on qualifying training for social workers. The UK clearly lags behind many other European countries. [. . .]

Implications for teachers and trainers

The knowledge that practitioners are willing to engage in the IT debate should, at least, encourage an examination of how we may include computer training on social work courses and how that curriculum can be structured to extract the underlying good will that clearly exists. [. . .]

Many social workers will need to adapt their attitude, and indeed their practice and this exploratory study suggested a willingness to do that. If they are to engage in the debate of how IT is used to benefit them and their service users, then qualifying training has to give them a minimum understanding of the technology and an ability to manipulate it in order to extract its benefits. In this capacity:

social workers will be capable of both identifying programmatic needs and exploring the practice dimensions of proposed technological solutions within a social work-oriented context.

(Rock *et al.*, 1993: 9)

Social work training and education should be preparing workers who are able to critically appraise IT in their future jobs. Qualifying training and in-house training needs to incorporate not only computer literacy on to courses, but also computer assisted learning and, most importantly, provide opportunities to discuss the ethical issues surrounding IT usage within the human services. Computers are not ethically neutral. As Glastonbury pointed out:

> we need go no further than the word processor on which this paper was written. The thesaurus has a quaint line in ethnic and gender 'neutrality'. 'Black' is described amongst others as 'evil, nefarious, wicked'; 'white' as 'pure, spotless, undefiled'. 'Man' is 'humanity, chap, guy'; 'woman' is 'handmaiden, housekeeper, maid' (1992: 21).

[...] Consequently, one of the main tasks of social work educators will be to help students become aware of the 'need to know'. The case must be made that tackling an IT module will improve their effectiveness as social workers and, most importantly, give significant added benefits to their clients. Students and practitioners may well learn best in the context of using computers to do what they want and need them to do. The study earlier showed how the local authority's attempt to teach social workers something they felt they did not need to know led to a poor competency level and may also have the additional effect of creating barriers to future learning.

In addition, the technique of teaching them to memorise commands failed because not only had the majority of the social workers no desire to use the machinery but also because adults are essentially person centred in their orientation to learning. In designing curriculum material we need to begin with the interest of the social worker and not with the computer.

Conclusion

This chapter has contended that, in general, the knowledge base and user take up of information technology is low in this particular group of social workers. This resistance to IT is possibly heightened by the perception that computerisation has little to offer social workers in their day to day practice. That, coupled with changes in child care practice, new legislation, child abuse scandals and lack of funding have all conspired to create an intolerable pressure which yet another doubtful innovation can only compound. Attempts at teaching computer skills, therefore, need a re-appraisal if we are not to continue alienating social workers from what is potentially a liberating and constructive additional tool which can reduce the burden of excessive caseloads and under resourcing. Without an opportunity to absorb what is, in effect, a new culture and take time to become socialised into new procedures and operations, social workers will remain frozen out of the debate and technology will remain a symbol of oppression by denying choices, chances, empowerment and, instead, information will be restricted, creating an even less democratic, more oppressive and less participatory society. We need to prepare students who are not only computer literate but who also have the confidence to critically evaluate and challenge IT in their jobs. Information technology has the potential to link together oppressed groups: women, disabled people and black people, if social workers, amongst others, are able to initiate that development. As Crawley (1992) suggests: 'young, non-disabled, white, heterosexual men are the only ones who do not justify a high priority in terms of access to new technology'. [. . .]

REFERENCES

Abels, P. (1972) 'Can computers do social work?', *Social Work*, 17.

Barnes, C. (1984) 'Questionnaire evaluation of the attitudes in respect of microcomputers within social services settings', *Computer Applications in Social Work*, 1(1): 13–23.

Cnaan, R.A. and Parsloe, P. (1989) 'The impact of information technology on social work practice', *Computers in Human Service*, 5.

Cockburn, C. (1991) *In the Way of Women: men's resistance to equality in organisations*, Basingstoke, Macmillan.

Downing, J. (1991) 'Computers for social change', *Computers in Human Services*, 8(1).

Ezell, M., Nurius, P. and Balassone, M. (1991) 'Preparing computer literate social workers: an integrative approach', *Journal of Teaching in Social Work*, 5(1): 81–99.

Finn, J. (1989) 'Microcomputers in private, non-profit agencies: a survey of trends and training requirements', *Social Work Research and Abstracts*, 24(1), Spring: 10–14.

Flynn, J.P. (1993) 'Survey of staff attitudes towards computer assisted instruction for staff orientation', in Glastonbury, B. (ed.) *Human Welfare and Technology*, Assen, Van Corcum.

Glastonbury, B. (1992) 'The integrity of intelligence', *New Technology in the Human Services*, 6(2).

LAMSAC (1982) *Survey of Local Authority Social Services Computer Applications*.

Marriot, R. (1953) 'Some problems in attitude survey methodology', *Occupational Psychology*, 27: 117–27.

Mutschler, E. and Hoefer, R. (1990) 'Factors affecting the use of computer technology in human service organisations', *Administration in Social Work*, 14(1): 87–102.

Nurius, P. and Nicoll, A. (1989) 'Computer literacy preparation: conundrums and opportunities for the social work educator', *Journal of Teaching in Social Work*, 3(2): 65–81.

Nurius, P., Hooyman, N. and Nicoll, A. (1989) 'The changing face of computer utilisation in social work settings', *The Journal of Social Work Education*, 86–197.

Reamer, F. (1986) 'The use of modern technology in social work: ethical dilemmas', *Social Work*, 31(6): 469–72.

Reinoehl, R. and Hannah, T. (1990) 'Computer literacy in human services', *Computers in Human Services*, 6(1).

Reinoehl, R. and Mueller, B. (1991) 'Computer literacy in human services education: parts 1 and 2', *Computers in Human Services*, 7(1/2).

Rock, B., Auerbach, C., Kaminsky, P. and Goldstein, M. (1993) 'Integration of computer and social work culture: a developmental model', in Glastonbury, B. (ed.) *Human Welfare and Technology*, Assen, Van Corcum.

Schön, D. (1983) *The Reflective Practitioner*, London, Temple Smith.

Sharma, A. and Hunter, T. (1992) 'Byte size chunks', *Community Care*, January.

Steyaert, J. (1993) 'Client information systems and their built in values', in Glastonbury, B. (ed.) *Human Welfare and Technology*, Assen, Van Corcum.

Streatfield, D. (1991) 'Social science information comes of age: or does it?', *Assignation*, 9(1): 15.

Thompson, N. (1990) 'The uncertainty principle in teaching social work and social science', *Social Sciences Teacher*, 19(2), Spring.

Williams, S. and Forrest, J. (1987) 'Embracing the future', *Social Services Insight*, May.

Zuboff, S. (1983) 'New worlds of computer mediated work', *Public Welfare*, 41(4): 36–44.

THIRTY-NINE

BECOMING A LEARNING ORGANISATION: A SOCIAL WORK EXAMPLE

Nick Gould

Source: *Social Work Education*, 2000, 19, 6.

Introduction

Within the worlds of commerce and industry there has been, since the mid-1980s, a strong interest in the concept of the learning organisation. Under conditions imposed by a globalising economy, where maintaining a competitive edge depends upon processes of continuous improvement, there has been an emerging view that this requires a commitment to continuous learning (Jarvis, 1999). Although short-term gains might be made by 'down-sizing' and other efficiency fixes, the most effective insurance against being left behind by rapid technological change and a volatile economic environment is to embed within the organisation processes which facilitate learning in order to keep abreast of change and to innovate (Senge, 1990). Much of this discourse and practice has been located within the spheres of management and business theory, and in the practices of commercial corporations, but there is an emerging realisation that personal social services are also finding themselves caught up in this globalising world of downward pressure on resources and rapidly changing patterns of social need where organisational change is not an occasional 'blip' but a continuous fact of life (Steyaert and Gould, 1999; Pugh and Gould, 2000). Despite this there has so far been no evident thinking about the transfer of learning organisation theory to social work organisations, perhaps because it is an approach normally associated with business culture, even though some proponents of the learning organisation write from within a commitment to humanist radicalism (Dovey, 1997) and reflective practice (Jarvis, 1999).

Indeed, within human service sectors such as social work, teaching and nursing, an interest in reflective learning has emerged broadly at the same time as the development of the concept of the learning organisation in industry (Gould and Taylor, 1996). Just as the philosophy of the learning organisation is that learning is not limited to training events or courses but is a set of processes located within the organisation, so the reflective learning paradigm rejects a view of learning as being solely the inductive application to practice of knowledge or techniques; learning is viewed as a process of purposive engagement with practice. This paper reports on an externally commissioned research study conducted by the author, a university-based social work academic, within a national, UK-based voluntary child care organisation. The inquiry sought to investigate with practitioners and their immediate managers their own understanding of how learning takes place within an organisational context, what existing strategies could be identified which supported learning, and what changes might be implemented which enhanced their and the organisation's capacity for learning?

The theory of the learning organisation

Although the literature on 'the learning organisation' is relatively recent, it builds on a longer sociological tradition of theorisation of the relationship between organisational structure and behaviour. In classic Weberian theory of bureaucracy, learning is strongly associated with traditional notions of professionalisation where stratification separates the educated and qualified 'thinkers' and 'deciders' from the 'doers'. The implications of this are that, primarily, learning for the job has taken place through qualifying education and any 'topping up' is focused on managerial levels of the organisation. In later scientific views of organisations, associated with Fordism and Taylorism, the emphasis was on the acquisition of technical skills for task efficiency. Individuals were trained to perform a segment of the production process within a highly standardised system. Over time a tension was to emerge between the dehumanising effects of Taylorism (see Beynon, 1973) and the human relations movement of the 1960s and 1970s within which writers such as Maslow (1968) and McGregor focused attention on meeting human needs through personal development, job enrichment and the quality of working life.

Contemporaneous with the development of human relations thinking was an identification of learning as a specific issue within management development, particularly as associated with the action learning theories of Revans (1980), that is the view that learning for management can be experiential, achieved through shared problem-solving (Margerison, 1994).

Revans had been responsible for training in the British mining industry during the Second World War. Scarcity of human resources made him realise that conventional training programmes were impractical because of the cost and interruptions to production resulting from taking managers away from the workplace to attend training events. Revans began to develop structured problem-based approaches to learning on the job, or 'action learning' (Revans, 1985). Revans's 'law' anticipates much of the theory of the learning organisation: 'For an organisation to survive its rate of learning must be equal to or greater than the rate of change in its external environment'.

Continuous change has been a theme of sociologists and futurologists such as Alvin Toffler and Daniel Bell, and it has emerged in the work of theorists of strategic management such as Charles Handy (1989) who challenged managers to accept that change had become a continuous reality and not something which temporarily interrupted periods of stability. Associated with this shift is an implicit change of metaphor for conceptualising organisational life, from the dominant Taylorist image of the organisation as a machine towards the metaphor of the organisation as a system, one which has to adapt through learning to the changing demands created by its environment.

At the heart of this progression of organisational theory is the problematic concept of learning; what it means, how it relates to organisational structure and behaviour, and whether there are real differences behind the managerialist slogans of 'organisational learning' (the processes through which learning takes place) and 'the learning organisation' (the characteristics of an organisation that learns). The overlap between these concepts seems to be large, and to make a rigid analytical distinction between them reifies academic turf wars rather than making a useful analytical distinction. What seems to be shared within these fields are two fundamental premises. First, individual learning is a necessary but not sufficient condition for organisational learning – the latter is a collective process which means that the organisation has not automatically learned as a result of an individual's learning. Second, the learning experience is more pervasive and distributed than that delivered through a specific, designated training or educational event; learning incorporates the broad dynamics of adaptation, change and environmental alignment of organisations, takes place across multiple levels within the organisation, and involves the construction and reconstruction of meanings and world views within the organisation.

This is not to suggest that a unified and uncontested field of enquiry exists within which there is a consensus as to what is meant by the learning organisation and organisational learning (Easterby-Smith *et al.*, 1998). Even between three seminal texts – Argyris and Schön (*Organisational Learning*, 1966), Pedler *et al.* (*The Learning Company*, 1991) and Senge (*The Fifth Discipline*, 1990), quite different projects can be identified. In a very useful review of this literature, Tsang (1997) points out that there is a fundamental tension between descriptive and prescriptive research in this area. The former tends to address the question, 'How does an organisation learn?' and is characterised by academically produced, technical research which has limited applicability to practice. The latter, prescriptive research raises the question, 'How should an organisation learn?' and is usually produced by consultants, and is in the form of descriptive case studies which are then over-generalised to make claims for applicability to all organisations. Clearly, research about learning organisations, if it is to produce useable theory, needs to aspire to achieve a level of integration between rigour and utility. Tsang provides some suggestions for such integration, primarily that inquiry should begin not from a normative theory of intervention (arguably a feature of Argyris and Schön's and Senge's work) but from empirical grounded research on the basis of which prescriptions can then be made. In turn, this can be the basis for a third stage of inquiry, to study the outcome of implementing the prescriptions in an organisation 'Descriptive studies in the form of action research are required' (Tsang, 1997: 86). This paper describes the methodology for such research within one social work agency, and the prescriptions which have emerged from it.

Methodology

[. . .] Two projects were approached and accepted an invitation to participate in the research. Although not selected by any systematic method of sampling, they were strongly contrasting in terms of their structure and size, which enabled comparisons to be constructed and explored. As one of the features of organisational learning is a concern with multiple organisational levels of learning, it was decided that staff should be involved from differing organisational levels. Two senior line managers participated; each had strategic responsibility for the organisation's services in a defined geographical area. The project managers were also interviewed. One project (project A) comprised a single team with a singleton manager, the other (project B) was the largest project in the UK incorporating several teams and the overall project manager and two team managers took part. Group interviews were also held with project workers, i.e. practitioners, two in project A and five workers and a student from project B. Thus, there was a total of 14 participants in the inquiry, representing regional management, local management and practitioner levels.

A preliminary letter was sent to participants explaining the purpose and design of the research. Interviews were of between 1 and 1.5 hours' duration. Contemporaneous notes were taken and the interviews were also tape-recorded. In the preliminary analysis the interviews were analysed using a process of continuous comparison; that is, in line with the principles of grounded theory (Glaser and Strauss, 1967), a qualitative research methodology which asserts that researchers should start from their own data and not from theoretically based pre-conceptions. Themes were identified from the interview material which were then coded manually to build up analytic categories against which the data could be sorted, compared and the categories refined. Thus, the categories were not a predetermined, theory-driven list, but emerged from the interview material. In order to address issues of reliability, this initial analysis was presented to a workshop of all the participants for comment. These comments were then incorporated in a report which was posted to all participants for further comment and refinement.

Findings

An inventory of 'learning'

Participants were initially asked how they felt that learning was integrated within their professional activity. A diverse range of activities were cited including:

- supervision provided through the chain of line management – in one project learning was a standing item on the supervision agenda;
- learning logs, although there was some uncertainty about the extent of the use of these;
- shadowing, this was the practice of accompanying others to see and learn from their practice;
- coaching, this was identified as something which 'democratised' the learning process as sometimes skills such as information technology use could be passed on between people in different sectors such as administrative support and practice;
- inter-team meetings were cited as something which were difficult to prioritise but were important opportunities for sharing experience;
- joint working was seen as an important element within the general development of a learning ethos, and went beyond shadowing (see above) to imply joint accountability and ownership of work;
- practice learning teaching involved not only practice teachers but also engaged co-workers in the integration of theory and practice; and
- courses and training events were readily cited as opportunities for learning, which might be expected, but these were also seen as problematic. There were cost-related and logistical obstacles to attending external events, and allocations of funding from a finite training budget produced issues of entitlement and equity. Nevertheless, there were creative responses to such opportunities such as cascade learning, where colleagues who attended events relayed material to colleagues or,

where the budget allowed, the whole team might attend a course so that learning was collective.

Models of learning

The interviews moved from this descriptive level of auditing discrete learning activities to a more open-ended discussion about how participants conceptualised the process of learning from practice. This produced a range of answers which were more discursive and yet indicated between projects clear distinctions over what might be called the model within which learning took place. Primarily, this was a distinction between learning which was integrated into a reflective cycle of action and inquiry, and learning as a more traditionally conceived activity which was discrete and separate from practice. [. . .]

Team learning

The team emerged from the interviews as being a critical context for learning. As we have seen, the inventory of learning already indicated team-based activities as learning opportunities, such as presentations within team meetings, sharing learning from external events, co-working with team colleagues as well as inter-team learning through secondments.

Managers were aware of the impacts of organisational variables which could impede the culture of learning within a team. For instance, one regional manager was able to identify examples of teams facing threats such as redundancy where there was an immobilisation of learning and an (understandable) pre-occupation with organisational survival. This same manager stressed the importance of 'culture' within the team, that is the practice of learning strategies such as hypothesis formulation and testing which took place independently of changes of personnel within the team. This meant that learning became independent of the leadership style of an individual team manager.

Participants were also frank in their judgement that just because a team met did not mean that learning was taking place. This was not necessarily seen as critical – the same individuals accepted that some team meetings had to deal with pressing business, in which case it became important to ensure that there were scheduled team opportunities which could be more learning-oriented, e.g. away-days. Conversely, a high premium was placed on opportunities for informal contact within which reflection could take place, the possibility of talking over a problematic situation over coffee or at other meeting points.

Dissemination of learning

It is a platitude in social work that the wheel is continuously reinvented because developments in learning and new knowledge are not effectively disseminated, whether it be horizontally between peers or vertically between hierarchical levels. This was readily identified in the interviews as a central problematic for the organisation:

> I would say that one of the things that the (organisation) is absolutely appalling about is sharing knowledge about what projects do. There is ... all that we have is a directory of (the organisation's) project names which means that we have to guess what projects do because there is nowhere that tells you what each project does.
>
> (Project worker)

[...]

Hierarchies of knowledge

Connected with the issue of the dissemination of learning, indeed a subset of that issue, was the emergence in the interviews of beliefs that a major inhibition of the dissemination of learning is a belief that there is an implicit hierarchy of knowledge within the organisation. Priority is perceived to be given to: (1) research which has been commissioned from external researchers; or (2) research which produces findings which have a public relations or marketing advantage for the agency. [...]

There was a perception that thresholds operate within the organisation which inhibit the circulation of findings from local projects if they are deemed to be insufficiently rigorous or too local to be generalised. This is seen to have an effect not only on whether work becomes known to the wider world, but whether it becomes available within the organisation itself.

Action research

Action research can be understood as a way of investigating professional experience which links practice and the analysis of practice into a single, continuously developing process. In their seminal discussion of action research, Carr and Kemmis (1986) define it as a form of self-reflective enquiry undertaken by participants in social situations in order to improve the rationality and justice of their own practices (p. 162). Action research and reflective practice are processes which have much in common and, as Jarvis has argued, may at times be simultaneous (Jarvis, 1999).

The interviews revealed that at all levels there was an awareness that action research is important, whether as part of learning from practice or as an element in the wider strategy of evaluation of projects. It was also understood that it was becoming a standard expectation of the organisation that action research should be incorporated within all project developments and this was reflected as a budget heading within project budgets. [...]

Learning laboratories and constant experimentation

[...]A constant theme within the learning organisation literature is the concept of the learning laboratory. Frequent reference is made to production plants which create 'micro-worlds' within which new processes can be tested and improved. This notion of experimentation under controlled circumstances is difficult to transfer to a social work context, where practice has to be by its nature in the 'real world', and where experimentation involving vulnerable people carries profound ethical difficulties.

Nevertheless, this was an issue which emerged strongly from the interviews and not from the perspective that might be expected – that is, that experimentation was too difficult or unethical – but that this was an important element of learning which was conducive to the improvement of practice. This was perceived as having two aspects, the necessity of the organisation to 'own' and be receptive to learning from unsuccessful activities, the other was the importance of allowing the local autonomy necessary to take risks with new ventures. One manager expressed the view that this required a cultural shift on the part of the organisation:

> The [organisation] is not very good at learning from mistakes and what hasn't gone well. It wants to focus on learning from success. It requires a supportive culture that allows people to experiment and innovate with security. A creative tension lies at the interface between established patterns of work and innovation. Failure becomes a 'guilty secret' within ... rather than a resource for learning. You need to take risks.
>
> (Project manager)

A regional manager, also agreeing that experimentation was important within social work, argued that this did, however, depend upon a shared organisational acceptance that innovation and learning involve risk-taking. This included empowering local projects to take initiatives so that innovation was not conducted in secret. A positive example of this in practice was the establishment of refuges for runaway children – which were contentious, operating in an uncertain legal context, but from which came powerful learning.

Technology and learning

A number of participants in the research had comments to make about the technologies which support learning and how these are embedded organisationally. In the contemporary climate, 'technology' tends to become equated with new information and communication technologies. However, some people readily identified that an important support for their learning

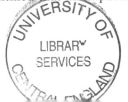

remained the older technology of the printed word. In particular, project workers spoke very positively about the support given by the organisation's central library. [. . .]

However, there was also substantial comment about new technology and how the organisation should move forward with the implementation of new technology in ways which could support learning. Comments tended to cluster around two issues: the general implementation of an information strategy within the organisation, and the exploitation of learning opportunities created by the Internet and World Wide Web. [. . .]

Many of those interviewed saw considerable potential for learning provided that the full possibilities of having a network were realised. [. . .]

Discussion

> Early work was concerned to find examples of good practice so that the learning organisation might be replicated . . . People who are looking for the right way have missed the point of the concept however. The right way is as elusive as any other idealised state of being – there is no perfect organisation, for they are all peopled by fallible human beings, therefore it is inevitable that organisations make mistakes, get things wrong and suffer setbacks.
>
> (Dale, 1994: 22)

One of the messages of postmodernism has been that there are no set blueprints for organisational structure and the attempt to impose one is likely to be counter-productive. Instead, diversity is an inevitable and desirable characteristic of social life. This small study has taken two projects within a national voluntary organisation and explored with staff the meaning for them of learning, and how that is supported or otherwise by the organisational context. Some responses were positive, such as the facilitation of learning by teamwork. It would be surprising not to find some aspects of the learning organisation reflected in social work agencies because of the centrality in social work of the core concepts within the learning organisation literature, particularly working in teams and systemic thinking. But the study also indicates areas needing more development if continuous learning is to be achieved at an organisational level.

The conventional model of learning from experience which has become fairly orthodox within social work literature on reflective learning suggests a cycle of action, reflection, conceptualisation and experimentation but is very much located in methodological individualism (Gould, 1989). As various critics have also pointed out, it has less to say about contexts of practice such as social work, which are not conducted in reflective settings such as design studios but in scenarios of direct engagement requiring rapid responses and improvisation (Eraut, 1995). The evidence from this study suggests that we need to adapt and relocate the individualistic experiential learning model to a more complex model which can incorporate some of the processes suggested by this study, without prescribing a specific organisational structure.

Three issues emerge from the data which need to be addressed within the module:

- **Knowledge.** The work of Schön and others has been important in redressing the balance between formal, research-based knowledge and personal knowledge generated from experience, but it may have swung too far in dismissing the part which continues to be played by formal knowledge. It was evident from the interviews that project workers are 'research-minded', they read to inform themselves by reading, particularly when engaging with new areas of work and this then becomes part of the background knowledge which informs intervention. Recognition of this, such as in continuing to support practitioners with library services, avoids some of the current sterile oppositions between 'evidence-based practice' and reflective learning.
- **Evaluation and action inquiry.** There is a significant development in the literature on learning organisations towards recognition of the need for continuous processes of evaluation to be embedded within organisational practices (Preskill and Torres, 1999). The organisation researched for this study has gone further than many agencies by requiring action research to be part of every initiative. One of the projects which participated in this inquiry had moved towards a model of intervention which incorporated research as part of the action cycle. However, it was also evident that even within this project, and more widely in the agency, there was a tension between the recognition that action research was important and the doubts they had about their competence to undertake this. This was also fuelled by the perception of hierarchies of knowledge so that local action research was always downgraded against commissioned externally conducted research.
- **Organisational memory.** Part of learning was not only the interrogation of the project's own experience, but a wish to identify where else in the organisation similar issues were being addressed, or where expertise lay that might be mobilised. This can be likened to the need to develop an organisational memory, one that is more systematic than the folk-knowledge of individuals within the organisation and less susceptible to the vagaries of staff turn-over.

Underpinning these three aspects of the social work agency as a learning organisation run the more generic concepts of power and empowerment – as Gherardi (1999) has argued, the learning organisation is not an abstract mental construct, it is produced in the social relations of the individuals within the organisation. The distribution of knowledge, the re-ordering of hierarchies of knowledge to give more voice to service users and practitioners, and the institutionalisation of bottom-up research methodologies, all require some decentralisation of power within an organisation. A potential contradiction within the theory and practice of the learning organisation is that grounded theory, such as pursued within this study, may uncover perspectives which are highly challenging for the organisation to embrace. At the same time, the very notion of the learning organisation carries dangers of becoming a slogan, the main purpose of which is to legitimise and mobilise top-down change:

> The literature on LO has been suspected of colluding with the 'ruling courts' which govern organizations and of employing, in an ideological manner, a discourse of democracy and liberation.
>
> (Gherardi, 1999: 105)

However, Dovey argues that the learning organisation does introduce a potentially radical strategic option, provided that those with executive control are also committed to forms of change which implicate power sharing (Dovey, 1997). The inquiry reported in this paper is modelling some of the processes of action research and participative inquiry which will engage with some of these power-sharing issues at a 'ruling court' executive level. . . . It is the first stage of an ongoing process which will test whether there will be progress from rhetoric into action. There has already been a workshop with the participants to consider and review the findings so far, as are reported in this paper, several dissemination events within the organisation, and meetings with members of the agency's national executive. Since this stage of the inquiry was completed the organisation's first strategic plan has been published, which makes an explicit commitment towards becoming a learning organisation. Other developments are taking place which endorse the findings of this study such as development of an intranet resource which will be an 'organisational memory' providing a database of current activities and an archive of project experience; collaboration with external initiatives to promote the dissemination of research to practitioners; and continuing development of evaluation and action research methods within projects. This is not to claim that these developments are unproblematic, or that they were entirely produced by this small research study conducted by an external university-based researcher; clearly, the study went 'with the grain' of emerging perspectives within the agency. However, the study does give one social work-based example of how the challenge presented from Tsang at the outset of this paper might be addressed – to produce learning organisation research which moves from a local, descriptive case study towards prescriptions for change.

REFERENCES

Argyris, C. and Schön, D. (1996) *Organizational Learning II: Theory, Method and Practice*, Reading, MA, Addison-Wesley.

Beynon, H. (1973) *Working for Ford*, London, Penguin.

Carr, W. and Kemmis, S. (1986) *Becoming Critical: education, knowledge and action research*, Geelong, Deakin University Press.

Dale, M. (1994) Learning organisations, in C. Mabey and P. Iles (eds) *Managing Learning*, London, International Thomson Publishing Co.

Dovey, K. (1997) The learning organization and the organization of learning: power, transformation and the search for form in learning organizations, *Management Learning*, 28(3): 331–49.

Easterby-Smith, M., Snell, R. and Gherardi, S. (1998) Organizational learning: diverging communities of practice? *Management Learning*, 29(3): 259–72.

Eraut, M. (1995) Schön shock: a case for reframing reflection-in-action? *Teachers and Teaching: Theory and Practice*, 1(1): 9–22.

Gherardi, S. (1999) Learning as problem-driven or learning in the face of mystery, *Organization Studies*, 20(1): 101–24.

Glaser, B. and Strauss, A. (1967) *The Discovery of Grounded Theory*, Chicago, Aldine.

Gould, N. (1989) Reflective learning for social work practice, *Social Work Education*, 8(2): 9–20.

Gould, N. and Taylor, I. (eds) (1996) *Reflective Learning for Social Work*, Aldershot, Arena.

Handy, C. (1989) *The Age of Unreason*, London, Business Books Ltd.

Jarvis, P. (1999) *The Practitioner Researcher: Developing Theory from Practice*, San Francisco, Jossey-Bass.

Margerison, C. (1994) Action learning and excellence in management development, in C. Mabey and P. Iles (eds) *Managing Learning*, London, International Thomson Publishing Co.

Maslow, A. (1968) *Towards a Psychology of Being*, New York, Van Nostrand.

Pedler, M., Boydell, T. and Burgoyne, J. (1991) *The Learning Company*, London, McGraw Hill.

Preskill, H. and Torres, R. (1999) *Evaluative Inquiry for Learning in Organizations*, Thousand Oaks, Sage.

Pugh, R. and Gould, N. (2000) Globalization, social welfare and social work, *European Journal of Social Work*, 3(2): 123–38.

Revans, R. (1980) *Action Learning*, London, Blond and Biggs.

Senge, P. (1990) *The Fifth Discipline*, London, Random Century.

Steyaert, J. and Gould, N. (1999) Social services, social work and information management: some European perspectives, *European Journal of Social Work*, 2(2): 165–75.

Tosey, P. (1998) The learning organisation, in P. Jarvis, J. Holford and C. Griffin (eds) *The Theory and Practice of Learning*, London, Kogan Page.

Tsang, E. (1997) Organisational learning and the learning organisation: a dichotomy between descriptive and prescriptive research, *Human Relations*, 50(1): 73–89.

INDEX